Drug Therapy

Articles from
The New England
Journal of Medicine on

Drug Therapy

1980–1984
Seventh in a series of reprint collections

Copyright © 1985 by Massachusetts Medical Society.

Library of Congress Cataloging in Publications Data:

Articles from the *New England Journal of Medicine* on Drug Therapy, 1980–1984.
   1. Chemotherapy — Addresses, essays, lectures. I. Massachusetts Medical Society. II. New England Journal of Medicine. (DNLM: 1. Drug Therapy — collected works. WB 330 A791)
RM262.A78   1985   615.5'8   85-7103

ISBN NUMBER: 0-910133-07-7

Printed in the United States of America
5 4 3 2

This book was set in Garamond type by the in-house typesetting department of the Massachusetts Medical Society.
Cover design by Jean LeGwin Design.

Introduction

OF the several categories of articles that appear in the *New England Journal of Medicine*, one of the most popular has consistently been the department devoted to Drug Therapy. Intended to be practical, up-to-date, clinically useful guides to timely issues in *materia medica*, the Drug Therapy articles are nonetheless selected according to the same rigorous standards of scientific accuracy that characterize the *Journal*'s famous Original Articles and Medical Progress reviews.

This volume presents a selection from the Drug Therapy articles published in recent years under the editorial guidance of Dr. Jan Koch-Weser, who initiated this series in 1971. Dr. Koch-Weser has now laid down his editorial pen, and we wish him well. This collection is a tangible manifestation of his service to the *Journal*, and he deserves our gratitude.

Following the tradition established by Dr. Koch-Weser, the *Journal* continues to publish authoritative assessments of current pharmacologic principles and practices under the Drug Therapy heading, as well as in other departments.

Contents

β-Adrenergic Blockade for Survivors of Acute Myocardial Infarction

William H. Frishman, M.D.,

Curt D. Furberg, M.D.,

and William T. Friedewald, M.D.

T HE β-adrenoceptor antagonists have been shown to be both safe and effective for the treatment of systemic hypertension, arrhythmia, angina pectoris, hypertrophic cardiomyopathy, thyrotoxicosis, and open-angle glaucoma, and for prophylaxis against migraine headache.[1] Recent clinical trials with one to four years of active treatment have demonstrated that some orally active β-blockers can reduce the risk of cardiovascular mortality in patients recovering from acute myocardial infarction.[2-15] On the basis of the results of the Norwegian Multicenter Study[10] and the Beta-Blocker Heart Attack Trial[11] in North America, the Food and Drug Administration has recently approved two nonselective β-blockers, timolol maleate (Blocadren) and propranolol (Inderal) for this indication. Metoprolol (Lopressor), a β_1-selective adrenergic blocker, is now under consideration for this same use. β-Blockers have also been suggested as a treatment for reducing the extent of myocardial injury and mortality during the acute phase of myocardial infarction,[16-18] but their role in this situation remains unclear.[19,20] This article assesses the current state of knowledge regarding the value of long-term β-blocker therapy in survivors of acute myocardial infarction and the implications for clinical practice.

The Clinical Problem

Despite a decline in the incidence of coronary heart disease, more than 600,000 patients a year are admitted to hospitals in the United States, with a diagnosis of acute myocardial infarction.[21] For patients having their first infarction,

From the Department of Medicine, Albert Einstein College of Medicine, Bronx, N.Y., and the Clinical Applications and Prevention Program of the National Heart, Lung, and Blood Institute, Bethesda, Md.

Dr. Frishman is a recipient of a Preventive Cardiology Academic Award (Grant HL-00653-4) from the National Institutes of Health.

Originally published on March 29, 1984 (310:830-837).

there is a 15 per cent mortality during hosptalization, and the figure is somewhat higher in patients with recurrent infarctions.[22] Upon discharge from the hospital, patients continue to have an increased risk of cardiovascular morbidity and mortality. Patients under 70 years of age who survive a myocardial infarction have a 10 per cent mortality rate in the first year, with the highest proportion of deaths occurring in the first three months.[22] Subsequently, there is a five per cent annual mortality rate, which is six times higher than the expected rate in an age-matched population without coronary disease.[22] Approximately 85 per cent of the deaths that occur after hospitalization for myocardial infarction are related to coronary heart disease, and almost half of these are sudden deaths. Ventricular fibrillation appears to be the primary mechanism for sudden death.

Prospective epidemiologic studies have identified subsets of patients who have survived a myocardial infarction with a high, intermediate, or low risk of mortality.[23,24] The high-risk subset represents 15 per cent of the postinfarction population. This patient group has a mortality ranging from 20 to 40 per cent in the first year after hospital discharge and is characterized by the presence of cardiac symptoms before the index coronary event, by frequent ventricular ectopy on in-hospital 24-hour ambulatory electrocardiographic recordings, and by left ventricular dysfunction on physical examination and radionuclide evaluation.[24] In contrast, the low-risk subgroup, which makes up 30 per cent of the postinfarction population, has a 2 per cent mortality in the first year after discharge. This subgroup is characterized by the absence of infarction or cardiac symptoms before the index cardiac event, the absence of high-grade ventricular ectopy and congestive heart failure during hospitalization, and a negative submaximal exercise test performed just before discharge.[23-26] Between these two subgroups is the remaining 55 per cent of the postinfarction population. This intermediate-risk subgroup has one or two characteristics of the high-risk subset and a first-year mortality rate of approximately 10 per cent.[24]

Prolonging life in this heterogeneous group of patients is a major goal of preventive therapy. To reach this goal, a variety of therapeutic approaches have been evaluated, including life-style measures (dietary modifications, weight reduction, cessation of smoking, and physical exercise) and coronary-artery reconstructive surgery.[22] Specific pharmacologic agents have included anticoagulants,[27] drugs that inhibit platelet aggregation,[28] lipid-lowering agents,[29] calcium-channel blockers,[30] and antiarrhythmic drugs.[22] Among the multiple interventions evaluated to date, only β-adrenergic blockade has been clearly demonstrated to be efficacious in reducing cardiovascular mortality in patients surviving the acute phase of myocardial infarction.[22]

β-Adrenergic Blockade in the Postinfarction Period

The presumed major mechanisms for increased cardiovascular mortality during the postinfarction period include persistent myocardial ischemia, cardiac arrhythmias, and left ventricular dysfunction.[22-24,31-33] Raised levels of circulating cate-cholamines or enhanced sympathetic drive can increase both the severity of myo-cardial ischemia[34] and the frequency of ventricular arrhythmias.[35] After the clinical introduction of propranolol for angina pectoris and arrhythmias in 1963, it was conceived that β-blocker administration might favorably influence the natural history of patients with myocardial infarction by attenuating the undesira-ble consequences of increased sympathetic-nervous-system activity.[36] However, since these drugs could also depress left ventricular function — the other major factor contributing to mortality after infarction — β-blockers were initially avoided in patients with myocardial infarction or were used in small doses for fear of causing congestive heart failure.[36-40] Only recently have the results of large long-term clinical trials conclusively demonstrated the efficacy and safety of β-blocker therapy.

The Long-Term β-Blocker Trials

Since 1974, 13 major randomized controlled trials with β-blockers after acute myocardial infarction have been reported, with treatment and mean patient fol-low-up extending from nine months to four years.[2-15,41,42] Over 16,000 survivors of acute myocardial infarction were studied in attempts to document reductions in total mortality, cardiovascular mortality, coronary mortality, sudden death, and nonfatal reinfarction.

Seven different β-blockers have been evaluated in these studies: alprenolol, oxprenolol, pindolol, practolol, propranolol, sotalol, and timolol (Table 1).[2-15,41,42] A long-term trial evaluating metoprolol has been completed, but the findings are not yet available.[43]

TABLE 1.   Pharmacologic Properties of the β-Adrenergic Blocking Drugs Tested in Long-Term Trials.

Drug	Relative β_1-Selectivity	Intrinsic Sympathomimetic Activity	Membrane-Stabilizing Activity
Alprenolol *	0	+	+
Metoprolol †	+	0	0
Oxprenolol *	0	+	+
Pindolol	0	+ +	0
Practolol *	+	+	0
Propranolol	0	0	+ +
Sotalol *	0	0	0
Timolol	0	0	0

*Not available for clinical use in the United States.
†Results of study not available.

The 13 trials met the following criteria for study design: a trial end point of total mortality or of a clearly defined cause-specific mortality, a total sample size of at least 200, and random assignment of patients to either the β-blocker group or a concurrently followed control group. The study populations of the 13 trials contained from 230 to 3837 patients.[2-15,41,42] Twelve of the 13 trials used a placebo-treated control group and had a double-blind design. The time between the infarction and the start of β-blocker or placebo treatment ranged from under 24 hours to 7½ years. In 11 trials, patients in the low-risk and intermediate-risk groups were predominantly studied,[2-11,13,14,41,42] and in two trials only high-risk patients were evaluated.[12,15]

The results from 11 of the 13 long-term trials showed a lower mortality rate in the β-blocker group than in the placebo group.[2-15] In the three largest studies, the reduction in mortality with β-blocker treatment was statistically significant.[8-11] In the remaining eight trials, the results were not conclusive with regard to overall mortality.

The most convincing long-term data emerged from the Norwegian timolol trial[10] and the Beta-Blocker Heart Attack Trial, which employed propranolol hydrochloride.[11,44] The Norwegian trial, involving 1884 patients, demonstrated that timolol maleate, given orally at a dosage of 10 mg twice daily for an average of 17 months and for up to 33 months, reduced total mortality by 36 per cent and reduced the rate of nonfatal reinfarction by 34 per cent. The benefit of timolol was evident regardless of the patient's age or heart size or the site of the infarct. The Beta-Blocker Heart Attack Trial, involving 3837 patients, indicated that propranolol, given orally at a dosage of 60 to 80 mg three times daily for an average of 25 months and for up to 39 months, reduced total mortality by 26 per cent, cardiovascular mortality by 26 per cent, sudden cardiac death by 28 per cent, and nonfatal reinfarction by 16 per cent.[11,44,45] The protective effect was primarily seen in the first 12 to18 months of intervention — an observation similar to the findings of the Norwegian timolol study. The first-year mortality rate of 11.3 per cent in the placebo group of the timolol study[10] was about twice the rate in placebo recipients in the propranolol study,[11] suggesting that a higher-risk population was studied in Norway. In spite of this difference in study populations, the treatment effect was similar: the reduction in the first-year mortality rate was approximately 33 per cent with timolol and 39 per cent with propranolol (in both trials, patients were followed for a minimum of one year).

The estimate of mortality benefit obtained after combining the results of all 13 β-blocker trials is 22 per cent. However, caution is advisable in interpreting such results, because in pooling data one disregards certain differences — for example, in the patient populations, the types of β-blocker and dosage, and the time of initiation and the duration of treatment.

Nine of the 10 trials[2,5,9,10,13-15,41,44,45] reporting on the incidence of nonfatal reinfarction showed lower rates in the actively treated group. In only one of the trials was this lower incidence statistically significant.[10,45] A comparison of the effect of treatment on the incidence of nonfatal reinfarction is complicated for many reasons. For example, the diagnostic criteria for infarction differed between the trials, resulting in large differences in incidence. However, a statistical test for homogeneity indicated that the result of each trial was consistent with those of the others. When all the findings from the nine placebo-controlled, double-blind trials are pooled, the reduction in nonfatal reinfarction is 22 per cent — a benefit almost identical to that for overall mortality.

Mechanisms of Benefit

An analysis of cause-specific mortality in the β-blocker trials indicates that the reductions in total mortality were due to a reduction in cardiovascular deaths.[2-15] Although different definitions of sudden death were employed in the trials, the benefit from β-blocker treatment appears to have stemmed particularly from the prevention of these deaths. In the seven trials that reported on sudden death,[2,5,8-13] pooled data revealed that treatment led to a 28 per cent reduction in mortality — a 33 per cent reduction in sudden cardiac death, and a 20 per cent reduction in nonsudden cardiac death. These figures suggest a primary anti-arrhythmic effect to explain the beneficial actions of β-blockers. However, the reduction in nonsudden cardiac death, coupled with the observed reduction in nonfatal reinfarctions with β-blocker therapy, cannot be explained by an anti-arrhythmic effect alone and raises questions about whether other protective mechanisms were also involved.

Antiarrhythmic Effects

The β-blockers as a group, although not powerful antiarrhythmic agents, can attenuate cardiac stimulation by the sympathetic nervous system and can perhaps attenuate the potential for reentrant ventricular arrhythmias and sudden death.[46,47] The β-blockers can also inhibit lipolysis and thereby reduce the stress-induced increase in free fatty acids — a metabolic factor capable of inducing ventricular arrhythmias in the ischemic myocardium.[48,49]

In experimental studies, β-blockers have been demonstrated to raise the ventricular-fibrillation threshold in the ischemic myocardium.[47] In placebo-controlled clinical trials, the drugs have reduced the number of episodes of ventricular fibrillation and cardiac arrest during the acute phase of myocardial infarction.[50,51] In studies of long-term β-blocker treatment after infarction and in other studies, the occurrence of complex ventricular arrhythmias has been reduced by these drugs.[13,52-55]

In the Beta-Blocker Heart Attack Trial, 24-hour ambulatory electrocardiographic monitoring was performed at base line in all patients and after six weeks of therapy in a subgroup of patients. In the placebo group, the incidence of ventricular arrhythmias was higher at six weeks than at the base line. This increase was blunted by propranolol therapy.[53] It was recently reported that among the placebo recipients in that study, patients with complex ventricular arrhythmias had a mortality rate almost 2.5 times that of patients without ventricular arrhythmias

(5.3 per cent vs. 6.4 per cent).[56] The placebo–propranolol difference in mortality rate was 4.5 per cent among patients with complex arrhythmias, but only 1.6 per cent among patients without arrhythmia.[56]

Antiischemic Effects

Since the incidences of nonsudden cardiovascular deaths and nonfatal reinfarction were reduced by β-blockers in the long-term trials, the antiischemic actions of the drugs may also have contributed to their beneficial effects in the postinfarction period.

Stimulation of cardiac β-adrenergic receptors by endogenous catecholamines increases myocardial oxygen consumption and can thereby aggravate the ischemic process. Drugs that block the β-adrenergic receptor reduce the effects of catecholamines and decrease myocardial oxygen requirements by reducing systemic arterial pressure, heart rate, and myocardial contractility at rest and during exercise.[17,57] The effects of these drugs on coronary blood flow are less well defined. β-Blockers may decrease coronary blood flow by allowing the unopposed influence of coronary vasoconstrictor impulses to prevail; however, the drugs may also augment or maintain overall coronary blood flow by slowing the heart rate and increasing diastolic perfusion time.[17,18,57,58] More controversial are studies reporting favorable effects of β-blockers on myocardial metabolism, the coronary microvasculature, collateral blood flow, the distribution of myocardial blood flow, oxygen–hemoglobin affinity, and platelet function.[17,57,59-61] One or several of these antiischemic mechanisms may underlie the beneficial effects of β-blocker therapy in survivors of myocardial infarction.

| Clinical Use

It has been demonstrated conclusively that β-blockers can prolong life in many patients who have had infarction, yet a number of important questions regarding the clinical application of these drugs remain to be answered: Should all patients receive β-blockers after myocardial infarction? When should therapy be instituted and for how long? Which β-blocker should be used and at what dose? What are the risks of therapy?

Which Patients Should Receive β-Blockers?

Results from recruitment efforts in long-term postinfarction trials have demonstrated that one to two weeks after the acute event, up to 20 per cent of survivors have absolute or relative contraindications to β-blockade, such as severe congestive heart failure, bronchial asthma, disorders of atrioventricular and sinus-node function, hypotension, vasospastic angina, and Raynaud's phenomenon.[62,63] It appears from the findings of the Norwegian timolol trial and the Beta-Blocker Heart Attack Trial that a large proportion of the remaining patients stand to benefit from β-blocker therapy.[10,11,44,64-66] A relative reduction of approximately 20 to 25 per cent in total mortality in this population can be expected during one to two years of such therapy. A trend toward an even greater benefit has been observed in patients 60 years of age or older and in patients with complicated infarctions (ventricular tachyarrhythmias or mild left ventricular dysfunction). [10,65-68]

In the subgroup of survivors of infarction in whom the risk of mortality is high (i.e., 30 per cent in the first year), β-blocker treatment of 100 such patients for at least one year would prolong the lives of 7, assuming a 25 per cent benefit from therapy. In the low-risk subgroup (2 per cent mortality in the first year), 1400 patients would have to be treated to prolong the lives of 7, assuming the same relative benefit. The clinician may therefore question the need to treat low-risk survivors of infarction, since the hazards and costs of β-blocker therapy may outweigh the potential reduction of cardiovascular mortality. [68,69] In making this decision, one must also consider that the risk of nonfatal reinfarction is favorably influenced by these drugs, and that the occurrence of this morbid event cannot be predicted as reliably as cardiovascular mortality.

The decision to start β-blocker treatment should probably not be based on any consideration of performing coronary arteriography for assessing the potential benefit of coronary-artery surgery. Information is not available to determine whether β-blockers are useful in patients who have undergone successful coronary-bypass surgery after their infarction. However, considering that the risk of mortality and morbidity in the postinfarction population has multiple causes that may not be altogether eliminated by coronary-artery surgery, it would seem reasonable to administer β-blockers to this population as well. The decision to treat patients who have had an infarction is certainly easiest when other proved indications for β-blockade exist (e.g., angina pectoris, hypertension, and supraventricular tachyarrhythmias).

When Should Treatment Be Started?

In most of the long-term trials, β-blocker treatment was initiated one to three weeks after the infarction. By that time patients had begun to recover and were in a relatively stable condition. It was clearly advantageous to begin treatment while patients were hospitalized. In two trials, the International Multicentre Study with practolol and the Beta-Blocker Heart Attack Trial with propranolol, the results of early and late initiation of treatment were compared in hospitalized patients. In both trials it appeared, though it was not proved, that therapy initiated early (six to nine days after acute infarction) was more advantageous than therapy initiated after two to three weeks. [70]

It has been suggested that β-blocker treatment should be started upon admission to the hospital to reduce the high rate of early mortality among inpatients. [17] It has also been argued that treatment started within 6 to 12 hours may limit infarct size and subsequent mortality. [17] An analysis of the reported trials of acute intervention with β-blockers can provide information on this matter.

There have been 18 controlled trials of the effects of acute intervention with a β-blocker on early (usually four-week) mortality.[6,7,37-40,51,52,71-80] In 10 trials, an oral treatment regimen was used, which was probably started too late to have a favorable effect on the size of the infarct or on the eventual development of acute infarction.[7,37-40,71-75] In 7 of these 10 trials, total mortality was higher in the β-blocker group than in the placebo group.[37-40,72,74,75]

In the remaining eight trials, intravenous β-blocker treatment was started immediately and followed by oral treatment, to assess whether early intervention could favorably affect mortality, presumably by limiting infarct size.[6,51,52,76-78] Three of these trials demonstrated a higher mortality in the β-blocker group than in the placebo group,[6,76,77] four showed a lower mortality in the β-blocker group,[51,52,78,80] and one showed no difference.[79] In one of the trials, using metoprolol, there was a statistically significant reduction in mortality,[52] predominantly in patients with anterior-wall infarcts. Metoprolol also appeared to reduce serum levels of lactate dehydrogenase isoenzyme, when treatment was started within 12 hours,[81] and to reduce the incidence of in-hospital ventricular fibrillation.[50] The effect on mortality was the same whether treatment was started before or after 12 hours, suggesting that a reduction of infarct size did not contribute to the benefit. Judging from the mortality curves, which did not start to diverge until after five to seven days of therapy, the benefit seen with metoprolol may have been related to the 90-day oral maintenance regimen rather than to early intravenous treatment. A second study of metoprolol at the same dosage, in which patients were enrolled within six hours after the onset of symptoms and were also treated for 90 days, did not show any clear benefit.[76] An acute-intervention trial using intravenous and oral atenolol showed a favorable effect on in-hospital mortality, a reduction in repetitive ventricular arrhythmias, and a reduction in serum levels of creatine kinase MB isoenzyme.[51] Despite these favorable findings, however, there was no significant difference in long-term mortality (up to two years of follow-up) between placebo-treated and atenolol-treated patients.[51] Two recent reports[79,80] have highlighted the importance of administering active treatment very early after the onset of infarction: the indexes of infarct size were favorably reduced when timolol was given within an average of four hours after the onset of symptoms,[80] whereas no such effect was observed when propranolol was given within an average of 8.9 hours after the onset of chest pain.[79]

The clinical value of treatment with a β-adrenergic blocker within 18 hours of a myocardial infarction is now being reexamined in three cooperative trials in Europe and in the United States.[43] One of these studies (the Metoprolol in Acute Myocardial Infarction trial) is assessing intravenous and oral metoprolol; the results should be available in late 1984. Another (the International Study of Infarct Survival) will be evaluating intravenous and oral atenolol in 18,000 patients.[43]

To date, β-blockers have not received FDA approval for early intravenous use in patients with myocardial infarction, except for the treatment of supraventricular tachyarrhythmias. Thus, on the basis of the evidence available, oral β-blocker therapy should be started six to nine days after acute myocardial infarction in patients who are hemodynamically stable and have no contraindications to this treatment.

No conclusive data are available regarding a benefit on long-term survival when β-blocker therapy is begun months to years after an acute infarction. Nonetheless, it seems reasonable to assume that a favorable effect on mortality and morbidity will occur if treatment is initiated within a few months after hospitalization. Support of this view arises from retrospective subgroup analyses of a trial of oxprenolol, which suggested a beneficial effect on survival if treatment was started within four months after myocardial infarction, but no benefit if treatment was started at four months or later.[14]

When to Stop Therapy?

Studies of timolol and propranolol treatment have demonstrated a continuously increasing effect on mortality over approximately 18 months.[10,11,44] Beyond that point, interpretation of the data is more difficult because there were fewer deaths. It should be noted that cumulative mortality curves can give misleading visual impressions and that a small number of late deaths in either treatment group can substantially change the slope of the curve. Nevertheless, the mortality curves for the control and intervention groups in the propranolol trial remained essentially parallel from 18 to 36 months. In addition, whether the accruing benefit over 18 months would disappear if treatment were stopped at that time is not known. It is possible that some members of the intervention group who were saved initially by β-blocker treatment would still receive benefit from continuous therapy. As Rose has asked, "Do β-blockers merely keep the wolf from the door, and when protection is withdrawn, does he return?"[82]

Considering the available evidence, any decision to continue β-blocker therapy beyond 18 months has to be based on clinical judgment rather than on hard scientific data. The limited information available from the trials shows more deaths in the placebo group than in the β-blocker group after as long as 48 months.[10,11,14] This suggests that there is sustained benefit from continued therapy. One may be concerned about the extended use of these drugs in the general postinfarction population. However, patients in the intermediate-risk and high-risk subsets, who could potentially benefit the most from β-blocker treatment, may be the group to consider for longer courses of therapy.

An argument for stopping β-blocker treatment after a fixed period is the recent observation that β-blockers can lower plasma levels of high-density-lipoprotein cholesterol and raise levels of triglycerides, potentially increasing the risk of accelerated atherogenesis.[83-85] Whether this should be a matter of concern in patients who already have advanced coronary-artery disease is debatable. Finally, in the long-term trials there was no evidence of a β-blocker "withdrawal reaction" in patients who discontinued active treatment — an early concern that has not been confirmed in the postinfarction population.[70]

Which β-Blocker and at What Dosage?

Each of the long-term postinfarction trials compared a single β-blocking drug with a placebo. Since no direct comparisons of drugs are available, it is not known whether any specific β-blocking compound has advantages over another when used after infarction. Some investigators have argued that the pharmacodynamic differences that these drugs manifest (such as $β_1$-selectivity, membrane-stabilizing properties, and partial agonist activity) may be important, so that β-blockers are not interchangeable. Other investigators believe that the benefit of β-blockers is conferred by the $β_1$-adrenergic blockade that is common to the class, rather than by a specific compound.[86] The results of the individual trials suggest that differences in clinical efficacy do exist among the various β-blocking drugs, but whether these differences are real is not clear. The most favorable effects on mortality in all subgroups of patients have been observed with nonselective β-blockers without partial agonist activity (e.g., propranolol and timolol).[10,11] The two largest trials using $β_1$-selective adrenergic blockers showed a benefit that was predominant in patients with anterior-wall myocardial infarction.[8,9,52] The results of three recent trials with β-blockers having partial agonist activity revealed little or no benefit.[14,15,42]

Evidence is strongest at present for the use of oral timolol or propranolol, which are both nonselective β-blockers with similar pharmacokinetics. Both drugs have been shown to reduce total mortality, cardiovascular mortality, sudden death, and nonfatal reinfarction. Timolol maleate was the first orally active β-blocker to be approved for reducing the long-term risk of cardiovascular mortality in hemodynamically stable survivors of acute myocardial infarction who had no contraindications to β-blockade; a fixed daily dosage of 20 mg should be given in two divided doses.[87] Propranolol was recently approved for this use, primarily because of the favorable findings from the Beta-Blocker Heart Attack Trial. In that study, 180 to 240 mg of oral propranolol was employed in three divided doses, and plasma levels were used to monitor the dosage regimen.[88] The 180-mg dosage was assigned to 82 per cent of the patients[88]; this amount is approximately equivalent in pharmacological potency to 20 mg of timolol.[87]

A regimen of three daily doses was evaluated in the propranolol study; however, there are pharmacologic studies supporting a twice-daily regimen in survivors of myocardial infarction.[89] Both timolol and propranolol have plasma half-lives of four to five hours and pharmacodynamic half-lives that are substantially longer, allowing for twice-daily doses in patients with angina pectoris or systemic hypertension.[87,88,90-92] Pharmacodynamic studies with propranolol in normal volunteers indicate that clinical β-blockade, as assessed by blunting of exercise-induced tachycardia, is well maintained whether the drug is administered twice or three times daily at a dosage of 160 to 240 mg per day.[89]

On the basis of these observations and data from the Beta-Blocker Heart Attack Trial, propranolol was approved for use in survivors of acute myocardial infarction at a dosage range of 180 to 240 mg per day in two or three divided doses. The Beta-Blocker Trial showed no significant correlation between trough plasma propranolol levels and beneficial effect, indicating that the lower trough level that occurred with two daily doses should not compromise drug efficacy. Whether the new sustained-release propranolol preparation (Inderal LA)[93] will allow effective single daily doses in postinfarction patients is not known.

The trials have still not indicated what the optimal dosage of a β-blocker is, or whether it is preferable to use a fixed-dosage regimen for all postinfarction patients or to titrate the dosage until clinical β-adrenergic blockade is achieved.[88] Neither issue was carefully assessed in the reported trials. In some acute-intervention and long-term trials with propranolol, there was evidence that with lower doses than those used in the Beta-Blocker Heart Attack Trial, no clinical benefit occurred.[41] In addition, up to 480 mg per day may be needed to treat coexisting conditions, such as hypertension, arrhythmia, and angina pectoris.[88] In determining clinical efficacy, following plasma drug levels is not helpful, except for monitoring patient compliance with the prescribed drug regimen.

Side Effects

In deciding whether or not to treat patients with β-blockers after infarction, the risks of therapy must be weighed against the potential benefits. In studies of patients with no absolute or relative contraindications to β-blocker treatment, severe adverse reactions leading to discontinuation of therapy were fairly infrequent. The proportion of patients taken off active treatment for medical reasons ranged from 5.7 to 20.7 per cent.[2-15,63] The composition of the patient populations, the drug dosages and durations of treatment, and the methods of ascertaining and reporting adverse effects are factors that need to be considered in comparing these numbers. A remarkable finding was the observation that side effects were common with placebo treatment; in fact, the frequencies were similar to those with active treatment.[10,11,63]

Cardiovascular problems accounted for the greatest number of severe reactions in the β-blocker groups. These included symptomatic congestive heart failure, hypotension with and without dizziness, bradycardia, and atrioventricular block.[63] Heart failure was much less common than expected, perhaps because most of the studies excluded patients with even moderate heart failure at entry.[94,95] Nonetheless, patients with a history of heart failure are more likely to have problems.[68] The high-risk patients assigned to the propranolol group in a Norwegian study had a transient increase in heart failure within the first two weeks of therapy.[12]

Caution should therefore be exercised when using β-blockers in patients whose myocardial and bronchial function may depend on adequate stimulation from the sympathetic nervous system. Overall, the different β-blockers used in these trials were remarkably well tolerated and demonstrated similar safety profiles[2-7,10-15,41]; the exception was practolol, which caused a unique set of adverse reactions leading to its removal from the world market.[9]

The trials also showed a high frequency of minor side effects with β-blockers, which did not lead to discontinuation of the treatment. These included cases of cold extremities, nausea, constipation, asthma, fatigue, mental depression, impotence, and dry eyes.[2-15] The excess reporting of these effects in the patients treated with β-blockers was relatively small.

Public-Health Impact

The reduction in cardiovascular mortality and recurrent infarction in survivors of myocardial infarction who are treated with β-blockers represents an important breakthrough in the treatment of coronary-artery disease.[96] For the first time, a pharmacologic therapy has had a clearly demonstrated favorable effect on survival in the period after infarction. This comes after years of testing different therapeutic regimens with benefits that remain unproved. β-Blockers act by delaying recurrent fatal and nonfatal coronary events. Patients who are "saved" by β-blockade have an uncertain prognosis, since their underlying atherosclerotic heart disease is generally progressive and most will ultimately die from it. β-Blockers appear to be of only partial and temporary benefit in preventing death from coronary-artery disease. The primary prevention of coronary-artery disease and the control of factors that precipitate coronary events remain our strongest hopes for the future.

References

1. Frishman WH. β-Adrenoceptor antagonists: new drugs and new indications. N Engl J Med 1981; 305:500-6.
2. Wilhelmsson C, Vedin JA, Wilhelmsen L, Tibblin G, Werkö L. Reduction of sudden deaths after myocardial infarction by treatment with alprenolol: preliminary results. Lancet 1974; 2:1157-60.
3. Vedin A, Wilhelmsson C, Werkö L. Chronic alprenolol treatment of patients with acute myocardial infarction after discharge from hospital: effects on mortality and morbidity. Acta Med Scand [Suppl] 1975; 575:1-40.
4. Ahlmark G, Saetre H, Korsgren M. Reduction of sudden deaths after myocardial infarction. Lancet 1974; 2:1563.
5. Ahlmark G, Saetre H. Long-term treatment with β-blockers after myocardial infarction. Eur J Clin Pharmacol 1976; 10:77-83.
6. Andersen MP, Bechsgaard P, Frederiksen J, et al. Effect of alprenolol on mortality among patients with definite or suspected acute myocardial infarction: preliminary results. Lancet 1979; 2:865-8.
7. Barber JM, Boyle DMcC, Chaturvedi NC, Singh N, Walsh MJ. Practolol in acute myocardial infarction. Acta Med Scand [Suppl] 1975; 587:213-9.
8. Improvement in prognosis of myocardial infarction by long-term beta-adrenoreceptor blockade using practolol: a multicentre international study. Br Med J 1975; 3:735-40.
9. Reduction in mortality after myocardial infarction with long-term beta-adrenoceptor blockade: multicentre international study. Supplementary report. Br Med J 1977; 2:419-21.

10. Norwegian Multicenter Study Group. Timolol-induced reduction in mortality and reinfarction in patients surviving acute myocardial infarction. N Engl J Med 1981; 304:801-7.

11. β-Blocker Heart Attack Trial Research Group. A randomized trial of propranolol in patients with acute myocardial infarction. I. Mortality results. JAMA 1982; 247:1707-14.

12. Hansteen V, Møinichen E, Lorentsen E, et al. One year's treatment with propranolol after myocardial infarction: preliminary report of Norwegian multicentre trial. Br Med J 1982; 284:155-60.

13. Julian DG, Prescott RJ, Jackson FS, Szekely P. A controlled trial of sotalol for one year after myocardial infarction. Lancet 1982; 1:1142-7.

14. Taylor SH, Silke B, Ebbutt A, Sutton GC, Prout BJ, Burley DM. A long-term prevention study with oxprenolol in coronary heart disease. N Engl J Med 1982; 307:1293-301.

15. Australian and Swedish Pindolol Study Group. The effect of pindolol on the two-year mortality after complicated myocardial infarction. Eur Heart J 1983; 4:367-75.

16. Frishman WH. Clinical pharmacology of the new beta-adrenergic blocking drugs. Part 12. Beta-adrenoceptor blockade in myocardial infarction: the continuing controversy. Am Heart J 1980; 99:528-36.

17. Braunwald E, Muller JE, Kloner RA, Maroko PR. Role of beta-adrenergic blockade in the therapy of patients with myocardial infarction. Am J Med 1983; 74:113-23.

18. Turi ZG, Braunwald E. The use of β-blockers after myocardial infarction. JAMA 1983; 249:2512-6.

19. Hampton JR. Should every survivor of a heart attack be given a beta-blocker? I. Evidence from clinical trials. Br Med J 1982; 285:33-6.

20. Long-term and short-term beta-blockade after myocardial infarction. Lancet 1982; 1:1159-61.

21. May GS, Furberg CD, Eberlein KA, Geraci BJ. Secondary prevention after myocardial infarction: a review of short-term acute phase trials. Prog Cardiovasc Dis 1983; 25:335-59.

22. May GS, Eberlein KA, Furberg CD, Passamani ER, DeMets DL. Secondary prevention after myocardial infarction: a review of long-term trials. Prog Cardiovasc Dis 1982; 24:331-52.

23. Davis HT, DeCamilla J, Bayer LW, Moss AJ. Survivorship patterns in the posthospital phase of myocardial infarction. Circulation 1979; 60:1252-8.

24. Multicenter Postinfarction Research Group. Risk stratification after myocardial infarction. N Engl J Med 1983; 309:331-6.

25. Théroux P, Waters DD, Halphen C, Debaisieux J-C, Mizgala HF. Prognostic value of exercise testing soon after myocardial infarction. N Engl J Med 1979; 301:341-5.

26. Fein SA, Klein NA, Frishman WH. Exercise testing soon after uncomplicated myocardial infarction: prognostic value and safety. JAMA 1981; 245:1863-8.

27. Frishman WH, Ribner HS. Anticoagulation in myocardial infarction: a modern approach to an old problem. Am J Cardiol 1979; 43:1207-13.

28. Persantine-Aspirin Reinfarction Study Research Group. Persantine and aspirin in coronary heart disease. Circulation 1980; 62:449-61.

29. The Coronary Drug Project Research Group. Clofibrate and niacin in coronary heart disease. JAMA 1975; 231:360-81.

30. Myocardial Infarction Study Group. Secondary prevention of ischaemic heart disease: a long-term controlled lidoflazine study. Acta Cardiol [Suppl] (Brux) 1979; 24:1-116.
31. Weinblatt E, Shapiro S, Frank CW, Sager RV. Prognosis of men after first myocardial infarction: mortality and first recurrence in relation to selected parameters. Am J Public Health 1968; 58:1329-47.
32. Coronary Drug Project Research Group. Factors influencing long-term prognosis after recovery from myocardial infarction — three-year findings of the Coronary Drug Project. J Chronic Dis 1974; 27:267-85.
33. Vedin A, Wilhelmsen L, Wedel H, et al. Prediction of cardiovascular deaths and non-fatal reinfarction after myocardial infarction. Acta Med Scand 1977; 201:309-16.
34. Vatner SF, McRitchie RJ, Maroko PR, Patrick TA, Braunwald E. Effects of catecholamines, exercise, and nitroglycerin on the normal and ischemic myocardium in conscious dogs. J Clin Invest 1974; 54:563-75.
35. Han J. Mechanisms of ventricular arrhythmias associated with myocardial infarction. Am J Cardiol 1969; 24:800-13.
36. Snow PJD. Effect of propranolol in myocardial infarction. Lancet 1965; 2:551-3.
37. Balcon R, Jewitt DE, Davies JPH, Oram S. A controlled trial of propranolol in acute myocardial infarction. Lancet 1966; 2:917-20.
38. Clausen J, Felsby M, Jørgensen FS, Nielsen BL, Roin J, Strange B. Absence of prophylactic effect of propranolol in myocardial infarction. Lancet 1966; 2:920-4.
39. Propranolol in acute myocardial infarction: a multicentre trial. Lancet 1966; 2:1435-7.
40. Norris RM, Caughey DE, Scott PJ. Trial of propranolol in acute myocardial infarction. Br Med J 1968; 2:398-400.
41. Baber NS, Wainwright-Evans D, Howitt G, et al. Multicentre post-infarction trial of propranolol in 49 hospitals in the United Kingdom, Italy, and Yugoslavia. Br Heart J 1980; 44:96-100.
42. European Infarction Study Group. European Infarction Study — a secondary beta-blocker prevention trial after myocardial infarction. Circulation 1983; 68: Suppl 3:III-294. abstract.
43. Cutler JA. A review of on-going trials of beta-blockers in the secondary prevention of coronary heart disease. Circulation 1983; 67 (6:Part 2):I-62-5.
44. Goldstein S. Propranolol therapy in patients with acute myocardial infarction: the Beta-Blocker Heart Attack Trial. Circulation 1983; 67 (6:Part 2):I-53-7.
45. Furberg CD, Bell RL. Effect of beta-blocker therapy on recurrent non-fatal myocardial infarction. Circulation 1983; 67 (6:Part 2):I-83-5.
46. Pratt C, Lichstein E. Ventricular antiarrhythmic effects of beta-adrenergic blocking drugs: a review of mechanism and clinical studies. J Clin Pharmacol 1982; 22:335-47.
47. Anderson JL, Rodier HE, Green LS. Comparative effects of beta-adrenergic blocking drugs on experimental ventricular fibrillation threshold. Am J Cardiol 1983; 51:1196-1202.
48. Opie LH. Myocardial infarct size. Part 1. Basic considerations. Am Heart J 1980; 100:355-72.
49. Hjalmarson Å. Myocardial metabolic changes related to ventricular fibrillation. Cardiology 1980; 65:226-47.
50. Rydén L, Ariniego R, Arnman K, et al. A double-blind trial of metoprolol in acute myocardial infarction: effects on ventricular tachyarrhythmias. N Engl J Med 1983; 308:614-8.

51. Yusuf S, Sleight P, Rossi P, et al. Reduction in infarct size, arrhythmias and chest pain by early intravenous beta-blockade in suspected acute myocardial infarction. Circulation 1983; 67 (6:Part 2):I-32-41.

52. Hjalmarson Å, Elmfeldt D, Herlitz J, et al. Effect on mortality of metoprolol in acute myocardial infarction: a double-blind randomised trial. Lancet 1981; 2:823-7.

53. Lichstein E, Morganroth J, Harrist R, Hubble E. Effect of propranolol on ventricular arrhythmia. The Beta-Blocker Heart Attack Trial experience: preliminary data from the Heart Attack Trial experience. Circulation 1983; 67 (6:Part 2):I-5-10.

54. Koppes GM, Beckmann CH, Jones FG. Propranolol therapy for ventricular arrhythmias 2 months after myocardial infarction. Am J Cardiol 1980; 46:322-8.

55. von der Lippe G, Lund-Johansen P, Kjekshus J. Effects of timolol on late ventricular arrhythmias after acute myocardial infarction. Acta Med Scand (Suppl) 1981; 651:253-63.

56. Capone R, Friedman L, Byington R. The effect of propranolol on mortality in patients following acute myocardial infarction with complex ventricular arrhythmias. Circulation 1983; 68: Suppl III:III-294. abstract.

57. Frishman WH. Multifactorial actions of β-adrenergic blocking drugs in ischemic heart disease: current concepts. Circulation 1983; 67 (6:Part 2):I-11-8.

58. Kirk ES, Sonnenblick EH. Newer concepts in the pathophysiology of ischemic heart disease. Am Heart J 1982; 103:756-67.

59. Opie LH. Myocardial infarct size. Part 2. Comparison of anti-infarct effects of beta-blockade, glucose-insulin-potassium, nitrates and hyaluronidase. Am Heart J 1980; 100:531-52.

60. Frishman WH, Weksler BB. Effects of β-adrenoceptor blocking drugs on platelet function in normal subjects and patients with angina pectoris. In: Roskamm H, Graefe KH, eds. Advances in β-blocker therapy: proceedings of an international symposium. Amsterdam: Excerpta Medica, 1980:164-90.

61. Schrumph JD, Sheps DS, Wolfson S, Aronson AL, Cohen LS. Altered hemoglobin-oxygen affinity with long-term propranolol therapy in patients with coronary artery disease. Am J Cardiol 1977; 40:76-82.

62. Frishman W, Silverman R, Strom J, Elkayam U, Sonnenblick E. Clinical pharmacology of the new beta-adrenergic blocking drugs. Part 4. Adverse effects: choosing a β-adrenoreceptor blocker. Am Heart J 1979; 98:256-62.

63. Friedman LM. How do the various beta-blockers compare in type, frequency and severity of their adverse effects? Circulation 1983; 67 (6:Part 2):I-89-90.

64. Pedersen TR. The Norwegian multicenter study of timolol after myocardial infarction. Circulation 1983; 67 (6:Part 2):I-49-53.

65. Furberg CD, Byington RP. What do subgroup analyses reveal about differential response to beta-blocker therapy: the Beta-Blocker Heart Attack Trial experience. Circulation 1983; 67 (6:Part 2):I-98-101.

66. Rodda BE. The Timolol Myocardial Infarction Study: an evaluation of selected variables. Circulation 1983; 67 (6:Part 2):I-101-6.

67. Hawkins CM, Richardson DW, Vokonas PS. Effect on propranolol in reducing mortality in older myocardial infarction patients: the Beta-Blocker Heart Attack Trial experience. Circulation 1983; 67 (6:Suppl 2):I-94-7.

68. Furberg CD, Hawkins CM, Lichstein E. Effect of propranolol in post-infarction patients with mechanical or electrical complications. Circulation (in press).

69. Griggs TR, Wagner GS, Gettes LS. Beta-adrenergic blocking agents after myocardial infarction: an undocumented need in patients at lowest risk. J Am Coll Cardiol 1983; 1:1530-3.

70. Baber NS, Lewis JA. Beta-adrenoceptor blockade and myocardial infarction: when should treatment start and for how long should it continue? Circulation 1983; 67 (6:Part 2):I-71-7.

71. Barber JM, Murphy FM, Merrett JD. Clinical trial of propranolol in acute myocardial infarction. Ulster Med J 1967; 36:127-30.

72. Briant RB, Norris RM. Alprenolol in acute myocardial infarction: double-blind trial. NZ Med J 1970; 71:135-8.

73. Wilcox RG, Roland JM, Banks DC, Hampton JR, Mitchell JRA. Randomised trial comparing propranolol with atenolol in immediate treatment of suspected myocardial infarction. Br Med J 1980; 280:885-8.

74. Wilcox RG, Rowley JM, Hampton JR, Mitchell JRA, Roland JM, Banks DC. Randomised placebo-controlled trial comparing oxprenolol with disopyramide phosphate in immediate treatment of suspected myocardial infarction. Lancet 1980; 2:765-9.

75. Coronary Prevention Research Group. An early intervention secondary prevention study with oxprenolol following myocardial infarction. Eur Heart J 1981; 2:389-93.

76. Evemy KL, Pentecost BL. Intravenous and oral practolol in the acute stages of myocardial infarction. Eur J Cardiol 1978; 7:391-8.

77. Johansson BW. A comparative study of cardioselective β-blockade and diazepam in patients with acute myocardial infarction and tachycardia. Acta Med Scand 1980; 207:47-53.

78. McIlmoyle L, Evans A, Boyle DMcC, et al. Early intervention in myocardial ischaemia. Br Heart J 1982; 47:189. abstract.

79. Muller J, Roberts R, Stone P, et al. Failure of propranolol administration to limit infarct size in patients with acute myocardial infarction. Circulation 1983; 68: Suppl 3:III-294. abstract.

80. International Collaborative Study Group. Reduction of infarct size with the early use of timolol in acute myocardial infarction. N Engl J Med 1984; 310:9-15.

81. Hjalmarson Å, Herlitz J. Limitation of infarct size by beta-blockers and its potential role for prognosis. Circulation 1983; 67 (6:Part 2):I-68-71.

82. Rose G. Prophylaxis with β-blockers and the community. Br J Clin Pharmacol 1982; 14:45S-48S.

83. Leren P, Foss PO, Helgeland A, Hjermann I, Holme I, Lund-Larsen PG. Effect of propranolol and prazosin on blood lipids: the Oslo study. Lancet 1980; 2:4-6.

84. Shulman RS, Herbert PN, Capone RJ, et al. Effects of propranolol on blood lipids and lipoproteins in myocardial infarction. Circulation 1983; 67 (6:Part 2):I-19-21.

85. Johnson BF. The emerging problem of plasma lipid changes during antihypertensive therapy. J Cardiovasc Pharmacol 1982; 4: Suppl 2:213s-21s.

86. Harrison DC. Beneficial effects of beta-blockers: a class action or individual pharmacologic spectrum? Circulation 1983; 67 (6:Part 2):I-77-82.

87. Frishman WH. Atenolol and timolol: two new systemic β-adrenoceptor antagonists. N Engl J Med 1982; 306:1456-62.

88. Shand DG. How should the proper dose of a beta blocker be determined? Circulation 1983; 67 (6:Part 2):I-86-8.

89. Mullane JF, Kaufman J, Dvornik D, Coelho J. Propranolol dosage, plasma concentration, and beta blockade. Clin Pharmacol Ther 1982; 32:692-700.

90. Thadani U, Parker JO. Propranolol in angina pectoris: comparison of therapy given two and four times daily. Am J Cardiol 1980; 46:117-23.

91. Berglund G, Andersson O, Hansson R, Olander R. Propranolol given twice daily in hypertension. Acta Med Scand 1973; 194:513-5.

92. MacLeod SM, Hamet P, Kaplan H, et al. Antihypertensive efficacy of propranolol given twice daily. Can Med Assoc J 1979; 121:737-40.

93. Leahey WJ, Neill JD, Varma MPS, Shanks RG. Comparison of the efficacy and pharmacokinetics of conventional propranolol and a long acting preparation of propranolol. Br J Clin Pharmacol 1980; 9:33-40.

94. Julian DG. Can beta-blockers be safely used in patients with recent acute myocardial infarction who also have congestive heart failure? Circulation 1983; 67 (6:Part 2): I-91.

95. Gundersen T. Influence of heart size on mortality and reinfarction in patients treated with timolol after myocardial infarction. Br Heart J 1983; 50:135-9.

96. Friedewald WT. Beta-adrenergic blockade after myocardial infarction: clinical and public health implications of the reported beta-blocker clinical trials. Circulation 1983; 67 (6:Part 2):I-110-1.

Correspondence

β-Adrenergic Blockade for Survivors of Acute Myocardial Infarction*

To the Editor:

In their review of β-adrenergic blockade for survivors of acute myocardial infarction (March 29 issue),[1] Frishman et al. note that a large proportion of patients stand to benefit from β-blockade therapy. In fact in the four placebo-controlled, randomized, double-blind clinical trials that provided population data,[2-5] the proportion of survivors of acute myocardial infarction found eligible for this therapy was only 13 per cent in the study by Hansteen et al., 23 per cent in the β-blocker heart attack trial, 45 per cent in the study by Julian et al., and 52 per cent in the Norwegian timolol study.

Since we had adopted the policy of long-term β-blockade after recent acute myocardial infarction, we were able to determine in our patients what proportion of survivors actually received this therapy. A total of 113 patients were hospitalized with acute myocardial infarction between February 1983 and March 1984. Of these, 15 (13 per cent) died in the acute phases of their illness before β-blockade therapy was initiated. Only 29 (30 per cent) of the survivors were suitable candidates for long-term prevention with a β-blocker. The remaining 69 (70 per cent) either had a contraindication to β-blockers (52 patients, 53 per cent) or were receiving the medication for another indication (17 patients, 17 per cent). The reasons for exclusion were congestive heart failure (40 patients), atrioventricular block (4), obstructive lung disease (4), insulin-treated diabetes mellitus (2),

*Originally published on September 6, 1984 (311:670-671).

symptomatic peripheral vascular disease (1), and poor compliance (1). Propranolol, 160 mg daily, was the agent most often prescribed, and the median follow-up period thus far has been six months. During this period the therapy was discontinued because of precipitation of severe side effects in 6 patients (20 per cent).

In this clinical survey we found that only a minority of patients (30 per cent) who survive acute myocardial infarction are in principle eligible for secondary prevention with β-blockade therapy. This figure is in the range obtained from the clinical trials cited above.[2-5] Moreover, the number of patients given long-term β-blockers for secondary prevention was diminished by an additional 20 to 30 per cent because of withdrawal after the development of serious side effects from these drugs.[2,4,5] Thus, although of proved benefit as a measure in secondary prevention of coronary heart disease, β-blockade therapy is restricted to only a limited number of survivors of acute myocardial infarction.

ODED SHALEV, M.D., NILI DROR, B.A.,
GALIA RAHAV, M.D., RAMI ELIAKIM, M.D.,
AND JACOB MENCZEL, M.D.
Hadassah University Hospital, Mt. Scopus
Jerusalem, Israel

1. Frishman WH, Furberg CD, Friedewald WT. Beta-adrenergic blockade for survivors of acute myocardial infarction. N Engl J Med 1984; 310:830-6.
2. Hansteen V, Møinichen E, Lorensten E, et al. One year's treatment with propranolol after myocardial infarction: preliminary report of Norwegian multicentre trial. Br Med J 1982; 284:155-60.
3. β-Blocker Heart Attack Trial Research Group. A randomized trial of propranolol in patients with acute myocardial infarction. II. Morbidity results. JAMA 1983; 250:2814-9.
4. Julian DG, Prescott RJ, Jackson FS, Szekely P. Controlled trial of sotalol for one year after myocardial infarction. Lancet 1982; 1:1142-7.
5. Norwegian Multicenter Study Group. Timolol-induced reduction in mortality and reinfarction in patients surviving acute myocardial infarction. N Engl J Med 1981; 304:801-7.

To the Editor:

Frishman et al. have nicely reviewed the use of β-adrenergic blockade in survivors of acute myocardial infarction. It is of interest that the most favorable effects on mortality have been observed with nonselective β-blockers.[1,2] The largest benefit from β-blockers was reduction of sudden death. One mechanism that was not discussed by Frishman et al. was the ability of nonselective β-blockers to block hypokalemia associated with epinephrine release. Levels of epinephrine consistent with the amount secreted during an acute myocardial infarction have been shown to decrease the serum potassium concentration by 0.8 mmol per liter. This phenomenon can be blocked by β_2 or nonselective β-blockers.[3,4] A possible series of events in some patients might start with stress leading to epinephrine release followed by rapid falls in potassium levels. Hypokalemia would lead to ventricular irritability in an ischemic heart, with subsequent fibrillation and sudden death. Non-selective β-blockers such as propranolol and timolol could prevent the hypokalemia and conceivably abort this sequence.

PHILIP ALTUS, M.D.
Tampa General Hospital
Tampa, FL 33606

1. Norwegian Multicenter Study Group. Timolol-induced reduction in mortality and reinfarction in patients surviving acute myocardial infarction. N Engl J Med 1981; 304:801-7.
2. β-Blocker Heart Attack Trial Research Group. A randomized trial of propranolol in patients with acute myocardial infarction. I. Mortality results. JAMA 1982; 247:1707-14.
3. Brown MJ, Brown DC, Murphy MB. Hypokalemia from beta$_2$-receptor stimulation by circulating epinephrine. N Engl J Med 1984; 309:1414-9.
4. Vincent HH, Man in't Veld AJ, Boomsma F, Derky FHM, Wenting GJ, Schalekamp MADH. Cardioprotection by blockade of beta$_2$-adrenoceptors. Eur Heart J 1983; 4 (Suppl D):109-15.

The above letters were referred to the authors of the article in question, who offer the following reply:

To the Editor:

We appreciate the comments of Dr. Shalev et al. and Dr. Altus regarding our recent paper.

The target population for β-blocker therapy consists of patients who have survived the acute phase of myocardial infarction — i.e., those alive and in stable condition one to two weeks after hospital admission. The data in the reported trials, based on more than 16,000 patients studied in 16 countries, indicate that 20 to 50 per cent of this target population had absolute or relative contraindications to β-blocker therapy. There are reasons to believe that patients excluded from trial participation because they were already taking β-blockers, were likely to be placed on them, or declined to participate would respond to β-blockers in a manner similar to those enrolled. Patients with congestive heart failure whose condition was controlled at the time of randomization were usually not excluded from participation. In fact, recent subgroup analysis suggests that patients with mechanical (pump) complications before enrollment responded very favorably to β-blocker treatment.[1]

Dr. Altus addresses a possible mechanism by which β-blockers may exert their protective effects in survivors of acute myocardial infarction. Although the prevention of catecholamine-induced hypokalemia may occur with nonselective β-blockers,[2] it is not known whether this effect actually contributed to the reduced mortality observed in the β-blocker postinfarction trials. The effect of β-blockade on serum potassium levels is now being analyzed from data obtained in the β-Blocker Heart Attack Trial. In addition to prevention of hypokalemia, other β-blocker actions[3] need to be studied for a better understanding of how these drugs reduce the risk of mortality, sudden death, and nonfatal reinfarction in survivors of acute myocardial infarction.

WILLIAM H. FRISHMAN, M.D.
Albert Einstein College of Medicine
Bronx, NY 10461

CURT D. FURBERG, M.D.
WILLIAM T. FRIEDEWALD, M.D.
National Heart, Lung, and Blood Institute
Bethesda, MD 20205

1. Furberg CD, Hawkins CM, Lichstein E. Effect of propranolol in postinfarction patients with mechanical or electrial complications. Circulation 1984; 69:761-5.
2. Vincent HH, Man in't Veld AJ, Boomsma F, Derkx FHM, Wenting GJ, Schalekamp MADH. Cardioprotection by blockade of beta$_2$-adrenoceptors. Eur Heart J 1983; 4 (Suppl D):109-15.
3. Frishman WH. Multifactorial actions of beta-adrenergic blocking drugs in ischemic heart disease: current concepts. Circulation 1983; 67: Suppl 1:I-11-8.

Drug Administration in Hepatic Disease

Roger L. Williams, M.D.

THE biologic processes that govern the absorption of a drug into the body and its elimination from it are important determinants of its pharmacologic effect and toxicity. Absorption occurs after administration of a drug parenterally or via the gastrointestinal tract, the skin, lung, eye, or other tissues and organs. Each route possesses certain characteristics that control the rate and extent of entry of a drug into the systemic circulation. Drugs are eliminated from the body through the excretion of unchanged drug or through biotransformation to one or more metabolites. Because absorption usually occurs more rapidly than elimination, the processes of elimination determine the concentration of drug and metabolite in the body at most times and are of prime importance in the maintenance of a desired drug concentration in the plasma or tissues. Elimination may occur in any tissue or organ of the body, but in most instances it is the result of active and passive processes within the kidney or liver. Although both organs metabolize drugs and both excrete drugs without biotransforming them, a primary function of the liver is to metabolize drugs to form metabolites that are more water soluble, and a primary function of the kidney is to excrete drugs without biotransformation.

Pharmacokinetics is one of the tools used by clinicians and investigators to measure hepatic and renal processes of elimination. It provides information about the time course of the amount of drug in the body (or concentration of drug in blood or plasma) in terms that can be used to design rational dosage regimens and to adjust those regimens in the presence of disease states that alter drug absorption and disposition. Clinicians now appreciate that alterations in renal function can affect the pharmacokinetic profile of a drug, and are accustomed to altering drug doses in the presence of renal impairment. The utility of altering the drug dose in renal impairment to improve efficacy and minimize toxicity depends on experimental observations that correlate alterations in drug disposition in the presence of renal disease with one or more indexes of renal function, such as creatinine level or creatinine clearance. These correlations, which are frequently expressed by means of a nomogram, provide a basis for altering the dose of a drug according to the degree of renal impairment.

From the Division of Clinical Pharmacology and Experimental Therapeutics, Department of Medicine, and the Department of Pharmacy, University of California, San Francisco.
Originally published on December 29, 1984 (309:1616-1622).

Current knowledge to provide a basis for altering dosage in the presence of hepatic disease is far less complete. Alterations in drug disposition in patients with hepatic impairment are not as consistent as in patients with renal impairment and do not always correlate well with biochemical indexes of hepatic function. Coupled with the complexities of hepatobiliary drug excretion and biotransformation, these facts may result in a certain degree of therapeutic nihilism. Clinicians have been admonished to avoid the use of drugs in patients with hepatic disease and to reduce the dose if a drug must be given. Although this approach is sometimes justified and the caution that it represents is always reasonable, it can also deny a patient access to beneficial drugs and can lead to the administration of drugs in amounts that are less than effective.

Hepatic structural and functional abnormalities not only occur in chronic cirrhosis and hepatitis but are factors common to a variety of pathophysiologic states, including congestive heart failure and metabolic, inflammatory, toxic, infectious, and neoplastic diseases. Many patient groups are therefore likely to receive drugs whose absorption and disposition may be altered by the presence of disease-induced morphologic and functional changes of the liver. In the past decade, a number of theoretical and experimental reports have appeared that extend our understanding of the role of the liver in the absorption and elimination of drugs and the ways in which alterations in hepatic disease can be reflected in changes in the pharmacokinetics of these drugs. This information may be used in turn to improve dosage regimens in patients with hepatic impairment. The interpretation and use of these studies in the clinical setting requires an understanding of certain pharmacokinetic precepts common to many of these reports, as well as an appreciation of specific elements of hepatic structure and function.

Pharmacokinetic Variables

Recent investigations of drug disposition in hepatic disease have relied on several fundamental pharmacokinetic variables to determine whether and to what degree hepatic dysfunction alters hepatic metabolism. These variables therefore serve a dual role: they can be used to determine dosage regimens for drugs that are administered to patients with hepatic impairment, and they also may reflect intrahepatic processes of biotransformation and excretion. The investigational use of pharmacokinetic variables to assess intrahepatic processes treats the liver as a "black box," whose detailed operations in vivo are beyond the scrutiny of the investigator but whose processes may be inferred from changes in output. Just as a problem in craftmanship or materials may be pinpointed through observation and analysis of the products of a factory, the use of pharmacokinetic variables to define alterations in hepatic function identifies defects in hepatic processes through observation and analysis of change in the pattern of drug and metabolite elimination.

Pharmacokinetic variables used in studies of hepatic alterations in drug disposition include clearance, volume of distribution, half-life, and fraction of drug unbound in blood and plasma. For drugs that exhibit monoexponential decline in the logarithm of the plasma-concentration–time curve, these variables are readily defined. Clinicians are familiar with concepts about clearance in renal physiology, in which renal clearance of an exogenous or endogenous (usually creatinine) compound is calculated through the use of the equation CL = UV/P. Like all expressions for clearance (CL), this equation relates a rate of elimination of a substance (U, or urinary concentration, times V, or urine flow rate) to a plasma or blood concentration (P). A more general expression for clearance of a drug by any eliminating organ (including the liver) is

$$\frac{\text{rate of elimination}_{\text{organ}}}{C} = CL_{\text{organ}}, \qquad (Eq.\ 1)$$

where C denotes the blood or plasma concentration of the drug whose clearance is being assessed, rate of elimination$_{\text{organ}}$ the rate at which the compound is eliminated by the organ, and CL_{organ} the clearance of a drug by the organ. An important and useful feature of clearance is that it is additive: If a drug is eliminated from the body by several organs, then total systemic clearance (CL_s) is equal to the sum of the individual organ clearances. If a drug is eliminated by a single organ (which is true of the liver for many drugs), systemic clearance is equal to organ clearance. The choice of concentration in Equation 1 defines the clearance: plasma clearance (CL_p), if C is plasma drug concentration (C_p); blood clearance (CL_b), if C is blood concentration (C_b); and clearance based on unbound-drug concentration (CL_f), if C is free-drug concentration (C_f) in plasma.

Volume of distribution (V) is a pharmacokinetic variable that relates the amount of drug in the body — A_b (rather than its rate of elimination, which is clearance) — to a concentration (C): $A_b/C = V$. As for clearance, the choice of concentration (C_b, C_p, or C_f) determines the volume (V_b, V_p, or V_f). Half-life ($t\frac{1}{2}$) is a variable that defines the time required for the amount of drug in the body (or the concentration of drug in the blood or plasma) to fall by half. It is calculated as the reciprocal of the rate constant of elimination (k) multiplied by 0.693 ($t\frac{1}{2} = k/0.693$). For a drug exhibiting monoexponential decline in plasma or blood, k is calculated as the slope of the log-linear portion of the concentration-versus-time curve. Protein binding is incorporated in expressions of volume and clearance (volume or clearance based on unbound-drug concentration) through the use of the term f, which is the ratio of unbound-drug concentration (C_f) to total concentration in blood ($f_b = C_f/C_b$) or plasma ($f_p = C_f/C_p$).

Although half-life is commonly used to characterize the pharmacokinetics of a drug, its utility in determining dosage regimens is less than that of clearance. At steady state, when the rate of drug administration equals the rate of drug elimination, clearance is used to calculate a dose that will achieve a desired plasma concentration of drug. According to Equation 1, the rate of administration (the desired dosage regimen) at steady state is the product of the plasma or blood clearance and the desired plasma or blood drug concentration. For example, if the clearance of a drug is 100 ml per minute (6 liters per hour) and the desired plasma concentration is 4 mg per liter, the dosage that will produce this concentration is 24 mg per hour (6 liters per hour × 4 mg per liter). Similarly, the volume of distribution may be used to calculate the amount of drug that must be administered to achieve a desired plasma or blood drug concentration. Because it takes approximately three to four half-lives to approach steady state, the half-life of a drug indicates the time it takes for the drug to reach a stable concentration in blood or plasma once a specific regimen is instituted, or for the concentration to fall to negligible amounts if a regimen is stopped.

Hepatic Physiology and Anatomy

Anatomically, the liver occupies a remarkable and in some ways unique position for an eliminating organ. Unlike the kidney, which "sees" a drug only after it has entered the systemic circulation, the liver is positioned, in terms of blood supply, between gastrointestinal sites of drug absorption and the systemic circuit (Fig. 1). Blood flowing to the liver is drawn primarily from the splanchnic vasculature that enters the liver through the portal system (about 80 per cent of total hepatic flow) and secondarily through the hepatic artery (20 per cent). After entering the liver, blood flows in the veins and arteries of the portal triads, enters the sinusoidal spaces of the liver, and exits via the central hepatic vein. Transfer of drug between the blood and the hepatocytes occurs within the sinusoids, with biotransformation or excretion (or both) of unchanged drug into the biliary system occurring at the level of the hepatocyte. As shown in Figure 1, drugs entering and leaving the liver in the bloodstream exist unbound (C_f) or bound (C_{bound}) to blood constituents, just as they exist in the liver and other tissues in the unbound ($C_{L,free}$) or bound ($C_{L,bound}$) state. Presumably, only drug that is unbound in blood or plasma enters the hepatocyte, and only unbound drug is subject to hepatic biotransformation or excretion. Recent evidence suggests that the entry of certain compounds into the hepatocyte can depend not only on passive diffusion of the unbound species, but also on a more active process involving a complex interaction between bound and unbound compound, albumin, and receptors on the surface of the hepatocyte.[1,2] The anatomic relation between the liver, the gastrointestinal tract, and the blood supply of these organs has important implications for drug absorption and dosage. Because the liver is situated between enteric sites of absorption and the systemic circulation, it can profoundly influence the bioavailability of a drug given orally — an action that has been described as the first-pass effect. If bioavailability (F) is defined as the fraction of the dose of a drug given orally that enters the systemic circulation, it is apparent that a drug that is efficiently removed by the liver from the bloodstream will have a low bioavailability. If the liver removes a drug completely from the blood on a single pass through the liver, the drug's bioavailability after an oral dose will be zero. After entry into the hepatocyte, a drug may be excreted without biotransformation, first into the biliary system and subsequently into the gastrointestinal tract, where reabsorption may occur. This entero-

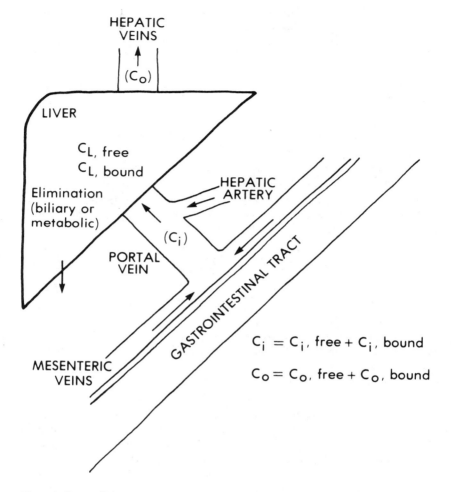

Figure 1. Routes of Transport in Hepatic Elimination of Drug.
For explanation of abbreviations, see text.

hepatic cycling may prolong the systemic availability of the drug. Alterations in hepatic blood flow through intrahepatic and extrahepatic shunts may also profoundly change drug absorption and disposition. Protein binding of a drug to plasma or blood constituents may influence the availability of drug to hepatic sites of biotransformation.

Because hepatic disease states may alter hepatic blood flow, enterohepatic cycling, drug protein binding, or intrahepatic functional processes, the influence of a particular disease on the elimination of a drug is highly variable and frequently unpredictable. A major conceptual advance in the past decade has been the use of the extraction ratio of a drug by the liver to categorize drugs according to whether they are highly or poorly extracted by this organ. This categorization provides a basis for determining the influence on drug disposition of specific hepatic variables, such as blood flow, protein binding, and intrahepatic elimination processes.

Extraction Ratio

At steady state, the rate of elimination of a drug by the liver may be defined as the difference between the rate at which the drug enters the organ and the rate at which it leaves. The rate of entry is equal to the flow of blood to the organ (Q) multiplied by the concentration of drug in the blood entering the organ (C_i), and the rate of exit of drug is equal to Q multiplied by the concentration of drug (C_o) in hepatic venous effluent (Fig. 1). According to the relation expressed in Equation 1, hepatic clearance (CL_H) is thus defined as

$$CL_H = \frac{QC_i - QC_o}{C_i}; \qquad (Eq.\ 2a)$$

$$CL_H = Q\left(\frac{C_i - C_o}{C_i}\right) \qquad (Eq.\ 2b)$$

The expression in parentheses in Equation 2b is defined as the extraction ratio. If the liver is highly efficient in removing a drug from the blood $(C_o \rightarrow 0)$, the extraction ratio approaches unity, and clearance of the drug by the liver approaches and becomes limited by hepatic blood flow:

$$CL_H = Q. \qquad (Eq.\ 3)$$

Equation 3 has important clinical implications. Elimination of highly extracted drugs by the liver is limited not by intrahepatic processes or protein binding but rather by the rate at which the hepatic portal system and hepatic artery can transport them to the liver. The metabolism of these drugs is therefore said to be perfusion, or flow-rate, limited. Hepatic metabolic processes and blood and tissue protein binding are factors that theoretically should not influence the hepatic clearance of highly extracted drugs, whereas changes in hepatic blood flow should be reflected directly in changes in hepatic clearance. Conditions in which hepatic blood flow may be reduced, such as congestive heart failure and cirrhosis, may result in decrements in clearance of highly extracted drugs — decrements that correspond directly with the reduction in flow. If a drug enters the hepatic-portal blood system intact after oral administration and is completely absorbed, the extraction ratio (ER) is related to bioavailability (F) by the following equation:

$$F = 1 - ER. \qquad (Eq.\ 4)$$

With highly extracted drugs, whose extraction ratio approaches unity, bioavailability will be correspondingly low $(F \rightarrow 0)$. Drugs that are efficiently removed from the bloodstream by the liver will have low systemic availability after oral administration. Furthermore, small changes in the extraction ratio will result in large changes in availability. If the extraction ratio declines only slightly (for example, from 0.95 to 0.90), the bioavailability doubles (from 0.05 to 0.10). This observation may explain why plasma drug concentrations of highly extracted drugs (for example, propranolol) differ widely among patients after oral administration. In patients in whom intrahepatic and extrahepatic shunts exist, particularly those with cirrhosis in whom portosystemic shunts have been surgically placed, bioavailability of highly extracted drugs will be dramatically increased.

Equations 2 and 3 demonstrate that measurements of hepatic clearance of highly extracted drugs do not reflect intrahepatic processes, but rather provide estimates of hepatic blood flow. Several theoretical attempts have been made to define hepatic clearance in the absence of flow limitations. All these attempts have relied on models that define a relation between the concentration of drug in the liver (a difficult if not impossible measure to perform in vivo) and the concentration of drug in blood leaving the liver. A widely used model, which postulates a direct relation between drug concentration in the liver and drug concentration in hepatic venous effluent, has produced the following general equation:

$$CL_H = Q\left(\frac{f_b CL_{intrinsic}}{Q + f_b CL_{intrinsic}}\right), \qquad (Eq.\ 5)$$

where $CL_{intrinsic}$ is defined conceptually as the intrinsic ability of the liver to clear a drug from the blood in the absence of flow limitations. Although the derivations and assumptions of Equation 5 are beyond the scope of this article (see references 3 through 5 for a more complete presentation), the equation is clinically pertinent. For highly extracted drugs ($f_b CL_{intrinsic} >> Q$), Equation 5 reduces, in accordance with the principles introduced in Equations 2a and 2b, to Equation 3 ($CL_H = Q$). For drugs that are poorly extracted ($f_b CL_{intrinsic} << Q$), Equation 5 reduces to

$$CL_H = f_b CL_{intrinsic}. \qquad (Eq.\ 6)$$

Equation 6 thus indicates that hepatic clearance of drugs that are poorly extracted by the liver is sensitive not to hepatic blood flow but to the unbound fraction of drug in blood (f_b) and to the intrinsic ability of the liver to clear a drug in the absence of flow limitations ($CL_{intrinsic}$). Changes in either variable should be reflected directly in changes in hepatic clearance.

Changes in blood flow, protein binding, and intrinsic ability of the liver to remove a drug are therefore all factors that can influence the elimination of a drug from the body by the liver. This influence varies depending on whether the drug is highly or poorly extracted by the liver. Clinical investigations of these variables in patients with liver disease have indicated that all three can be altered in the presence of hepatic impairment. The influence of hepatic disease on drug disposition will thus depend on the importance of the liver in the elimination of the drug (that is, the fraction of total systemic clearance represented by hepatic clearance), the degree to which the drug is extracted by the liver, and the type and extent of

Table 1. Pharmacokinetics of Highly Extracted Drugs in Liver Disease.*

Drug	Disease	Volume †	Half-Life	Clearance	Reference
Lidocaine	Cirrhosis	2.22±0.94 liters/kg (1.70±0.21) (Vd$_\beta$)	343±234 min ‡ (108±7.0)	5.2±2.1 ml/min/kg ‡ (9.2±0.8)	10
	Acute hepatitis	3.10±1.80 liters/kg (2.00±0.5) (Vd$_{ss}$)	160 min (90)	13.0±3.9 ml/min/kg (20.0±3.9)	11
Meperidine	Cirrhosis	263±28 liters (232±53) (Vd$_{ss}$)	359±77 min ‡ (213±25)	573±158 ml/min ‡ (900±316)	12
	Acute hepatitis	5.56±1.8 liters/kg (5.94±2.65) (V)	6.99±2.74 hr ‡ (3.37±0.82)	649±228 ml/min ‡ (1261±527)	13
Metoprolol	Cirrhosis	4.0±0.94 liters/kg (3.2±0.49) (Vd$_{ss}$)	7.2±3.79 hr (4.2±2.69)	0.61±0.41 liter/min (0.80±0.27)	14
Morphine	Cirrhosis	2.3±1.3 liters/kg (2.9±2.4) (V)	2.2±1.3 hr (2.5±1.5)	1.15±0.35 liters/min (1.23±0.43)	15
Pentazocine	Cirrhosis	356±94 liters (415±107) (Vd$_\beta$)	396±115 min ‡ (230±28)	675±296 ml/min ‡ (1246±236)	12
Propranolol	Cirrhosis	380±108 liters ‡ (290±54) (Vd$_\beta$)	11.2±8.47 hr ‡ (4.0±0.9)	580±370 ml/min (860±270)	16
Verapamil	Cirrhosis	481±141 liters ‡ (296±67) (V)	815±516 min ‡ (170±72)	0.545±0.181 liter/min ‡ (1.571±0.405)	17

*Values are expressed as means ±S.D.; those in parentheses were observed in healthy controls.

†V denotes volume of distribution (one-compartment model), Vd$_\beta$ volume of distribution calculated as [clearance × 0.693]/half-life, and Vd$_{ss}$ volume of distribution at steady state.

‡Significantly different from control value (P<0.05).

derangement of the three variables. In discussing clinical investigations of drug disposition in hepatic disease, it is useful to distinguish studies of highly extracted drugs from studies of poorly extracted drugs.

Highly Extracted Drugs

Because the clearance of highly extracted drugs is sensitive to changes in hepatic blood flow (Equation 3), knowledge of derangements in the flow of blood to the liver is clinically useful. Although measurement of hepatic blood flow has proved difficult in human beings,[6] several studies have suggested that hepatic blood flow, although highly variable, is generally reduced in patients with chronic liver disease.[7-9] In accord with this observation, clinical studies have documented that the clearance of highly extracted drugs is also generally reduced in patients with chronic alcoholic liver disease (Table 1). For these drugs, the reduction (ratio of average clearance in cirrhotic subjects to average clearance in healthy controls) ranges between 0.35 and 0.94. Most of the clinical studies cited in Table 1 did not estimate hepatic blood flow or intrinsic clearance and thus were not able to determine whether the decrease in clearance was attributable to a reduction in blood flow (as expected) or to a reduction in intrinsic clearance. One study that did, however, concluded that the reduction in the systemic clearance of the highly extracted drug D-propranolol could be attributed as much to a reduction in intrinsic clearance as to a reduction in hepatic blood flow.[18]

The data in Table 1 suggest that the dosage of highly extracted drugs should be reduced by at least 50 per cent in patients with chronic liver disease. In patients with cirrhosis, an additional reason for reducing the dose is the high degree of intrahepatic and extrahepatic shunting that may occur in the presence of this disease. Because shunts reduce drug contact with hepatic sites of elimination, shunting can result in dramatic increases in oral bioavailability. Groszmann et al. estimated that more than 50 per cent of portal blood flow may be shunted through mesenteric and splenic vascular beds in patients with chronic liver disease.[19]

Changes in the volume of distribution and half-life of highly extracted drugs in patients with hepatic disease are not as consistent as changes in clearance. With several drugs, a substantial reduction in clearance occurs without a change in volume (Table 1). Because of the relation of half-life to clearance and volume ($t\frac{1}{2} - 0.693$ V/CL), decrements in clearance — without changes in volume — will produce proportional increases in half-life. This prediction has been confirmed for several of the drugs listed in Table 1. The absence of a change in volume of distribution indicates that the amount of drug to be given to achieve a desired plasma concentration does not change on average in patients with chronic liver disease, although the rate of drug administration to maintain this concentration (defined by the clearance) should be reduced. Because half-lives of highly extracted drugs are frequently prolonged in patients with liver disease, the time required to attain and fall from a steady-state concentration (usually

TABLE 2. Pharmacokinetics of Poorly Extracted Drugs in Liver Disease.*

Drug	Disease †	Volume ‡	Half-Life	Clearance	Reference
Ampicillin	Cirrhosis	59.1±43.1 liters § (19.5±4.6) (Vd_{ss})	1.90±0.56 hr § (1.31±0.15)	280±136 ml/min (3.24±80)	20
Chloramphenicol	Cirrhosis	50.0±9.96 liters § (65.9±11.3) (V)	10.45±2.79 hr § (4.61±0.93)	59.2±20.6 ml/min § (169±25.6)	21
Chlordiazepoxide	CAH	428±108 ml/kg (321±77) (Vd_{ss})	40.1±5.1 hr § (16.5±3.6)	7.6±1.08 ml/hr/kg (13.8±1.2)	22
	Cirrhosis	0.48±0.14 liter/kg (0.33±0.06) (Vd_{ss})	62.7±27.3 hr § (23.8±11.6)	7.7±2.1 ml/min § (15.4±4.4)	23
Cimetidine	Cirrhosis	1.4±0.6 liters/kg (1.10±4) (V)	2.9±1.1 hr (2.3±0.7)	463±145 ml/min (511±93)	24
Diazepam	Cirrhosis	1.74±0.21 liters/kg § (1.13±0.23) (Vd_{ss})	105.6±15.2 hr § (46.6±14.2)	13.8±2.4 ml/min § (26.6±4.1)	25
Furosemide	Cirrhosis	12.0±3.5 liters (9.3±3.7) (Vd_{ss})	129±75 min § (74±18)	120±36 ml/min (142±42)	26
Lorazepam	Cirrhosis	2.01±0.82 liters/kg § (1.28±0.34) (Vd_{β})	31.9±9.6 hr § (22.1±5.4)	0.81±0.48 ml/min/kg (0.75±0.23)	27
	Acute hepatitis	1.52±0.61 liters/kg (1.28±0.34) (Vd_{β})	25.0±6.4 hr (22.1±5.4)	0.74±0.34 ml/min/kg (0.75±0.23)	

*Values are expressed as means ±S.D.; those in parentheses were observed in healthy controls.

‡See second footnote to Table 1.

†CAH denotes chronic active hepatitis.

§Significantly different from control value (P<0.05).

TABLE 2. (continued)

Drug	Disease †	Volume ‡	Half-Life	Clearance	Reference
Naproxen	Cirrhosis	16.8±4.79 liters/hr § (1.21±1.73) (Vd$_\beta$)	— —	0.556±0.102 liter/hr (0.547±0.083)	28
Oxazepam	Cirrhosis	60.9±23.3 liters (61.2±34.5) (Vd$_\beta$)	5.8±2.69 hr (5.6±2.26)	155.5±70.4 ml/min (136.0±13.1)	29
	Acute hepatitis	51.7±17.2 liters (47.7±16.7) (Vd$_\beta$)	5.3±0.7 hr (5.1±1.3)	137.4±51.4 ml/min (113.5±30.7)	
Prednisone	CAH	69±13 liters (70±8) (V)	3.0±1.0 hr (3.3±1.0)	278±78 ml/min (256±56)	30
Theophylline	Cirrhosis	0.563±0.08 liter/kg (0.482±0.08) (V)	28.8±14.3 hr § (6.0±2.1)	18.8±11.3 ml/hr/kg § (63.0±28.5)	31
Tolbutamide	Cirrhosis	0.15±0.03 liter/kg (0.15±0.03) (V)	4.0±0.9 hr § (5.9±1.4)	26±5.4 ml/hr/kg § (18±2.8)	32
Warfarin	Acute hepatitis	0.19±0.04 liter/kg (0.21±0.02) (V)	23±5 hr (25±3)	6.1±0.9 liters/hr (6.1±0.7)	33

three to four drug half-lives) may be lengthened in patients with hepatic impairment. For example, according to the data of Thompson et al. on lidocaine,[10] the time required to reach steady-state concentrations of lidocaine after institution of a constant rate of infusion will be about 24 hours in patients with hepatic impairment, in comparison to about 10 hours in persons without hepatic disease.

Because the disposition of a highly extracted drug is relatively insensitive to changes in protein binding, variations in drug binding are not of primary importance in the pharmacokinetic analysis of highly extracted drugs in liver disease. Changes in protein binding of highly extracted drugs, however, may alter their pharmacologic effect. The following equations may be derived from the clearance relations defined in Equation 1:

$$\text{Rate of elimination} = \ CL_fC_f = CL_pC_p; \qquad (Eq.\ 7)$$
$$CL_pC_p = CL_fC_f; \qquad (Eq.\ 8a)$$
$$CL_p = CL_fC_f/C_p; \qquad (Eq.\ 8b)$$
$$CL_p = CL_ff_p \qquad (Eq.\ 8c)$$

If plasma or blood clearance of a highly extracted drug is not changed but protein binding is decreased in the presence of liver disease, the net effect will be a decrease in CL_f (clearance based on unbound-drug concentration) and, at a constant rate of drug administration, an increase in C_f (Equation 8c). Because the unbound-drug concentration (C_f) is the concentration that equilibrates with the drug concentration at the site of pharmacologic effect, C_f presumably determines pharmacologic effect. The relations expressed in Equations 7 and 8a through 8c provide the theoretical basis for the statement that changes in plasma or blood binding of highly extracted drugs will not change drug disposition but may alter pharmacologic effect.

Poorly Extracted Drugs

The disposition of poorly extracted drugs is more sensitive to changes in the intrinsic ability of the liver to eliminate a drug $(CL_{intrinsic})$ and in binding of drug to blood constitutents than it is to hepatic blood flow. Changes in blood flow and intrahepatic and extrahepatic shunting of blood past functioning hepatocytes are not likely to alter either the clearance or the bioavailability of poorly extracted drugs. Because numerous physiologic factors can influence both drug binding and intrahepatic processes of biotransformation and biliary excretion, the influence of acute and chronic hepatic disease on the disposition of poorly extracted drugs is predictably more variable than their influence on the disposition of highly extracted drugs. Data from clinical investigations support this prediction: unchanged, decreased, or even increased drug clearance has been reported for poorly extracted drugs in patients with hepatic impairment (Table 2). Some patterns are nevertheless apparent in the data that appear in Table 2. The disposition of benzodiazepines that are eliminated from the body primarily through glucuronidation (e.g., lorazepam and oxazepam) appears to be unaffected by chronic hepatic disease, whereas the disposition of benzodiazepines (e.g., diazepam and chlordiazepoxide) that require nonconjugative (Type I) pathways for elimination is reduced in the presence of hepatic disease.

The influence of protein binding on the disposition of poorly extracted compounds has been documented for several drugs in patients with hepatic disease. For example, the increase in tolbutamide clearance in patients with acute viral hepatitis (Table 2) has been attributed primarily to a decrease in tolbutamide binding to plasma proteins without a change in clearance based on unbound-drug concentration (Equation 8c). The influence of cirrhosis on plasma binding and clearance of naproxen is more complex. Total steady-state plasma clearance of naproxen was not significantly altered in patients with cirrhosis as compared with healthy controls (Table 2). However, determination of plasma binding and estimation of clearance based on unbound-drug concentration indicated that both were substantially reduced in the cirrhotic subjects as compared with the controls. The net effect of these changes on total plasma clearance was minimal.

In contrast to the changes in plasma or blood binding of highly extracted drugs, changes that may influence pharmacologic effect but not alter drug clearance, the changes in plasma binding of poorly extracted drugs may alter drug clearance but not pharmacologic effect. At a given rate of drug administration, clearance based on unbound-drug concentration will determine the steady-state plasma or blood unbound-drug concentration. This concentration presumably determines the pharmacologic effect of a drug. In the absence of changes in CL_f, changes only in plasma binding (f_p) will result in changes in plasma clearance and total plasma drug concentration but not in changes in unbound-drug concentration (because CL_f does not change — see Equation 7). Thus, with tolbutamide, if hepatic impairment produces only changes in drug binding, no dose adjustment is necessary because C_f does not change and this concentration determines pharmacologic effect. With naproxen, if CL_f is decreased by more than 50 per cent in the presence of chronic alcoholic liver disease, a corresponding reduction in dose of 50 per cent or more may be required to maintain a given unbound-drug concentration. These observations indicate the importance of determining protein binding in assessing the disposition of both highly extracted and poorly extracted drugs in the presence of liver disease. The influence of hepatic disease on drug binding has been reviewed by Blaschke.[34]

Conclusions

Theoretical analyses have defined hepatic blood flow, protein binding, and the intrinsic capacity of the liver to eliminate a drug ($CL_{intrinsic}$) as primary determinants of hepatic drug clearance. The importance of these factors in drug disposition and pharmacologic effect differs according to whether a drug is highly extracted or poorly extracted by the liver. These theoretical concepts provide a basis for understanding and using clinical pharmacokinetic data now available in order to define the absorption and disposition of many drugs in the presence of hepatic impairment. These data can influence the selection of a drug for a patient with hepatic dysfunction and may also determine an initial dosage regimen and estimate when steady-state conditions will be reached under this regimen. Subsequent dosage adjustments may then be based on clinical response and, when indicated, determination of plasma or blood drug concentrations.

Several caveats about these general statements are necessary. The variance in the mean estimates of clearance is substantial for drugs that have been studied in patients with hepatic disease. Although an average clearance is a reasonable basis for a dosage regimen, subsequent increments or decrements in dose in the individual patient will almost certainly be necessary to achieve a desired plasma drug concentration. In addition, alteration in the pharmacologic effects of drugs in patients with liver disease, in the presence or absence of changes in drug pharmacokinetics, has not been considered. Only a few reports have appeared to document changes in drug response occurring in association with hepatic disease.[35,36] These studies have generally confirmed the clinical impression that the effects of agents that act on the central nervous system are more pronounced in patients with hepatic impairment, particularly those with hepatic encephalopathy. Finally, virtually all investigations of drug disposition in chronic liver disease have focused on disposition in chronic alcoholic cirrhosis. Drug disposition in other forms of liver disease, either primary or secondary, has seldom been investigated, and few studies have been performed to assess how longitudinal variation in the activity of acute or chronic hepatic disease influences drug disposition. The data in Tables 1 and 2 should be regarded as approximations on which to base initial dosage regimens. These observations emphasize the importance of clinical judgment and the availability of drug-concentration measurements in selecting dosages in patients with hepatic impairment.

References

1. Forker EL, Luxon BA. Albumin helps mediate removal of taurocholate by rat liver. J Clin Invest 1981; 67:1517-22.
2. Weisiger R, Gollan J, Ockner R. Receptor for albumin on the liver cell surface may mediate uptake of fatty acids and other albumin-bound substances. Science 1981; 211:1048-51.
3. Wilkinson GR, Shand DG. A physiological approach to hepatic drug clearance. Clin Pharmacol Ther 1975; 18:377-90.
4. Rowland M, Benet LZ, Graham GG. Clearance concepts in pharmacokinetics. J Pharmacokinet Biopharm 1973; 1:123-36.
5. Pang KS, Rowland M. Hepatic clearance of drugs. I. Theoretical considerations of a "well-stirred" model and a "parallel tube" model: influence of hepatic blood flow, plasma and blood cell binding, and the hepatocellular enzymatic activity on hepatic drug clearance. J Pharmacokinet Biopharm 1977; 5:625-53.
6. Williams RL, Benet LZ. Drug pharmacokinetics in cardiac and hepatic disease. Annu Rev Pharmacol Toxicol 1980; 20:389-413.
7. Richardson PDI, Withrington PG. Liver blood flow. II. Effects of drugs and hor-

mones on liver blood flow. Gastroenterology 1981; 81:356-75.

8. Nies AS, Shand DG, Wilkinson GR. Altered hepatic blood flow and drug disposition. Clin Pharmacokinet 1976; 1:135-55.

9. Daneshmend TK, Jackson L, Roberts CJC. Physiological and pharmacological variability in estimated hepatic blood flow in man. Br J Clin Pharmacol 1981; 11: 491-6.

10. Thompson PD, Melmon KL, Richardson AJ, et al. Lidocaine pharmacokinetics in advanced heart failure, liver disease, and renal failure in humans. Ann Intern Med 1973; 78:499-508.

11. Williams RL, Blaschke TF, Meffin PJ, Melmon KL, Rowland M. Influence of viral hepatitis on the disposition of two compounds with high hepatic clearance: lidocaine and indocyanine green. Clin Pharmacol Ther 1976; 20:290-9.

12. Neal EA, Meffin PJ, Gregory PB, Blaschke TF. Enhanced bioavailability and decreased clearance of analgesics in patients with cirrhosis. Gastroenterology 1979; 77:96-102.

13. McHorse TS, Wilkinson GR, Johnson RF, Schenker S. Effect of acute viral hepatitis in man on the disposition and elimination of meperidine. Gastroenterology 1975; 68:775-80.

14. Regårdh CG, Jordö L, Ervik M, Lundborg P, Olsson R, Rönn O. Pharmacokinetics of metoprolol in patients with hepatic cirrhosis. Clin Pharmacokinet 1981; 6:375-88.

15. Patwardhan RV, Johnson RF, Hoyumpa A Jr, et al. Normal metabolism of morphine in cirrhosis. Gastroenterology 1981; 81:1006-1011.

16. Wood AJJ, Kornhauser DM, Wilkinson GR, Shand DG, Branch RA. The influence of cirrhosis on steady-state blood concentrations of unbound propranolol after oral administration. Clin Pharmacokinet 1978; 3:478-87.

17. Woodcock BG, Rietbrock I, Vöhringer HF, et al. Verapamil disposition in liver disease and intensive-care patients: kinetics, clearance, and apparent blood flow relationships. Clin Pharmacol Ther 1981; 29:27-34.

18. Pessayre D, Lebrec D, Descatoire V, Peignoux M, Benhamou J-P. Mechanism for reduced drug clearance in patients with cirrhosis. Gastroenterology 1978; 74:566-71.

19. Groszmann R, Kotelanski B, Cohn JN, Khatri IM. Quantitation of portasystemic shunting from the splenic and mesenteric beds in alcoholic liver disease. Am J Med 1972; 53:715-22.

20. Lewis GP, Jusko WJ. Pharmacokinetics of ampicillin in cirrhosis. Clin Pharmacol Ther 1975; 18:475-84.

21. Narang APS, Datta DV, Nath J, Mathur VS. Pharmacokinetic study of chloramphenicol in patients with liver disease. Eur J Clin Pharmacol 1981; 20:479-83.

22. Morgan DD, Robinson JD, Mendenhall CL. Clinical pharmacokinetics of chlordiazepoxide in patients with alcoholic hepatitis. Eur J Clin Pharmacol 1981; 19:279-85.

23. Roberts RK, Wilkinson GR, Branch RA, Schenker S. Effect of age and parenchymal liver disease on the disposition and elimination of chlordiazepoxide (Librium). Gastroenterology 1978; 75:479-85.

24. Schentag JJ, Cerra FB, Calleri GM, Leising ME, French MA, Bernhard H. Age, disease and cimetidine disposition in healthy subjects and chronically ill patients. Clin Pharmacol Ther 1981; 29:737-43.

25. Klotz U, Avant GR, Hoyumpa A, Schenker S, Wilkinson GR. The effects of age and liver disease on the disposition and elimination of diazepam in adult man. J Clin Invest 1975; 55:347-59.

26. Allgulander C, Beermann B, Sjögren A. Furosemide pharmacokinetics in patients with liver disease. Clin Pharmacokinet 1980; 5:570-5.
27. Kraus JW, Desmond PV, Marshall JP, Johnson RF, Schenker S, Wilkinson GR. Effects of aging and liver disease on disposition of lorazepam. Clin Pharmacol Ther 1978; 24:411-9.
28. Upton RA, Williams RL, Nierenberg D, et al. Naproxen disposition in cirrhosis. Clin Pharmacol Ther 1982; 31:276-7. abstract.
29. Shull HJ Jr, Wilkinson GR, Johnson R, Schenker S. Normal disposition of oxazepam in acute viral hepatitis and cirrhosis. Ann Intern Med 1976; 84:420-5.
30. Schalm SW, Summerskill WHJ, Gi VLW. Prednisone for chronic active liver disease: pharmacokinetics, including conversion to prednisolone. Gastroenterology 1977; 72: 910-3.
31. Mangione A, Imhoff TE, Lee RV, Shum LY, Jusko WJ. Pharmacokinetics of theophylline in hepatic disease. Chest 1978; 73:616-22.
32. Williams RL, Blaschke TR, Meffin PJ, Melmon KL, Rowland M. Influence of acute viral hepatitis on disposition and plasma binding of tolbutamide. Clin Pharmacol Ther 1977; 21:301-9.
33. Williams RL, Schary WL, Blaschke TF, Meffin PJ, Melmon KL, Rowland M. Influence of acute viral hepatitis on disposition and pharmacologic effect of warfarin. Clin Pharmacol Ther 1976; 20:90-7.
34. Blaschke TF. Protein binding and kinetics of drugs in liver diseases. Clin Pharmacokinet 1977; 2:32-44.
35. Read AE, Laidlaw J, McCarthy CF. Effects of chlorpromazine in patients with hepatic disease. Br Med J 1969; 3:497-9.
36. Maxwell JD, Carrrella M, Parkes JD, Williams R, Mould GP, Curry SH. Plasma disappearance and cerebral effects of chlorpromazine in cirrhosis. Clin Sci 1972; 43:143-51.

| Correspondence

Is Drug Administration in Hepatic Disease Really So Complicated?*

To the Editor:

On reading the article by Williams in the December 29 issue,[1] one may come away discouraged. A physician who wants to treat patients according to the standards set by Dr. Williams must know at least the hepatic clearance, volume of distribution, half-life, first-pass elimination, and free fraction of a drug in order to administer it safely to any patient with cirrhosis. In most instances this goal cannot be reached. I believe that simpler concepts are sufficient and have a much greater chance of being applied in practice. After teaching about this topic for many years I have learned that at the bedside most physicians find it easier to implement intuitive notions than to handle mathematical formulas. On the basis of this experience, our group has developed a classification of pharmacokinetic risk

*Originally published on May 17, 1984 (310:1331-1332).

TABLE 1. A Classification of Pharmacokinetic Risks.

Risk Group	Hepatic Elimination	Dosage Implications	Examples
"High" risk	High extraction, flow limitation	Reduction of initial and maintenance dosages	Propoxyphene, pentazocine, verapamil
"Limited" risk	Low extraction, capacity limitation	Reduction of maintenance dosage only	Diazepam, theophylline, pentobarbital
"Low" risk	Little change in liver disease	No reduction in dosage	Oxazepam, digoxin, furosemide

(Table 1) and already classified more than 50 drugs, many of them in common use.[2] Obviously, pharmacodynamic aspects such as therapeutic ratio and responsiveness of the organ system being treated need additional attention. Nevertheless, the proposed concept is easy to implement. To those who missed practical conclusions for the bedside in Dr. Williams' article, it is suggested that they consider the risk-concept approach.[2]

JOHANNES BIRCHER, M.D.
University of Berne
CH-3010 Berne, Switzerland

1. Williams RL. Drug administration in hepatic disease. N Engl J Med 1983; 309:1616-22.
2. Bircher J. Altered drug metabolism in liver disease — therapeutic implications. In: Thomas HC, Macsween RNM, eds. Recent advances in hepatology. London: Churchill Livingstone, 1983:1, 101-13.

To the Editor:

There is an error in the article by Williams (page 1619, column 2, last paragraph, line 7 [page 29]). The statement "t½ − 0.693 V/CL" makes no sense; I am sure that he meant "t½ = 0.693 V/CL."

This is apparently a typographic error, but it is still very confusing to someone who is not an expert in pharmacodynamics. The formula is correctly stated on page 1617.

K. LEO BUXBAUM, M.D.
6315 S. Greenleaf Ave.
Whittier, CA 90601

To the Editor:

Dr. Williams has provided us with an excellent review on hepatic drug metabolism in health and disease. However, there is one error in his text. He correctly states on page 1617 [page 23], "It [half-life] is calculated as the reciprocal of the rate constant of elimination (k) multiplied by 0.693." The expression in parentheses that follows his statement should read $(t\frac{1}{2} = 0.693/k)$.*

RICHARD H. GANNON, PHARM.D.
Yale–New Haven Hospital
New Haven, CT 06540

The above letters were referred to Dr. Williams, who offers the following reply:

To the Editor:

Dr. Bircher raises a common pedagogical issue — namely, whether it is better for clinicians to learn concepts or memorize lists. In my article I hoped to present relatively simple equations and concepts that would allow clinicians to understand why and how drug-dosage regimens may be altered in patients with hepatic impairment. I do not believe that these concepts are beyond the grasp of the practicing physician. Many of the equations and relationships in the article are widely applied in other areas of medicine, including cardiology and renal physiology. If clinicians cannot apply these kinetic concepts at the bedside, it may be that clinical pharmacologists and pharmacokineticists need to do a better job in transmitting their skills to the practicing physician, instead of concluding that the practicing physician is incapable of understanding kinetic principles and must be directed instead to rote memorization.

Both Drs. Buxbaum and Gannon are correct. I apologize for the typographic errors.

ROGER L. WILLIAMS, M.D.
UCSF Drug Studies Unit
San Francisco, CA 94143

*Wagner JG. Fundamentals of clinical pharmacokinetics. Hamilton, Ill.: Drug Intelligence Publication, 1975:23.

Ranitidine: A New H_2-Receptor Antagonist

Jerome B. Zeldis, M.D., Ph.D.,

Lawrence S. Friedman, M.D.,

and Kurt J. Isselbacher, M.D.

OVER the past six years the treatment of peptic-ulcer disease has been dramatically altered by the introduction and use of cimetidine. This substituted imidazole compound is an effective H_2-receptor antagonist, which acts on the gastric parietal cell to inhibit gastric acid production. Cimetidine is prescribed worldwide, and on the basis of numerous controlled clinical trials, it is considered effective in the healing of both duodenal[1] and gastric ulcers.[2] Recently, ranitidine, another H_2-receptor antagonist, has undergone extensive clinical studies and has been approved by the U.S. Food and Drug Administration for the short-term treatment of duodenal ulcers and hypersecretory states such as the Zollinger–Ellison syndrome. Although other antiulcer agents, including other H_2-receptor blockers, are now undergoing clinical investigation, this review will focus on the pharmacology and clinical use of ranitidine as compared with cimetidine. In view of the vast literature on ranitidine and its clinical effects, reference citations for this review have had to be limited and selective. The reader is referred to a recent symposium[3] and several reviews[4-6] for a more extensive citation of the pertinent literature.

Mechanism of Action

Because the chemical structures of the older H_2-receptor antagonists, including cimetidine, are similar to that of histamine, the imidazole ring has been considered essential for H_2-receptor binding. However, this is not the case, since ranitidine, which has a furan rather than an imidazole structure (Fig. 1), is a very potent competitive inhibitor of the binding of histamine to H_2-receptors. Furthermore, unlike cimetidine, ranitidine binds minimally if at all to such other sites as androgen receptors, the hepatic mixed-function oxidase system, and peripheral lymphocytes. This greater binding specificity of ranitidine probably

From the Gastrointestinal Unit (Medical Services), Massachusetts General Hospital, and the Department of Medicine, Harvard Medical School, Boston.

Originally published on December 1, 1983 (309:1368-1373).

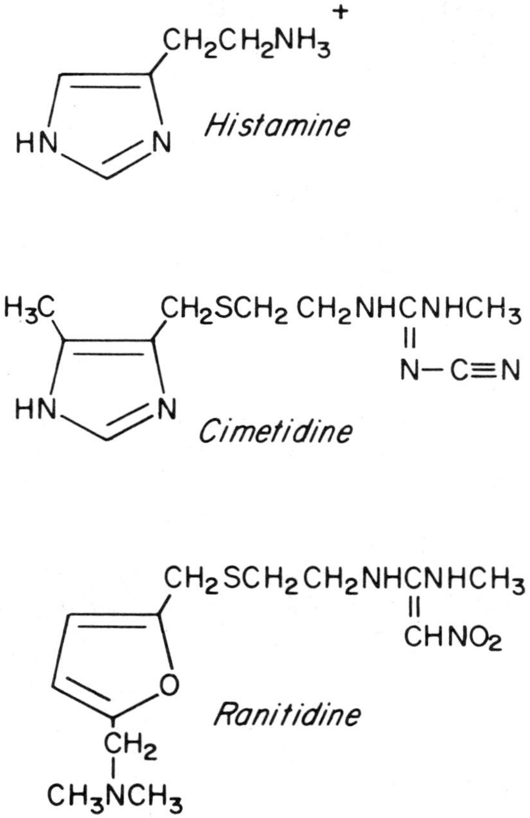

Figure 1. *The Chemical Structures of Histamine, Cimetidine, and Ranitidine.*

accounts for the fact that it appears to lack some of the serious side effects seen clinically with cimetidine (see below).

Despite the presence of H_2 receptors throughout the body, inhibition of histamine binding to the receptors of gastric parietal cells is the major beneficial clinical effect of H_2-receptor antagonists. Secretion of acid by the stomach depends on the binding of gastrin, acetylcholine, and histamine to their respective receptors on the parietal-cell surface. Blocking any one of these binding sites leads to a reduction in acid secretion. Thus, H_2-receptor blockade is effective in inhibiting the gastric secretion that follows stimulation by gastrin, acetylcholine (i.e., vagal stimulation), or histamine itself. Studies with ranitidine indicate that it is 5 to 12 times as potent as cimetidine (on a molar basis) in inhibiting stimulated gastric acid secretion in human beings.[5] Both ranitidine and cimetidine decrease gastric blood flow and the volume of gastric secretion. There is also a decrease in pepsin output; however, this appears to be secondary to the reduced volume of gastric secretion, since the pepsin concentration in the gastric juice remains unchanged.[7] Although it has been suggested that H_2-receptor antagonists may also have some cytoprotective function,[8] evidence to support this is inconclusive at best.

Pharmacokinetics

When given orally, ranitidine is rapidly absorbed from the gastrointestinal tract, and absorption is not influenced by food ingestion. After an oral dose of 150 mg, peak plasma concentrations occur within one to three hours, but the duration of inhibition of pentagastrin-induced acid secretion may last from 8 to 12 hours.[9] After a 150-mg oral dose of ranitidine, the mean peak plasma concentration is about 400 ng per milliliter; however, the range in peak concentrations is quite broad — from 200 to 600 μg per milliliter. In most persons a 50 per cent inhibition of gastric acid output can be achieved with plasma ranitidine concentrations of 100 to 200 ng per milliliter,[10] but because of the considerable variation of response in both normal subjects and patients with peptic-ulcer disease, determination of blood concentrations in persons taking ranitidine may be of limited value in adjusting the drug dose. It is noteworthy from a practical standpoint that in patients with duodenal ulcer who are receiving 150 mg of ranitidine twice daily, the mean inhibition of gastric acid secretion is 70 per cent over 24 hours and 90 per cent over a 6-hour nocturnal period.[11,12] Under similar conditions, 1000 mg of cimetidine produces a 48 per cent reduction in acid output over 24 hours and a 70 per cent decrease in nocturnal acid secretion.[11]

The serum half-life of orally administered ranitidine, like that of cimetidine, is approximately two to three hours. The bioavailability of ranitidine is about 50 per cent, as compared with 70 per cent for cimetidine. The bioavailability of ranitidine is influenced by hepatic function, since the drug is taken up and metabolized by the liver by "first-pass" kinetics. Up to 30 per cent is metabolized by the liver to become nitrogen oxide, sulfuric oxide, and desmethyl derivatives,[13,14] but 50 per cent or more of the drug is excreted by the kidney unchanged. In geriatric patients the half-life of ranitidine is prolonged by about 50 per cent, presumably because of a decrease in the glomerular filtration rate. As expected, the bioavailability of ranitidine in patients with liver disease is increased, and the serum half-life is slightly prolonged because of decreased hepatic metabolism and a slightly reduced glomerular filtration rate.[15] It is probably not necessary to change the usual therapeutic dose of ranitidine (i.e., 150 mg twice daily) in patients with liver disease. However, in patients with serious renal disease (e.g., creatinine levels higher than 4.0 mg per deciliter), therapeutic levels can be achieved with lower doses of ranitidine; thus, 75 mg twice daily is recommended for such patients.

Clinical Effectiveness

Ranitidine appears to be as effective as cimetidine in the treatment of a variety of acid-peptic disorders, but with the advantages of a more prolonged period of action and fewer adverse side effects. Most of the studies to date have compared ranitidine at a dosage of 150 mg twice daily with cimetidine at a dosage of 1000 mg daily (200 mg three times daily and 400 mg at bedtime) or with placebo.

Peptic-Ulcer Disease

In most clinical trials ranitidine (150 mg twice daily) has been shown to be as effective as cimetidine in accelerating the healing of acute duodenal ulcers.[3,16] These studies have consisted of "open" trials as well as controlled comparisons of ranitidine with placebo or cimetidine (usually 1000 mg daily) or both. On the basis of endoscopic evidence, ulcer healing has been demonstrated in about 70 per cent of patients by the end of four weeks and in 85 to 90 per cent by the end of eight weeks.[4,16] A nighttime dose of 150 mg of ranitidine has been shown to be comparable to 400 mg of cimetidine in preventing the recurrence of duodenal ulcers.[17] Approximately 15 to 25 per cent of patients who are maintained on a nighttime dose of ranitidine or cimetidine have had a recurrence of their duodenal ulcer within one year, as compared with 55 per cent of those maintained on placebo.[18,19]

Initially, a regimen of 150 mg of ranitidine twice daily was used in studies of duodenal-ulcer healing because pharmacokinetic data showed that maximal inhibition of acid output persisted for more than eight hours after a single dose of 150 mg. However, a number of investigators[6,20,21] have demonstrated equal clinical effectiveness at six to eight weeks with a dose of 100 mg twice daily. Nevertheless, it would appear that duodenal-ulcer healing may occur somewhat earlier with the higher dose of ranitidine. Mangiameli et al.[22] conducted a four-week randomized double-blind study of patients with duodenal ulcer who were receiving daily doses of 300 or 200 mg of ranitidine or placebo. At four weeks both ranitidine-treated groups had a markedly greater disappearance of abdominal pain than placebo-treated patients. However, the healing of ulcers as determined by endoscopy occurred in 83.3 per cent of patients receiving 300 mg of ranitidine daily, as compared with 52.2 per cent of those receiving 200 mg and 36.4 per cent of those receiving placebo. In other studies, however, lower doses of ranitidine have been reported to be quite effective. For example, in one study 40 mg of ranitidine twice daily plus 80 mg at bedtime (i.e., 160 mg per day) produced a four-week healing rate of 83 per cent and an eight-week healing rate of 94 per cent.[23] In general, it would seem that a thrice-daily dosing regimen is unnecessary and that the standard ranitidine dose of 150 mg twice a day is maximally effective without an increased incidence of side effects.

The data permitting assessment of ranitidine in the treatment of gastric ulcer are somewhat limited. Available studies suggest that the cumulative percentage of gastric ulcers that are healed at eight weeks is similar to that observed with duodenal ulcers, but the healing rate of gastric ulcers appears slower.[24-26] In a major comparative study of ranitidine (300 mg daily) and cimetidine (1000 mg daily), gastric-ulcer healing rates were similar. At four weeks, the healing rate with ranitidine was 58 per cent, as compared with 57 per cent with cimetidine; at eight weeks the rates were 77 and 76 per cent, respectively.[26] A nighttime ranitidine dose of 150 mg has also been shown to be beneficial in preventing the recurrence of gastric ulcers. In a double-blind placebo-controlled study of 33 patients, the relapse rate after one year was 6.7 per cent for those receiving ranitidine and 44 per cent for those receiving placebo.[27]

Acute Upper-Gastrointestinal-Tract Bleeding

There has been widespread use of cimetidine in the treatment of acute upper-gastrointestinal-tract bleeding and in attempts to prevent gastrointestinal bleeding in critically ill hospitalized patients. However, the role of H_2-receptor blockers in these settings remains controversial, especially since a major study showed that the continuous infusion of liquid antacids was more effective than cimetidine in the prevention of stress ulcers.[28] Moreover, the diversity of causes of gastrointestinal bleeding hampers interpretation of the results of many published studies.

In a study of acutely ill patients who were admitted to an intensive-care unit, Macchi et al.[29] demonstrated that an intravenous dose of 20 mg of ranitidine administered every four or eight hours raised the intragastric pH level and decreased acid output by more than 90 per cent. In none of these patients did stress gastritis or gastrointestinal bleeding develop during the trial. The authors concluded that ranitidine may be effective in preventing the stress ulcerations that are often seen in severely ill patients, but no comparison of ranitidine with oral infusions of liquid antacids was made. In a double-blind study,[30] 158 consecutive patients hospitalized for acute gastrointestinal bleeding were randomly assigned to therapy with either ranitidine (150 mg orally twice daily) or placebo after the cessation of bleeding. Although the overall incidence of subsequent bleeding in the two groups was not statistically different (14 of 76 for the ranitidine group and 21 of 75 for the placebo group), there was a significant decrease in the incidence of subsequent bleeding in the subgroup of patients with duodenal ulcer who were treated with ranitidine as compared with those who were treated with placebo (3 of 27 vs. 11 of 26, $P<0.05$). The available data thus suggest that ranitidine may be effective therapy for patients with acute gastrointestinal bleeding due to duodenal ulcers. However, the role of ranitidine in the management of acute upper-gastrointestinal-tract bleeding due to other causes remains to be determined.

Reflux Esophagitis

In several studies of patients with reflux esophagitis, the administration of 150 mg of ranitidine twice daily resulted in decreased frequency and severity of heartburn and retrosternal pain as compared with treatment with placebo.[3] Despite improvement in the endoscopic appearance of the esophagus, in most studies treatment with ranitidine has not resulted in greater histologic improvement than with placebo. These results are comparable to those in studies of cimetidine therapy in patients with reflux esophagitis. It is possible that the beneficial effects of ranitidine in reflux esophagitis may be related to other factors in addition to the inhibition of gastric acid secretion. Thus, one study showed a dose-related increase in lower-esophageal-sphincter pressure when ranitidine was given intravenously in doses of 0.5 to 1.0 mg per kilogram of body weight to healthy subjects,[31] but these findings have been questioned.[32] Alternatively, the failure of both ranitidine and cimetidine to result in histologic improvement of esophagitis may indicate that in the presence of free reflux a greater reduction in gastric acid secretion may be required to heal the esophageal mucosa than is usually obtained with standard doses of ranitidine; this explanation remains unproved.

Hypersecretory States and "Cimetidine-Resistant" Acid Secretion

Ranitidine has been shown to be effective in clinical situations in which very high doses of cimetidine have failed to produce significant improvement or in which cimetidine has had to be discontinued because of intolerable side effects. In addition, several reports indicate that ranitidine appears to be highly effective in hypersecretory states such as the Zollinger–Ellison syndrome.

In one study of 11 patients with the Zollinger–Ellison syndrome in whom cimetidine proved ineffective, satisfactory control of symptoms and suppression of gastric secretion were achieved with high doses of ranitidine (600 to 1200 mg daily).[33] Moreover, a dose of 900 mg of ranitidine daily raised the gastric pH level above 2.0 for a longer time than did a dose of 2400 mg of cimetidine daily.

Recently, Jensen et al.[34] described nine male patients with the Zollinger–Ellison syndrome in whom gynecomastia and impotence developed while they were taking high doses of cimetidine. When these patients were switched to ranitidine in equipotent doses, symptoms due to gastric hypersecretion were well controlled and suppression of gastric acid secretion was maintained. Furthermore, gynecomastia and impotence disappeared in all nine patients.

Danilewitz et al.[35] reported on three postsurgical patients with cimetidine-resistant, life-threatening gastric hypersecretion (1400 to 6000 ml per day, pH 1.0 to 1.2). Despite the administration of intravenous cimetidine in doses of up to 2.4 g daily for two to seven weeks, each patient's condition deteriorated. Cimetidine was replaced with intravenous ranitidine, and complete inhibition of acid secretion was achieved in each case with a dose of 300 μg per kilogram. Inhibition of gastric secretion was subsequently maintained with oral ranitidine (300 mg daily). It is noteworthy that in one patient with cimetidine-associated leukopenia this complication did not develop with ranitidine.

A small number of patients (approximately 8.0 per cent)[36] with peptic-ulcer disease do not respond symptomatically or as determined by endoscopic examination to cimetidine in standard doses (1000 to 1200 mg daily). In one report the majority of such patients responded to a standard regimen of ranitidine (150 mg twice daily).[36] Although higher doses of cimetidine might also have been effective, it is evident that ranitidine provides an alternative approach to the treatment of patients with ulcers that are resistant to current standard antiulcer therapy.

Side Effects

Ranitidine appears to be a safe drug; only minor side effects have been reported to date. However, the experience with this drug is still much more limited than that with cimetidine, and any effects of long-term administration of higher than usual doses have yet to be studied. The minor side effects that have been observed include headache in 1.8 per cent of users; less than 1 per cent of users have reported malaise, dizziness, constipation, nausea, and skin rash.[37] Headaches are usually mild and resolve or subside despite continued therapy. Skin rashes, pruritic or nonpruritic, also usually resolve with continued therapy. As with cimetidine, transient increases in serum aminotransferase levels have been observed,[38] and one case of possible anicteric hepatitis was reported in a 63-year-old woman two weeks after she began receiving 150 mg of ranitidine twice daily.[39] There have been no adverse cardiac effects from oral therapy in animals or human beings,[40,41] but two cases of bradycardia have been reported after intravenous infusion of ranitidine.[42] Bradycardia may have resulted from a rise in plasma histamine, which has been shown to occur after rapid infusions of either ranitidine or cimetidine.[43] There has been one report of glaucoma exacerbated by ranitidine in a patient who had a similar response to cimetidine.[44]

In contrast to cimetidine, ranitidine does not elevate basal levels of testosterone and seems devoid of antiandrogenic activity, presumably because it does not bind to androgen receptors.[45] Furthermore, oral administration of ranitidine has not been associated with a rise in prolactin secretion. Moreover, as indicated above, a study of patients with the Zollinger–Ellison syndrome in whom gynecomastia and impotence developed with high doses of cimetidine showed that, when these patients were switched to ranitidine, there was prompt reversal of these side effects. There has been only one report of gynecomastia in a patient receiving ranitidine (150 mg daily for eight days); the condition disappeared when the drug was stopped and recurred after treatment was resumed.[46]

The dose-dependent confusion and mental depression that may occur with cimetidine,[47,48] particularly in elderly patients and those with uremia or cirrhosis, have thus far not been reported with ranitidine. It is conceivable that this is due to the fact that ranitidine, in contrast to cimetidine, is distributed minimally into the central nervous system and does not bind to certain brain receptors.[49] Ranitidine also appears to lack the renal side effects of cimetidine. Elevations in serum creatinine levels and rare instances of interstitial nephritis that have been attributed to cimetidine[50,51] have thus far not been reported with ranitidine.

Ranitidine also differs from cimetidine in its effects on the immune system. For example, human lymphocytes have receptors for cimetidine but not for ranitidine,[52] and cimetidine has been demonstrated to have effects on cell-mediated immunity[53] and possibly to aid in the immunologic therapy of cancer.[54,55] If such properties of cimetidine result from its binding to lymphocyte receptors, similar effects from ranitidine would not be expected and have not so far been observed. Thrombocytopenia and agranulocytosis, which occur rarely with cimetidine,[56] have not been reported to date with ranitidine.

Ranitidine binds much less avidly than cimetidine to the drug-metabolizing microsomal P-450 enzyme system in hepatocytes. Therefore, in the usual therapeutic doses, ranitidine does not appear to contribute to the type of adverse drug interactions that may occur with cimetidine. For example, ranitidine does not alter the hepatic detoxification of diazepam, warfarin, or propranolol. Although both cimetidine and ranitidine decrease hepatic blood flow, only cimetidine has been shown to prolong the hepatic clearance of such drugs as propranolol[57] and lidocaine,[58,59] for which the rate-limiting step of elimination depends on hepatic blood flow. Ranitidine appears to be safer than cimetidine in patients taking drugs that are metabolized by the hepatic microsomal oxidase system.

An important and controversial issue relating to prolonged H_2-receptor blockade is the long-term consequence of gastric achlorhydria. Besides predisposing the patient to bezoar formation,[60] achlorhydria resulting from H_2-receptor blockade may weaken the gastric barrier to systemic infection, and at least one case of systemic brucellosis has been associated with cimetidine therapy.[61] Some investigators[62,63] but not others[64,65] have observed the proliferation of enteric and nitrate-reducing bacteria in the stomachs of patients taking H_2-receptor antagonists. There has also been great concern that prolonged elevation of the gastric pH level results in the production of N-nitroso compounds[63,65] as a result of an increase in nitrate-reducing bacteria in the stomach. Compounds such as the N-nitroso–conjugated bile acids (e.g., N-nitroso glycocholate and N-nitroso taurocholate) that are produced by bacterial metabolism are potent mutagens in vitro.[66] However, the N-nitroso derivatives of ranitidine that are formed in the stomachs of patients taking ranitidine have not been found to be mutagenic,[67] nor have cimetidine or ranitidine been found to be carcinogenic in various animal species.[68] Moreover, although the N-nitroso derivative of cimetidine that is formed in the stomachs of cimetidine users is mutagenic in vitro, there has been no increased incidence of cancer that could be attributed to prolonged cimetidine use.

Conclusion

Ranitidine is a more potent H_2-receptor antagonist on a molar basis than cimetidine, and on the basis of current data, appears to lack some of the important side effects that may occur with cimetidine. However, extensive clinical experience with and careful study of cimetidine have confirmed its efficacy and safety.

Moreover, drugs other than H_2-receptor blockers are effective in treating many of the disorders for which cimetidine or ranitidine are used. At the present time the choice of either cimetidine or ranitidine in various clinical situations appears to be arbitrary. Situations that would seem to favor the use of ranitidine over cimetidine include the treatment of patients who are taking multiple drugs (especially drugs metabolized by the cytochrome P-450 mixed-oxygenase system or drugs for which metabolism is otherwise affected by cimetidine [e.g., diazepam, warfarin, lidocaine, and propranolol]); elderly patients and patients with cirrhosis or uremia who are prone to become confused and depressed while taking cimetidine; men who have fertility problems or who require large doses of cimetidine; patients who do not respond to cimetidine or who cannot tolerate its side effects; and possibly, patients whose compliance might be improved with a drug taken twice rather than four times daily.

Finally, it should be noted that other potent inhibitors of gastric acid secretion have been developed and are currently undergoing clinical trials. These include prostaglandin-E derivatives, other substituted imidazole H_2-receptor antagonists with durations of action much longer than that of ranitidine, and substituted benzimidazoles that decrease gastric acid production by inhibiting hydrogen–potassium ATPase in the parietal cell. Undoubtedly, one or more of these drugs will join cimetidine and ranitidine as agents useful in the treatment of acid-peptic disease.

References

1. Binder HJ, Cocco A, Crossley RJ, et al. Cimetidine in the treatment of duodenal ulcer; a multicenter double blind study. Gastroenterology 1978; 74:380-8.
2. Isenberg JI, Peterson WL, Elashoff JD, et al. Healing of benign gastric ulcer with low-dose antacid or cimetidine: a double-blind, randomized, placebo-controlled trial. N Engl J Med 1983; 308:1319-24.
3. Misiewicz JJ, Wormsley KG, eds. The clinical use of ranitidine. Oxford: Medicine Publishing Foundation, 1982.
4. Berner BD, Conner CS, Sawyer DR, Siepler JK. Ranitidine: a new H_2-receptor antagonist. Clin Pharm 1982; 1:499-509.
5. Brogden RN, Carmine AA, Heel RC, Speight TM, Avery GS. Ranitidine: a review of its pharmacology and therapeutic use in peptic ulcer disease and other allied diseases. Drugs 1982; 24:267-303.
6. Konturek SJ. Pharmacology and clinical use of ranitidine. Mt Sinai J Med 1982; 49:370-82.
7. Konturek SJ, Obtulowicz W, Kwiecień N, Sito E, Oleksy J, Miszczuk-Jamska B. Effect of ranitidine, a new H_2-antagonist, on gastric and pancreatic secretion in duodenal ulcer patients. Dig Dis Sci 1980; 25:737-43.
8. Konturek SJ, Kwiecień N, Obtulowicz W, Polanski M, Kopp B, Oleksy J. Comparison of prostaglandin E_2 and ranitidine in prevention of gastric bleeding by aspirin in man. Gut 1983; 24:89-93.
9. Konturek SJ, Obtulowicz W, Kwiecień N, Kopp B, Oleksy J. Kinetics and duration of action of ranitidine on gastric secretion and its effect on pancreatic secretion in duodenal ulcer patients. Scand J Gastroenterol [Suppl] 1981; 69:91-9.

10. Peden NR, Saunders JHB, Wormsley KG. Inhibition of pentagastrin-stimulated and nocturnal gastric secretion by ranitidine: a new H_2-receptor antagonist. Lancet 1979; 1:690-2.

11. Walt RP, Malé P-J, Rawlings J, Hunt RH, Milton-Thompson GJ, Misiewicz JJ. Comparison of the effects of ranitidine, cimetidine and placebo on the 24 hour intragastric acidity and nocturnal acid secretion in patients with duodenal ulcer. Gut 1981; 22:49-54.

12. Walt RP, Malé P-J, Hunt RH, Rawlings J, Milton-Thompson GJ, Misiewicz JJ. The effect of ranitidine and cimetidine on the twenty-four hour intragastric acidity profile and nocturnal acid secretion in duodenal ulcer patients. Scand J Gastroenterol [Suppl] 1981; 69:33-7.

13. Martin LE, Bell JA, Carey PF, Dallas FAA, Dixon GT, Jenner WN. A review of pharmacokinetics and metabolism of ranitidine in animals and man. In[3], pp. 23-31.

14. Martin LE, Oxford J, Tanner RJN. Use of high-performance liquid chromatography-mass spectrometry for the study of the metabolism of ranitidine in man. J Chromatogr 1982; 251:215-24.

15. Young CJ, Daneshmend TK, Roberts CJC. Effects of cirrhosis and ageing on the elimination and bioavailability of ranitidine. Gut 1982; 23:819-23.

16. Langman MJS, Henry DA, Bell GD, Burnham WR, Ogilvy A. Cimetidine and ranitidine in duodenal ulcer. Br Med J 1980; 281:473-4.

17. Alstead EM, Ryan FP, Holdsworth CD, Ashton MG, Moore M. Ranitidine in the prevention of gastric and duodenal ulcer relapse. Gut 1983; 24:418-20.

18. Hunt RH, Walt RP, Trotman IF, et al. Comparison of ranitidine 150 mg nocte, with cimetidine, 400 mg nocte, in the maintenance treatment of duodenal ulcer. In[3], pp. 192-5.

19. Gough K. Different doses of ranitidine in the long-term treatment of duodenal ulcer: interim analysis. In[3], pp. 196-200.

20. Barbier P, Dumont A, Adler M. Evaluation en étude de la ranitidine dans la thérapeutique de 40 ulcérations gastro-duodénales. Acta Gastroenterol Belg 1979; 42:268-74.

21. Berstad A, Kett K, Aadland E, et al. Treatment of duodenal ulcer with ranitidine, a new histamine H_2-receptor antagonist. Scand J Gastroenterol 1980; 15:637-9.

22. Mangiameli A, Monaco S, Catalano F, Blasi A. Ranitidine in short-term treatment of duodenal ulcer. Ital J Gastroenterol 1982; 14:5-6.

23. Dobrilla G, Barbara L, Bianchi Porro G, et al. Placebo controlled studies with ranitidine in duodenal ulcers. Scand J Gastroenterol [Suppl] 1981; 69:101-7.

24. Ashton MG, Holdsworth CD, Ryan FP, Moore M. Healing of gastric ulcers after one, two, and three months of ranitidine. Br Med J 1982; 284:467-8.

25. Gibinski K, Nowak A, Gabryelewicz A, et al. Multicentre double blind clinical trial on ranitidine for gastroduodenal ulcer. Hepatogastroenterology 1981; 28:216-7.

26. Wright JP, Marks IN, Mee AS, et al. Ranitidine in the treatment of gastric ulceration. S Afr Med J 1982; 61:155-8.

27. Cockel R, Dawson J, Jain S. Ranitidine in the long-term treatment of gastric ulcers. In[3], pp. 232-8.

28. Priebe HJ, Skillman JJ, Bushnell LS, Long PC, Silen W. Antacid versus cimetidine in preventing acute gastrointestinal bleeding: a randomized trial in 75 critically ill patients. N Engl J Med 1980; 302:426-30.

29. Macchi H, Fiasse R, Reynaert M, Desager JP, Dive Ch. Effect of intravenous raniti-dine on gastric acid secretion in severely ill patients admitted to an intensive care unit. In[3], pp. 269-74.

30. Dawson J, Cockel R. Ranitidine in acute upper gastrointestinal haemorrhage. Br Med J 1982; 285:476-7.

31. Bertaccini G, Molina E, Bobbio P, Foggi E. Ranitidine increases lower oesophageal sphincter pressure in man. Ital J Gastroenterol 1981; 13:147-50.

32. Wallin L, Madsen T, Boesby S. Gastro-oesophageal function in normal subjects after oral administration of ranitidine. Gut 1983; 24:154-7.

33. Mignon M, Vallot T, Bonfils S. Use of ranitidine in the management of Zollinger-Ellison syndrome. In[3], pp. 281-2.

34. Jensen RT, Collen MJ, Pandol AJ, et al. Cimetidine-induced impotence and breast changes in patients with gastric hypersecreting states. N Engl J Med 1983; 308: 883-7.

35. Danilewitz M, Tim LO, Hirschowitz B. Ranitidine suppression of gastric hypersecre-tion resistant to cimetidine. N Engl J Med 1982; 306:20-2.

36. Brunner G, Losgen H, Harke U. Ranitidine in the treatment of cimetidine-resistant ulcerations of the upper intestinal tract. In[3], pp. 254-6.

37. Simon B, Muller P, Dammann H-G, Kommerell B. Adverse effects of cimetidine and safety profile of ranitidine. In[3], pp. 58-64.

38. Cohen A, Fabre L. Tolerance to repeated intravenous doses of ranitidine HCl and cimetidine HCl in normal volunteers. Curr Ther Res (in press).

39. Barr GD, Piper DW. Possible ranitidine hepatitis. Med J Aust 1981; 2:421.

40. Jack D, Richards DA, Granata F. Side-effects of ranitidine. Lancet 1982; 2:264-5.

41. Jack D, Smith RN, Richards DA. Histamine H_2 antagonists and the heart. Lancet 1982; 2:1281.

42. Camarri E, Chirone E, Fanteria G, Zocchi M. Ranitidine induced bradycardia. Lancet 1982; 2:160.

43. Parkin JV, Ackroyd EB, Glickman S, Hobsley M, Lorenz W. Release of histamine by H_2-receptor antagonists. Lancet 1982; 2:938-9.

44. Dobrilla G, Felder M, Chilovi F, de Pretis G. Exacerbation of glaucoma associated with both cimetidine and ranitidine. Lancet 1982; 1:1078.

45. Edwards CRW, Riley AJ. Endocrine effects of ranitidine: comparison with cimeti-dine. In[3], pp. 65-9.

46. Tosi R, Cagnoli M. Painful gynaecomastia with ranitidine. Lancet 1982; 2:160.

47. Kimelblatt BJ, Cerra FB, Calleri G, Berg MJ, McMillen MA, Schentag JJ. Dose and serum concentration relationships in cimetidine-associated mental confusion. Gastro-enterology 1980; 78:791-5.

48. Schentag JJ, Cerra FB, Calleri G, DeGlopper E, Rose JQ, Bernhard H. Pharmaco-kinetic and clinical studies in patients with cimetidine-associated mental confusion. Lancet 1979; 1:177-81.

49. Smith IR, Cleverby MT, Ganellin CR, Metters KM. Binding of [^{3}H]cimetidine to rat brain tissue. Agents Actions 1980; 10:422-6.

50. Rudnick MR, Bastl CP, Elfenbein IB, Sirota RA, Yudis M, Narins RG. Cimetidine-induced acute renal failure. Ann Intern Med 1982; 96:180-2.

51. Richman AV, Narayan JL, Hirschfield JS. Acute interstitial nephritis and acute renal failure associated with cimetidine therapy. Am J Med 1981; 70:1272-4.

52. Peden NR, Robertson AJ, Boyd EJS, et al. Mitogen stimulation of peripheral blood lymphocytes of duodenal ulcer patients during treatment with cimetidine or ranitidine. Gut 1982; 23:398-403.

53. Jorizzo JL, Sams WM Jr, Jegasothy BV, Olansky J. Cimetidine as an immunomodulator: chronic mucocutaneous candidiasis as a model. Ann Intern Med 1980; 92: 192-5.

54. Borgström S, von Eyben FE, Flodgren P, Axelsson B, Sjögren HO. Human leukocyte interferon and cimetidine for metastatic melanoma. N Engl J Med 1982; 307:1080-1.

55. Hill NO, Pardue A, Khan A, et al. Interferon and cimetidine for malignant melanoma. N Engl J Med 1983; 308:286.

56. de Galocsy C, van Ypersele de Strihou C. Pancytopenia with cimetidine. Ann Intern Med 1979; 90:274.

57. Heagerty AM, Castleden CM, Patel L. Failure of ranitidine to interact with propranolol. Br Med J 1982; 284:1304.

58. Feely J, Wilkinson GR, McAllister CB, Wood AJJ. Increased toxicity and reduced clearance of lidocaine by cimetidine. Ann Intern Med 1982; 96:592-4.

59. Feely J, Gay E. Lack of effect of ranitidine on the disposition of lignocaine. Br J Clin Pharmacol 1983; 15:378-9.

60. Nichols TW Jr. Phytobezoar formation: a new complication of cimetidine therapy. Ann Intern Med 1981; 95:70.

61. Cristiano P, Paradisi F. Can cimetidine facilitate infections by oral route? Lancet 1982; 2:45.

62. Reed PI, Smith PLR, Haines K, House FR, Walters CL. Effect of cimetidine on gastric juice N-nitrosamine concentration. Lancet 1981; 2:553-6.

63. Stockbrugger RW, Cotton PB, Eugenides N, Bartholomew BA, Hill MJ, Walters CL. Intragastric nitrites, nitrosamines, and bacterial overgrowth during cimetidine treatment. Gut 1982; 23:1048-54.

64. Muscroft TJ, Youngs DJ, Burdon DW, Keighley MRB. Cimetidine is unlikely to increase formation of intragastric N-nitroso-compounds in patients taking a normal diet. Lancet 1981; 1:408-10.

65. Milton-Thompson GJ, Lightfoot NF, Ahmet Z, et al. Intragastric acidity, bacteria, nitrite, and N-nitroso compounds before, during, and after cimetidine treatment. Lancet 1982; 1:1091-5.

66. Tannenbaum SR. N-nitroso compounds: a perspective on human exposure. Lancet 1983; 1:629-31.

67. Brittain RT, Harris DM, Martin LE, Poynter D, Price BJ. Safety of ranitidine. Lancet 1981; 2:1119.

68. Poynter D, Pick CR, Harcourt RA, et al. Evaluation of ranitidine safety. In[3], pp. 49-57.

| Correction*

Ranitidine — A New H_2-Receptor Antagonist (Dec. 1, 1983; 309:1368-73). On page 1369 [page 41] under the "Pharmacokinetics" heading, the tenth line should read " . . . 200 to 600 ng . . . " (not μg, as printed).

*Originally published on April 5, 1984 (310:932).

Correspondence

Ranitidine*

To the Editor:

In the recent article by Zeldis et al. concerning ranitidine, the section addressing side effects is of particular interest (Dec. 1 issue).[1]

Only incidental skin rashes, pruritic and nonpruritic, have been reported, and these rashes are said to resolve despite continued therapy.[2] In sharp contrast to reported side effects of ranitidine, I would like to share an interesting brief case experience.

A 33-year-old woman presented with a long history of substernal and midepigastric burning pain, bloating, and increased frequency of belching. These symptoms increased approximately one hour after eating and would occasionally awaken her at night. The results of an upper-gastrointestinal series were normal. Biopsies of the distal esophagus and stomach revealed chronic esophagitis and acute gastritis. I recommended ranitidine, 150 mg by mouth twice a day for one month. She was taking no other medications and had no known allergies. She took her first dose of ranitidine later that day at approximately 12:30 p.m. One hour later she noted increasing difficulty with inspiration, which progressed to moderate upper-airway stridor. Over the next hour (to 2:30 p.m.), the stridor persisted and a diffuse urticarial rash developed over the abdomen and both flanks. The blood pressure was found to be 120/64 mm Hg, the pulse 100 and regular, and the respiratory rate 25. The patient was afebrile, with notable upper-airway stridor. The lung fields were clear. An urticarial rash involved the abdomen, lower chest, and both flanks. Epinephrine (USP [1:1000]), 0.5 ml, was given subcutaneously. Over the next 30 minutes the stridor resolved, as did the rash over the next two hours. Diphenhydramine hydrochloride (Benadryl), 50 mg, was given every six hours, for a total of four doses. The patient was advised not to use ranitidine or nitrofurantoin in the future. She had an otherwise uneventful course.

Only as clinical experience increases can the true safety of any new agent be assessed.

CRAIG M. BRAYKO, M.D.
401 15th Ave. S.
Great Falls, MT 59405

1. Zeldis JB, Friedman LS, Isselbacher KJ. Ranitidine: a new H_2-receptor antagonist. N Engl J Med 1983; 309:1368-73.
2. Misiewicz JJ, Wormsley KG, eds. The clinical use of ranitidine. Oxford: Medicine Publishing Foundation, 1982:58-64.

To the Editor:

Zeldis et al. may be premature in dismissing so quickly the neurologic side effects of ranitidine. Mental confusion has been reported with ranitidine,[1-3] even at the

*Originally published on June 14, 1984 (310:1601-1606).

level of clinical trials; at a similar stage in the use of cimetidine, neurologic complications were equally uncommon. Although penetration of the central nervous system by ranitidine is low in healthy subjects,[4] penetration by cimetidine was thought to be nonexistent,[5] until it was assayed in seriously ill patients with renal and hepatic failure.[6] The statement that "Headaches are usually mild and resolve or subside despite continued therapy" stands in contrast to reports of severe headaches that required reduction of dosage or total cessation of therapy.[7,8] Such a case is described below.

A 47-year-old man was in excellent health except for a history of peptic-ulcer disease and reflux esophagitis, for which he was taking cimetidine intermittently. His wife obtained samples of ranitidine, 150 mg, which he began taking twice a day. After one week a severe, throbbing, bifrontal headache developed, which occurred daily and was worst in the afternoon. The patient stopped taking ranitidine, and the headache remitted in two days. Three days later he restarted the drug; in two or three days the severe throbbing headache recurred but again remitted quickly after ranitidine was discontinued. The patient considered these headaches incapacitating. He had no previous history of severe headaches, although his mother had migraine; he was taking no other drugs and rarely used caffeine or alcohol; and there was no change in his dietary habits or known occupational exposures during this time.

On the basis of sporadic reports it is difficult to determine which of the available H_2 antagonists might have more neurologic side effects. At present, however, the evidence fails to justify claims that ranitidine is superior in this regard.

CHARLES M. EPSTEIN, M.D.
Emory University School of Medicine
Atlanta, GA 30322

1. Albano O, Francavilla A, Meduri B, et al. Ranitidine in the treatment of duodenal ulcer: double-blind comparison of several methods of administration. Glaxo International Symposium — ranitidine: the new H_2 antagonist. Farmacologia e Clinica — Cefalu, 1981.
2. Hughes JD, Reed WD, Serjeant CS. Mental confusion associated with ranitidine. Med J Aust 1983; 2:12-3.
3. Francavilla A, Panella C, Ierardi E, et al. Effects of ranitidine: a short-term clinical trial for duodenal ulcer treatment using two different types of oral administration: serum prolactin stimulation after bolus injection. Ital J Gastroenterol 1983; 15(1):39-42.
4. Walt RP, LaBrooy SJ, Avgerinos A, Oehr T, Riley A, Misiewicz JJ. Investigations on the penetration of ranitidine into the cerebrospinal fluid and a comparison of the effects of ranitidine and cimetidine on male sex hormones. Scand J Gastroenterol [Suppl] 1981; 69:19-24.
5. Brimblecombe RW, Duncan WAM. The relevance to man of pre-clinical data for cimetidine. Cimetidine: Proceedings of the second international symposium on histamine H_2-receptor antagonists. Excerpta Medica, Amsterdam — ICS (Netherlands), 1977; no. 416, 54-66.

6. Schentag JJ, Cerra FB, Calleri G, DeGlopper E, Rose JQ, Bernhard H. Pharmacokinetic and clinical studies in patients with cimetidine-associated mental confusion. Lancet 1979; 1:177-81.

7. Morgan AG, McAdam WAF, Pacsoo C. A comparison of ranitidine with Caved-S in duodenal ulcer treatment. In: Misiewicz JJ, Wormsley KG, eds. The clinical use of ranitidine. Symposium series 5. Proceedings of the 2nd International Symposium on Ranitidine. Oxford: Medicine Publishing Foundation, 1982:168-71.

8. Lishman AH, Record CO. Ranitidine in the management of duodenal ulceration: controlled and open comparison with cimetidine. In: Misiewicz JJ,[7] pp. 163-7.

To the Editor:

In the article by Zeldis et al. there are omissions and misstatements concerning both ranitidine and cimetidine.

Determination of the safety profile of a drug is a continuous process necessitating years of experience and millions of patients. Even at this early stage, ranitidine has been reported to interact with a number of drugs, including warfarin, metoprolol, fentanyl, and midazolam.[1-4] Case reports of gynecomastia,[5] mental confusion,[6] and impotence[7] have appeared in the literature. In addition, the prescribing information for ranitidine mentions the occurrence of slight elevations of serum creatinine and decreases in platelet counts. Recent evidence indicates that neither ranitidine nor cimetidine decreases hepatic blood flow, although both may interfere with the clearance of indocyanine green.[8-10] Although H_2-receptor antagonists will reduce gastric circulation that has been stimulated by histamine, there is little evidence that this occurs under unstimulated conditions.[11]

Although cimetidine binds weakly to androgen receptors,[12] many studies have demonstrated that it has no influence on basal levels of testosterone.[13-15] Likewise, in a six-month double-blind placebo-controlled trial in 30 male volunteers, cimetidine did not influence sperm count, sperm morphology or motility, or sperm penetration in zona-free hamster ova.[14] There is no foundation for the statement of concern over the use of cimetidine in men who have fertility problems.

Omitted from the Zeldis review is any mention of the limitation of the dosage form of ranitidine to the 150-mg tablet. Thus, difficulty would be encountered if a dose of 75 mg twice daily were given to patients with renal impairment. In addition, the authors cite one of the few negative studies on the use of cimetidine in stress-related mucosal damage,[16] omitting reference to over 30 favorable reports.

T.J. Humphries, M.D.
William O. Frank, M.D.
John J. Seaman, Pharm.D.
Ralph M. Myerson, M.D.
Smith Kline and French Laboratories
Philadelphia, PA 19101

1. Desmond PV, Breen KJ, Harman PJ, Mashford ML, Morphett BJ. Decreased clearance of warfarin after treatment with cimetidine or ranitidine. Aust NZ J Med 1983; 13:327. abstract.

2. Spahn H, Mutschler E, Kirch W, Ohnhaus EE, Janisch HD. Influence of ranitidine on plasma metoprolol and atenolol concentrations. Br Med J 1983; 286:1546-7.

3. Lee HR, Gandolfi AJ, Sipes IG, Bentley J. Effect of histamine H_2-receptors on fentanyl metabolism. Pharmacologist 1982; 24:145. abstract.

4. Elwood RJ, Hildebrand PJ, Dundee JW, Collier PS. Ranitidine influences the uptake of oral midazolam. Br J Clin Pharmacol 1983; 15:743-5.

5. Tosi S, Cagnoli M. Painful gynecomastia with ranitidine. Lancet 1982; 2:160.

6. Hughes JD, Reed WD, Serjeant CS. Mental confusion associated with ranitidine. Med J Aust 1983; 2:12-3.

7. Viana L. Probable case of impotence due to ranitidine. Lancet 1983; 2:635-6.

8. Tyden G, Thulin L, Myberg B. The effect of cimetidine on liver blood flow in anesthetized men. Acta Chir Scand 1983; 149:303-5.

9. Estampes B, Volter F, Beaugrand M, Ferrier J-P. Cimetidine and portal hypertension: study of different hemodynamic parameters in eight cirrhotic subjects [in French]. Gastroenterol Clin Biol 1982; 6:512-3.

10. Dunk AA, Jenkins WJ, Burroughs AK, et al. The effect of ranitidine on the plasma clearance and hepatic extraction of indocyanine green in patients with chronic liver disease. Br J Clin Pharmacol 1983; 16:117-20.

11. Delaney JP, Michel HM, Bond J. Cimetidine and gastric blood flow. Surgery 1978; 84:190-3.

12. Winters SJ, Lee J, Troen P. Competition of the histamine H_2 antagonist cimetidine for androgen binding sites in man. J Androl 1980; 1:111-4.

13. Carlson HE, Ippoliti AF, Swerdloff RS. Endocrine effects of acute and chronic cimetidine administration. Dig Dis Sci 1981; 26:428-32.

14. Enzmann GD, Leonard JM, Paulsen CA, Rogers J. Effect of cimetidine on reproductive function in man. Clin Res 1981; 29:26A. abstract.

15. Spona J, Weisz W, Rudiger E, et al. Hormone serum levels during oral cimetidine treatment of patients with peptic ulcers. Hepatogastroenterology 1981; 28:165-8.

16. Priebe HJ, Skillman JJ, Bushnell LS, Long PC, Silen W. Antacid versus cimetidine in preventing acute gastrointestinal bleeding: a randomized trial in critically ill patients. N Engl J Med 1980; 302:426-30.

To the Editor:

Zeldis et al. state that ranitidine differs from cimetidine in its effects on the immune system because human lymphocytes have been shown to have receptors for cimetidine but not for ranitidine.[1] Thus the antitumor activity of cimetidine in mice[2-4] and in human beings,[5-7] which is probably due to the inhibition of T-suppressor-lymphocyte activity, would not be expected with ranitidine. Our experimental results on lymphocyte proliferation and survival of tumor-bearing mice are not in accordance with this hypothesis.

We have recently studied the suppressive effect of histamine and Dimaprit (an H_2-receptor agonist) on the proliferation in vitro of murine lymphocytes induced by phytohemagglutinin or allogeneic spleen cells. Three H_2-receptor antagonists — metiamide, cimetidine, and ranitidine — equally blocked suppression by histamine and Dimaprit.[8] In 3LL tumor-bearing mice, cimetidine slowed metastatic development and prolonged survival.[3] In fibrosarcoma-bearing C57BL/6 mice, daily intraperitoneal injections of metiamide increased survival.[4] We compared the effects of cimetidine and ranitidine in mice of this strain (daily intraperitoneal injections of 0.5 mg per mouse); control mice received saline solution. The preliminary results show that ranitidine is as potent as cimetidine in increasing survival in these fibrosarcoma-bearing mice (Table 1). This antitumor activity was not due to direct cytotoxic activity on tumor cells. Indeed, like cimetidine,[3] metiamide, cimetidine, and ranitidine added to 3LL-cell cultures at concentrations from 10^{-12} to 10^{-3} M had no influence on the incorporation of [^{3}H]thymidine.

TABLE 1.   Survival among Fibrosarcoma-Bearing Mice Given Cimetidine or Ranitidine and Controls.*

Study Group (No.)	Percentage Surviving							
	Day 21	Day 23	Day 25	Day 28	Day 30	Day 32	Day 34	Day 36
Controls (12)	100	92	58	50	33	33	33	25
Cimetidine (12)	100	100	92	92	83	62	58	58
Ranitidine (12)	100	100	100	100	100	83	66	58

*Day denotes number of days after tumor-cell graft.

Thus, metiamide, cimetidine, and ranitidine share at least four common properties: inhibition of gastric secretion, blockade of the suppressive activity of histamine and Dimaprit on lymphocyte proliferation, increase in survival of fibrosarcoma-bearing mice, and absence of direct cytotoxicity on tumor cells.

CLAUDE BURTIN, PH.D., PIERRE SCHEINMANN, M.D.,
ANTOINETTE FRAY, PH.D., GENEVIEVE LESPINATS, M.D.,
CHRISTIAN NOIROT, M.D., AND JEAN PAUPE, M.D.
Faculté Medecine Necker Enfants Malades
75730 Paris Cedex 15, France

1. Peden NR, Robertson AJ, Boyd EJS, et al. Mitogen stimulation of peripheral blood lymphocytes of duodenal ulcer patients during treatment with cimetidine or ranitidine. Gut 1982; 23:398-403.
2. Gifford RRM, Ferguson RM, Voss BV. Cimetidine reduction of tumour formation in mice. Lancet 1981; 1:638-40.
3. Osband ME, Hamilton D, Shen Y-J, et al. Successful tumour immunotherapy with cimetidine in mice. Lancet 1981; 1:636-8.
4. Burtin C, Scheinmann P, Salomon JC, Lespinats G, Canu P. Decrease in tumour growth by injections of histamine or serotonin in fibrosarcoma-bearing mice: influence of H_1 and H_2 histamine receptors. Br J Cancer 1982; 45:54-60.

5. Armitage JO, Sidner RD. Antitumour effect of cimetidine? Lancet 1979; 1:882-3.
6. Borgstrom S, von Eyben FE, Flodgren P, Axelsson B, Sjogren HO. Human leucocyte interferon and cimetidine for metastatic melanoma. N Engl J Med 1982; 307:1080-1.
7. Burtin C, Scheinmann P, Noirot C, Taboury J, Paupe J. Combination of cimetidine with other drugs for treatment of cancer. N Engl J Med 1983; 308:591-2.
8. Bonnet M, Lespinats G, Burtin C. Histamine and serotonin suppression of lymphocyte response to phytohemagglutinin and allogeneic cells. Cell Immunol (in press).

To the Editor:

The article by Zeldis et al. refers to possible hepatic side effects of ranitidine therapy. The authors point out that transient increases in serum aminotransferase levels have occurred in patients receiving ranitidine,[1] as well as in a patient with possible anicteric hepatitis (described in the Australian literature).[2] There have been additional reports of liver-enzyme abnormalities after oral ranitidine therapy (described in the Canadian literature).[3]

A 66-year-old man presented with fever, malaise, and a history of chronic ulcer disease. He had been taking ranitidine, 150 mg by mouth at night, for four to five weeks before admission. He had taken quinine in the past for nocturnal leg cramps but had not taken any for three months before admission. Laboratory data obtained on admission were notable for an erythrocyte sedimentation rate of 97 mm per hour, a serum glutamic oxaloacetic transaminase (aspartate aminotransferase) of 128 U per liter, a serum glutamic pyruvic transaminase (alanine aminotransferase) of 145 U per liter, an alkaline phosphatase of 466 U per liter, and a gamma-glutamyl transpeptidase of 535 U per liter. The coagulation profile and white-cell count were normal. A workup for fever was negative, and a liver biopsy revealed granulomatous inflammation with eosinophilia. Ranitidine therapy was discontinued in the hospital, after which the patient became afebrile and his liver functions became normal over one week.

Because of the aminoalkyl furan ring structure of ranitidine, investigators have anticipated an increase in reports of hepatic toxicity in patients treated with oral ranitidine.[4] Studies have shown dose-related increases in live chemistries after intravenous ranitidine administration (manufacturer's prescribing information [Glaxo, 1983]). Potential hepatotoxicity secondary to oral therapy may be related to the endogenous availability of reduced glutathione and partly related to cytochrome P-450 activity.[4] It is true that quinine has recently been observed to produce granulomatous hepatitis,[5] but our patient had stopped taking quinine several months before admission.

Because of the recent availability and rapidly increasing use of ranitidine, physicians should be aware of possible adverse hepatic effects of oral ranitidine therapy.

KENNETH OFFIT, M.D., M.P.H.
DONNA ASKIN SOJKA, B.S., R.PH.
Lenox Hill Hospital
New York, NY 10021

1. Cohen A, Fabre L. Tolerance to repeated intravenous doses of ranitidine HCL and cimetidine HCL in normal volunteers. Curr Ther Res (in press).
2. Barr GD, Piper DW. Possible ranitidine hepatitis. Med J Aust 1981; 2:421.
3. Cleator IGM. Adverse effects of ranitidine therapy. Can Med Assoc J 1983; 129:405.
4. McCarthy DM. Ranitidine or cimetidine. Ann Intern Med 1983; 99:551-3.
5. Katz B, Weetch M, Chopra S. Quinine-induced granulomatous hepatitis. Br Med J 1983; 286:264-5.

To the Editor:

Histamine H_2-receptor antagonists have been linked to granulocytopenia in the past.* Zeldis et al. state that "Thrombocytopenia and agranulocytosis . . . have not been reported to date with ranitidine." We report here a case of aplastic anemia associated with ranitidine.

A 58-year-old man was admitted with melena, coffee-grounds emesis, and fever. There was a history of chronic alcohol use and of constrictive pericarditis treated by pericardiectomy. The patient had a temperature of 38°C (101°F) and ascites. The hematocrit was 15 per cent, the reticulocyte count 345,000 per cubic millimeter, and the white-cell count 30,000 per cubic millimeter, with 60 per cent polymorphonuclear leukocytes, 7 per cent band forms, 19 per cent lymphocytes, 12 per cent monocytes, 1 per cent myelocytes, 1 per cent metamyelocytes, and 4 per cent nucleated red cells. Esophagoscopy revealed no source of bleeding; however, an upper-gastrointestinal series showed esophageal varices. The patient was given a transfusion with packed red cells and treated with gentamicin and cefoxitin, spironolactone, and cimetidine, and gradually improved. All cultures were negative, and the gentamicin and cefoxitin were discontinued. Because of restlessness, the patient was placed on oxazepam.

On the fifth hospital day he become lethargic. The serum ammonia level was 172 μmol per liter (normal, up to 26) though results of other liver-function tests were nearly normal. On the seventh hospital day, because of the lethargy, oxazepam and cimetidine were discontinued and ranitidine tablets, 150 mg, were given twice daily. Within a week the total granulocyte count had fallen to 110 per cubic millimeter, the platelet count to 55,000 per cubic millimeter, and the reticulocyte count to 19,200 per cubic millimeter; the fever recurred (Fig. 1). Serum folate and vitamin B_{12} levels were normal. The ranitidine was discontinued on the 14th hospital day, and blood-cell counts gradually improved. The fever resolved with antibiotic therapy. On the 30th hospital day a bone-marrow biopsy performed for prognostic purposes showed that the marrow was recovering.

Initially this patient's bone marrow was healthy, as shown by the elevation of the white-cell, platelet, and reticulocyte counts in response to stress. The first drop in these counts was to a plateau at normal levels (the platelet count was slightly lower because of dilution by red-cell transfusions). The next dramatic drop coincided with the addition of ranitidine (spironolactone and acetamino-

*Forrest JA, Shearman DJ, Spence R, Celestin LR. Neutropenia associated with metiamide. Lancet 1975; 1:392-3.

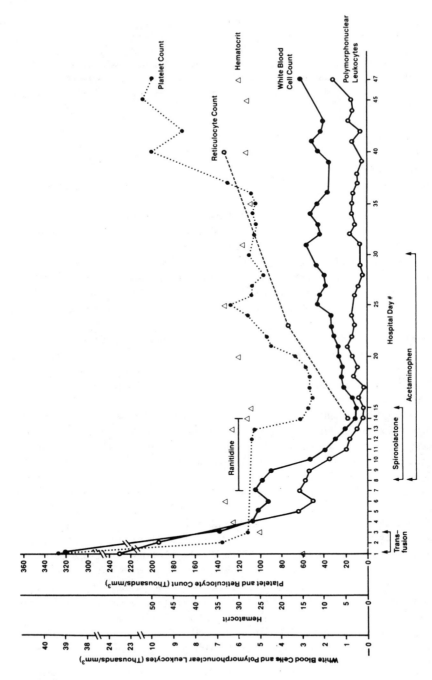

Figure 1. Effect of Ranitidine on Hematologic Values of a Patient with Melena and Fever.

phen) and reached nadirs associated with severe aplastic anemia. Marrow recovery followed discontinuation of ranitidine (and spironolactone) despite continuation of acetaminophen.

Thus, although we cannot absolutely exclude virus, spironolactone, or other drugs as causes of bone-marrow suppression, we believe that ranitidine should be viewed with suspicion in this case. At least in situations such as this, it should not be assumed that ranitidine has fewer side effects than cimetidine.

DAVID C. HARMON, M.D.
RICHARD SHUMAN, M.D.
Massachusetts General Hospital
Boston, MA 02114

To the Editor:

Zeldis et al. mention that myeloid toxicity due to ranitidine has never been reported. This, however, is not true of cimetidine treatment, which has caused such toxicity.* We observed a patient in whom neutropenia developed during ranitidine treatment. The toxicity of ranitidine on progenitor cells was confirmed by bone-marrow culture.

A 50-year-old patient had been taking cimetidine for a duodenal ulcer since 1980. In May 1983, when he was taking 400 mg daily, gastroscopy showed a benign gastric ulcer. Cimetidine treatment was stopped, and ranitidine treatment, 300 mg per day, was initiated.

Before the ranitidine was begun, blood counts were normal (4.7×10^9 white cells per liter with 3.0×10^9 polymorphonuclear cells per liter) (Fig. 1). After 30 days of treatment, white cells were 5.1×10^9 and polymorphonuclear cells 1.4×10^9 per liter, but hemoglobin levels and platelet counts were normal. On Day 40, although neutropenia persisted, the cellularity was normal according to a bone-marrow smear; a bone-marrow culture in soft agar, to which placenta-conditioned medium had been added as stimulant, showed a very low number of myeloid progenitor cells (CFU-GM) — 10 colonies per 2×10^5 mononucleated cells and 110 clusters per 2×10^5 mononucleated cells after eight days. Ranitidine treatment was stopped. Three days later there were 2.15×10^9 polymorphonulear cells per liter. Since the symptoms recurred and the bone-marrow cellularity was normal, and since ranitidine-induced myeloid toxicity had never previously been reported, ranitidine was tried again nine days later. After eight days of treatment, the polymorphonuclear-cell counts dropped from 3.9×10^9 to 1.2×10^9 per liter, and ranitidine treatment was stopped again. Ten days later the count was 2.7×10^9 per liter. A bone-marrow culture performed three months later, when blood counts were normal, showed an increased number of CFU-GM, with 95 colonies and more than 1000 clusters per 2×10^5 mononucleated cells on Day 10.

---

*De Galocsy C, Van Ypersele de Strihou C. Pancytopenia with cimetidine. Ann Intern Med 1979; 90:274.

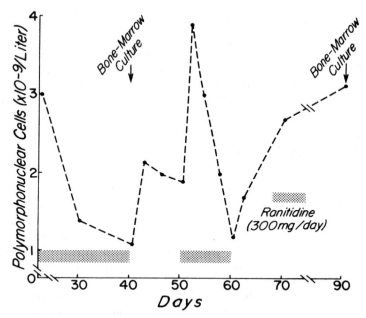

Figure 1. Effect of Ranitidine on the Polymorphonuclear-Cell Count of a Patient with Gastric Ulcer.

When ranitidine was added to the culture medium at a concentration of 300 μg per milliliter — approximately equal to the ranitidine serum concentration during treatment with 300 mg per day (as stated by Zeldis et al.) — there was a dramatic decrease in the number of colonies (22 per 2×10^5 cells) and clusters (108 per 2×10^5 cells) on Day 10. This effect was not observed when ranitidine was added to the medium and the cells were washed before plating.

These results suggest that ranitidine may have myeloid toxicity, even in a patient who has had no neutropenia during several months of cimetidine treatment.

A. HERRERA, AND P. SOLAL-CELIGNY
Hôpital Beaujon
F 92118 Clichy, France

C. DRESCH
Hôpital Saint Louis
F 75010 Paris, France

J VALLIN, AND P. BERNADES
Hôpital Beaujon
F 92118 Clichy, France

The above letters were referred to the authors of the article in question and to Glaxo, Inc., who offer the following replies:

To the Editor:

We indicated in our review that, as with any new drug, continued experience with ranitidine may result in the identification of as yet unknown adverse reactions. Dr. Herrera and colleagues provide convincing evidence that ranitidine may cause neutropenia, an effect not previously reported. In contrast, in the case reported by Drs. Harmon and Schuman, it is difficult to ascribe the marrow depression to ranitidine with any degree of certainty. The patient's blood-cell counts fell to subnormal levels several days before the introduction of ranitidine, the patient was receiving many drugs, and information about the underlying medical illness was insufficient. It is also difficult to implicate ranitidine as the cause of granulomatous hepatitis in the patient described by Drs. Offit and Sojka. The known causes of granulomatous hepatitis were not excluded. Moreover, a follow-up liver biopsy to document histologic resolution was not performed, and (understandably) re-challenge with ranitidine was not undertaken.

Dr. Brayko describes urticaria and stridor in a patient receiving oral ranitidine. This reaction may have been due to a sudden rise in the serum histamine level. Ranitidine and cimetidine have both been found to displace histamine from H_2 receptors and to cause a rise in the serum histamine level after rapid intravenous infusion.[1] It is postulated that a similar phenomenon may follow oral administration of ranitidine, and that this may account for both urticaria and headaches caused by ranitidine (Bauman JH: personal communication).

Dr. Epstein's report is consistent with our statement that about 1.8 per cent of patients taking ranitidine experience headaches.

The letter of Dr. Burtin et al. is provocative. However, we are not aware of any current evidence that ranitidine binds to human lymphocytes or modulates the human immune response; therefore, the murine model may not mimic the human situation. The small number of mice in each group limits the power of the study to detect a significant difference between ranitidine and cimetidine and between either group given an H_2 antagonist and the control group.

In view of what has been published on ranitidine, the statements made by Dr. Humphries and colleagues are somewhat surprising. Ranitidine has been shown to bind less avidly than cimetidine to the P-450 enzyme system in the hepatocyte. Consistent with this, the clearance of metoprolol has been shown to be affected to a much greater extent by cimetidine than by ranitidine (Janisch H: personal communication). In fact, steady-state serum concentrations of metoprolol are not affected by ranitidine treatment.[2] The effect of ranitidine on the metabolism of fentanyl has been demonstrated only in vitro and with high, nonpharmacologic concentrations of ranitidine.[3] Published data on the effect of ranitidine on warfarin clearance are conflicting.[4-6] Increased absorption of midazolam (a drug not available in the United States) in patients taking ranitidine is due to increased gastric pH and would be expected to occur with any agent that raises the gastric pH, including cimetidine and liquid antacids.[7]

Humphries et al. reiterate our statement that only a single case of ranitidine-associated unilateral gynecomastia has been reported.[8] The one report of mental confusion attributed to ranitidine concerned an elderly woman who had pulmonary edema and was taking several other drugs.[9] The single case of impotence attributed to ranitidine has been adequately refuted.[10,11] Although the prescribing information for ranitidine states that in clinical trials some patients have had increases in serum creatinine levels and decreases in platelet counts, in no case were these changes clinically important. Moreover, a similar incidence of the same abnormalities was seen in the placebo-control group (Eschelman FN: personal communication). Finally, cimetidine has been demonstrated in some studies to increase the basal level of testosterone[12,13] and decrease the sperm count[14] and penile tumescence.[15] Because these findings have not been reported with ranitidine to date, we still consider it prudent to use ranitidine rather than cimetidine in men with fertility problems.

JEROME B. ZELDIS, M.D., PH.D., LAWRENCE S. FRIEDMAN, M.D., AND KURT J. ISSELBACHER, M.D.
Massachusetts General Hospital
Boston, MA 02114

1. Parkin JV, Ackroyd EB, Glickman S, Hobsley M, Lorenz W. Release of histamine by H_2-receptor antagonists. Lancet 1982; 2:938-9.
2. Kelly JG, Shanks RG, McDevitt DG. Influence of ranitidine on plasma metoprolol concentrations. Br Med J 1983; 287:1218-9.
3. Lee HR, Gandolfi AJ, Sipes IG, Bentley J. Effect of histamine H_2-receptors on fentanyl metabolism. Pharmacologist 1982; 24:145. abstract.
4. Desmond PV, Breen KJ, Harman PJ, Mashford ML, Morphett BJ. Decreased clearance of warfarin after treatment with cimetidine or ranitidine. Aust NZ J Med 1983; 13:327. abstract.
5. Serlin MJ, Sibeon RG, Breckenridge AM. Lack of effect of ranitidine on warfarin action. Br J Clin Pharmacol 1981; 12:791-4.
6. O'Reilly RA. Comparative interaction of cimetidine and ranitidine with racemic warfarin in man. Fed Proc 1983; 42:1175. abstract.
7. Elwood RJ, Hildebrand PJ, Dundee JW, Collier PS. Ranitidine influences the uptake of oral midazolam. Br J Clin Pharmacol 1983; 15:743-5.
8. Tosi R, Cagnoli M. Painful gynaecomastia with ranitidine. Lancet 1982; 2:160.
9. Hughes J, Reed WD, Serjeant CS. Mental confusion associated with ranitidine. Med J Aust 1983; 2:12-3.
10. Smith RN, Elsdon-Dew RW. Alleged impotence with ranitidine. Lancet 1983; 2:798.
11. Peden NR, Wormsley KG. Alleged impotence with ranitidine. Lancet 1983; 2:798.
12. Peden NR, Boyd EJS, Browning MCK, Saunders JHB, Wormsley KG. Effects of two histamine H_2-receptor blocking drugs on basal levels of gonadotrophins, prolactin, testosterone and oestradiol-17β during treatment of duodenal ulcer in male patients. Acta Endocrinol (Copenh) 1981; 96:564-7.

13. Wang C, Lai CL, Lam KC, Yeung KK. Effect of cimetidine on gonadal function in man. Br J Clin Pharmacol 1982; 13:791-4.
14. Van Thiel DH, Gavaler JS, Smith WI Jr, Paul G. Hypothalamic-pituitary-gonadal dysfunction in men using cimetidine. N Engl J Med 1979; 300:1012-5.
15. Jensen RT, Collen MJ, Pandol SJ, et al. Cimetidine-induced impotence and breast changes in patients with gastric hypersecretory states. N Engl J Med 1983; 308: 883-7.

To the Editor:

Since the editorial policy of the *Journal* limits responses to 40 typed lines, our comments on these seven letters are necessarily terse. Five of the letters deal with clinical events that were not reported to us or to the Food and Drug Administration by the correspondents, who, however, subsequently provided more information at our request.

Harmon and Schuman describe pancytopenia in a patient whose bone marrow was affected by hemorrhage and fever. A log-plot shows a sharp fall in white cells and platelets that started seven days before ranitidine was given. Clearly, on a temporal basis, one must exclude ranitidine as a cause. Moreover, cimetidine was given intravenously for the first seven days, and cefoxitin and gentamicin were given for two days, and each of these has occasionally produced blood dyscrasias.

Herrera et al. report a clinically unimportant, reversible neutropenia occurring twice after ranitidine treatment. The bone-marrow morphology was normal, unlike the maturation arrest that has been described with cimetidine.[1] Judgment of the marrow-culture assay is difficult because the facts given are insufficient, and the incubation test is irrelevant because the ranitidine level used was about 1000 times higher than therapeutic concentrations of the drug.

In Offit and Sojka's patient, the granulomatous hepatitis associated with an acute febrile illness resolved rapidly with three antibiotics — an improvement coincident with ranitidine withdrawal. Drug-induced granulomatous hepatitis is rare and has never been reported with ranitidine, but it can occur with quinine, which this patient had taken. Many cases are idiopathic.

Severe headaches occur occasionally and anaphylactoid reactions occur rarely with ranitidine as well as cimetidine, so the reports by Drs. Epstein and Brayko are not surprising. We will add a notice about these adverse reactions to the package insert; we had already proposed this to the FDA.

The laboratory findings of Dr. Burtin and colleagues are in conflict with virtually all other information about the actions of ranitidine on human lymphocytes. Their work cannot be judged properly because not enough facts are given.

Dr. Humphries and colleagues suggest that it is too early to assess the safety of ranitidine. They must therefore be unaware that more than 8 million patients have now been treated with the drug in developed countries during the past five years — a volume of clinical experience that must have detected all but the rarest of adverse events likely to occur. So far as we are aware, no validated clinically important interference with endocrine function or drug interaction has been reported in patients treated with ranitidine. Accordingly, we believe that any objective assessment of the available evidence would, like the reviews by Zeldis et al. and Strum,[2] inevitably conclude that the histamine H_2-blocking action of ranitidine is more selective than that of cimetidine. Since most of the controversy about their relative selectivities of action has concerned the possibility that ranitidine may, like cimetidine, inhibit the hepatic cytochrome P-450 mixed-function oxygenase enzyme system, a review of all the evidence concerning ranitidine and this enzyme, and drugs that are substrates of it, is available from Glaxo Inc. to enable interested readers to make their own judgments. In our view, there is no valid evidence of inhibition of this enzyme system by therapeutic doses of ranitidine.

DAVID JACK, PH.D.
ROBERT N. SMITH, M.D.
Glaxo Group Research Limited
Greenford, England

PETER J. WISE, M.D.
Glaxo Inc.
Research Triangle Park, NC 27709

1. Pariente EA, Nouel O. Cimetidine-induced bone marrow suppression. Dig Dis Sci 1980; 25:396.
2. Strum WB. Ranitidine. JAMA 1983; 250:1894-6.

Treatment of Herpesvirus Infections

(In Two Parts)

Martin S. Hirsch, M.D.,
and Robert T. Schooley, M.D.

HERPESVIRUS infections remain among the most troublesome afflictions facing patients and clinicians. Although "remedies" for herpes infections have long been with us, until recently none has withstood close scrutiny. Since this subject was last reviewed in the *Journal,* [1] a number of well-controlled clinical trials of anti-herpes agents have been conducted. Moreover, both topical and intravenous preparations of acyclovir have been licensed in the United States, and licensure of oral acyclovir is on the horizon. Other anti-herpes nucleoside derivatives and a multitude of different interferon preparations are under trial. Physicians have gone from a situation in which there was no treatment for herpes infections to one in which, for certain conditions, choices must be made between effective alternatives.

We will review the currently licensed anti-herpes compounds and other promising agents under investigation, summarize recent clinical trials, and offer specific guidelines for the management of individual infections. The guidelines for management are offered with the recognition that they may soon be outdated. The licensure of oral acyclovir is likely to alter many current recommendations. Although we cannot recommend unlicensed drugs, we will attempt to anticipate future developments in this area. In the first part of this review we will cover varicella zoster and Epstein–Barr viruses, and in the second part, cytomegalovirus and herpes simplex Types 1 and 2.

Vidarabine

Vidarabine (9-β-D-arabinofuranosyladenine, adenine arabinoside, Ara-A, Vira-A) has now become the established standard for first-generation anti-herpes agents.

From the Infectious Disease Unit, Department of Medicine, Massachusetts General Hospital and Harvard Medical School, Boston.

Supported in part under a contract (1-CP-43222) with the National Cancer Institute, by a grant (AI 17057) from the National Institute of Allergy and Infectious Disease, and by the Mashud A. Mezerhane B. Fund.

Originally published in two parts on October 20, 1983 (309:963-970) and October 27, 1983 (309:1034-1039).

It is a purine nucleoside analogue with some antiviral activity against all members of the human herpesvirus group. Within cells, vidarabine is phosphorylated by cellular kinases to a triphosphate form, which acts as a relatively selective competitive inhibitor of DNA polymerase.[2-4] In addition, vidarabine may be incorporated into the viral DNA molecule at different positions, producing chain termination,[3] although this hypothesis has been challenged.[5] In vivo, vidarabine is readily deaminated to arabinosyl hypoxanthine, which has less antiviral activity than the parent compound. The plasma half-life is three to four hours, and nearly 60 per cent of a dose is recovered in the urine, principally as arabinosyl hypoxanthine. The agent is widely distributed in the body, with levels in cerebrospinal fluid approximately one third to one half those in serum.[4]

Vidarabine is relatively insoluble, and its intravenous administration requires a large fluid load. It is usually dissolved at a concentration of less than 0.5 mg per milliliter and given by 12-hour infusion once each day. This large fluid requirement may pose a problem in patients with herpes encephalitis and cerebral edema. Although vidarabine monophosphate is more soluble and has similar in vitro activity, its use in herpes simplex encephalitis has recently been curtailed because of an apparent lack of efficacy or because of increased toxicity in collaborative trials.

The most common adverse effects of intravenous vidarabine have been gastrointestinal (nausea, vomiting, and diarrhea) and neurologic (tremors, paresthesias, ataxia, and seizures).[5,6] The neurologic side effects may appear many days after the beginning of therapy and are usually reversible. Preexisting neurologic, hepatic, or renal disease may predispose patients to vidarabine neurotoxicity, as may the concomitant use of allopurinol.[7] Allopurinol inhibition of xanthine oxidase may result in increased levels of arabinosyl hypoxanthine. The drug should be used cautiously in patients with renal insufficiency, with dose reductions of at least 25 per cent. At high doses (20 to 30 mg per kilogram of body weight per day), megaloblastic anemia, leukopenia, and thrombocytopenia may occur. Inappropriate secretion of antidiuretic hormone has also been described.[8] In some experimental models, vidarabine has teratogenic, mutagenic, and carcinogenic properties. Its use in pregnant women and infants should thus be limited to those with life-threatening illnesses.

Acyclovir

Acyclovir (9-2(2-hydroxyethoxymethyl)guanine; acycloguanosine) is a recently licensed nucleoside analogue with a high degree of specificity against herpes simplex and varicella zoster viruses. It is available in the United States in both intravenous and topical preparations; oral formulations are licensed in Britain and will probably be available here shortly. Acyclovir's limited toxicity and great specificity in numerous clinical trials make it a major advance in herpesvirus therapy.

Infection of cells with herpes simplex virus results in the production of a viral thymidine kinase that phosphorylates acyclovir to acyclovir monophosphate.[9] Acyclovir is phosphorylated much more rapidly and effectively by viral thymidine kinase than by cellular enzymes, resulting in a 40-fold to 100-fold increase in acyclovir monophosphate in infected cells. Subsequent phosphorylation by cellular enzymes causes production of acyclovir triphosphate, a potent and selective inhibitor of herpesvirus DNA polymerase.[10-12] Acyclovir triphosphate may also inhibit DNA synthesis by serving as a substrate for this enzyme, causing early chain termination of viral DNA.[13]

Acyclovir is approximately 160 times more active than vidarabine against herpes simplex Type 1.[12] Herpes simplex Type 2 and varicella zoster are also quite sensitive to acyclovir. Epstein–Barr virus is less sensitive but can be inhibited by achievable serum levels (6 to 7 μM), despite the absence of a virus-coded thymidine kinase. Epstein–Barr-virus DNA polymerase appears to be 100 times more sensitive to the inhibitory effects of acyclovir triphosphate than is cellular polymerase alpha.[14] Most clinical isolates of cytomegalovirus are resistant.[15]

Herpes simplex virus may become resistant to the antiviral effects of acyclovir by several mechanisms. Most commonly, viral mutants develop that fail to induce appreciable levels of thymidine kinase.[16,17] Thymidine kinase–deficient mutants have been isolated from patients receiving acyclovir.[18-20] Although these mutants may be less pathogenic in animals,[20,21] it is premature to conclude that development of such resistance will not cause clinical problems. Thymidine kinase may also be generated with diminished affinity for acyclovir,[22] or a DNA polymerase may be produced that is less sensitive to the effects of acyclovir triphosphate.[16,17,23] These latter forms of resistant mutants may be more pathogenic,[23] but they have not yet been observed clinically.

After intravenous administration of 0.5 to 15.0 mg of acyclovir per kilogram, the serum half-life is two to four hours. Peak plasma levels after an intravenous dose of 5 mg per kilogram are 30 to 40 μM, whereas after oral administration of 200 mg, peak levels of 1.4 to 4.0 μM (mean, 2.5 μM) are reached after one to two hours.[24-26] The drug is widely distributed, and cerebrospinal-fluid levels are approximately half of plasma levels.[25] Acyclovir is largely excreted by the kidney, primarily by glomerular filtration and partly by tubular secretion.[24] Dose reductions and interval prolongations are suggested in patients with renal insufficiency. Hemodialysis removes about 60 per cent of acyclovir.[27]

To date, the toxicity of acyclovir has been minimal. Local irritation has been noted during intravenous administration if extravasation occurs, since the pH of diluted drug is 10 to 11. Reversible elevations of serum creatinine have occasionally developed, usually after rapid bolus injections.[28] At therapeutic concentrations, no effects on the immune system or hematopoietic precursor cells are observed,[29-31] and studies of teratogenicity and mutagenicity in animals have been largely negative.

Other Antivirals

A variety of other agents have received attention as potential anti-herpes agents. Only those currently licensed or of possible clinical use will be covered here.

Interferons

These broad-spectrum antiviral proteins have recently been extensively reviewed.[32-34] Three major types are currently recognized, of which interferon alpha has received the greatest attention. Interferons act indirectly to induce other antiviral enzymes and to modulate host immune responses.

Interferon alpha is cleared from the circulation after intravenous administration, with a half-life of two to three hours; after intramuscular injection, the half-life is four to six hours.[35-36] It does not penetrate well into the cerebrospinal fluid and is not removed by hemodialysis.[37] Toxic effects have included fever, local pain, anorexia, fatigue, confusion, malaise, alopecia, and hematologic toxicity.[38,39] The hematologic toxicity (lymphocytopenia, granulocytopenia, and thrombocytopenia) is dose dependent and readily reversible.

Recently, human interferon genes have been cloned into bacterial and yeast clones, allowing the production of large quantities of relatively pure interferon preparations. The pharmacology and toxicity of these clones appear similar to those of the native interferons from which they are derived.[40,41]

Phosphonoformate

Phosphonoformate has been extensively studied in Sweden and to a lesser extent elsewhere.[42,43] It inhibits herpes simplex virus DNA polymerase more efficiently than cell alpha or beta DNA polymerase, and is being studied in clinical trials as a topical treatment for cutaneous herpes infections in Europe.[43]

Bromovinyldeoxyuridine

Bromovinyldeoxyuridine — E-5-(2-bromovinyl)-2'-deoxyuridine (BVDU) — is active against herpes simplex Type 1 and varicella zoster virus, but it is less active against herpes simplex Type 2 in vitro than acyclovir.[44,45] It is phosphorylated to the 5'-monophosphate by a virus-coded thymidine kinase in a fashion similar to the phosphorylation of acyclovir. The monophosphate (BVDU-MP) is subsequently converted to diphosphates and triphosphates intracellularly. The triphosphate derivative (BVDU-TP) competes with deoxythymidine triphosphate for viral DNA polymerase more effectively than with cellular DNA polymerases.[46] The greater sensitivity of herpes simplex Type 1 to bromovinyldeoxyuridine appears to result from the greater affinity of herpes simplex Type 1 thymidine kinase than that of Type 2. Several in vitro and animal studies have suggested that bromovinyldeoxyuridine is an effective antiviral agent.[47] Trials in patients are under way in Europe,[48] and tolerance trials have begun in the United States.

Fluoroiodoaracytosine

Fluoroiodoaracytosine (2'-fluoro-5-iodo-aracytosine, FIAC) is a nucleoside antiviral agent with potent antiviral properties in vitro, particularly against herpes simplex Type 1 but also against cytomegalovirus.[49,50] This agent is phosphorylated preferentially by herpes simplex–induced thymidine kinase in a fashion similar to phosphorylation of acyclovir and bromovinyldeoxyuridine, and thymidine kinase–negative herpes simplex mutants are resistant. Trials of this agent are currently under way in patients.

Trifluorothymidine and Idoxuridine

Ophthalmic preparations of trifluorothymidine and idoxuridine have been licensed for some time and used widely in herpes simplex keratitis. Both agents inhibit herpes DNA synthesis by mechanisms not totally elucidated. Trifluorothymidine (trifluridine, Viroptic) is available as a 1 per cent aqueous solution, and idoxuridine as a 0.5 per cent ointment (Stoxil) or a 0.1 per cent solution (Stoxil, Dendrid, Herplex).

| Varicella Zoster Virus

For most children, varicella is a relatively benign disease. Chickenpox, however, may be associated with serious morbidity or mortality in neonates, immunocompromised patients, or adults.[51-54] After a primary infection, varicella zoster virus resides in dorsal-nerve-root ganglia in latent form. The virus may emerge from this location in later years either spontaneously or in association with immunosuppression, to cause herpes zoster. This condition is associated with considerable acute morbidity and, especially in older patients, may result in prolonged postherpetic neuralgia. In addition, in a minority of immunocompromised patients the virus may disseminate to other areas of the skin or to the viscera, causing the syndrome of disseminated zoster. Although most patients recover from disseminated zoster, the condition is associated with considerable morbidity and often results in prolonged hospitalization.[55]

Varicella zoster virus is susceptible in vitro to a number of antiviral agents, including vidarabine, acyclovir, bromovinyldeoxyuridine, fluoroiodoaracytosine, and several other nucleoside analogues.[56-61]

Varicella

Because of the severity of primary varicella zoster infection in immunocompromised patients, considerable efforts have been expended in the development of a live attenuated-virus vaccine.[62,63] At present the vaccine remains experimental in the United States. Post-exposure prophylaxis with zoster immune plasma or zoster immune globulin in susceptible, high-risk persons ameliorates primary infection.[64-67] Since many exposures are unrecognized, primary infection develops in a relatively large number of high-risk persons who have not received post-exposure prophylaxis.

Both vidarabine and acyclovir have been tested in placebo-controlled trials in the therapy of varicella in immunosuppressed patients.[68,69] Whitley et al. demonstrated that vidarabine (10 mg per kilogram per day for five days) decreased the time of appearance of new cutaneous lesions, the daily mean lesion count, and the mean duration of fever, as compared with placebo. Complications of visceral dissemination were reduced from 55 to 5 per cent by vidarabine therapy. In a smaller study comprising only 20 children with varicella who were receiving immunosuppressive therapy, benefits of intravenous acyclovir in terms of time to healing, time to attainment of culture negativity, or days of fever were not demonstrable. Even in this small study, however, acyclovir exhibited a clearcut benefit in preventing the development of pneumonitis (acyclovir vs. placebo recipients, 0 vs. 45 per cent). The toxicity of the drug was minimal.

The efficacy of interferon alpha in the treatment of varicella in children with cancer has been studied in two prospective randomized placebo-controlled studies.[70,71] In the initial study, involving only 18 subjects, patients received placebo or interferon alpha (Cantell) (4.2×10^4 to 2.5×10^5 U per kilogram daily) until no new cutaneous lesions had appeared for 24 hours. Although no differences could be demonstrated between the two groups in the time to cessation of new cutaneous lesions, interferon recipients were less likely than placebo recipients to have severe complications of varicella (meningoencephalitis, pneumonia, hepatitis, or hemorrhagic complications). In the subsequent study, in which 44 children were enrolled, patients received either placebo or interferon alpha (3.5×10^5 U per kilogram per day for two days, followed by 1.75×10^5 U per kilogram per day for three days). In this larger study, the mean number of days of new lesion formation was shortened by interferon from 5.3 to 3.8 days. In addition, the overall incidence of mortality or life-threatening dissemination was reduced from 29 to 9 per cent by interferon administration. Although the drug was reasonably well tolerated in both studies, the recently demonstrated efficacy of vidarabine and acyclovir suggests that interferons may have a relatively limited use for this indication.

Vidarabine and acyclovir have not yet been compared directly in a randomized trial of therapy for varicella in immunocompromised patients. It is clear that patients are benefited by treatment with either drug. Until trials are completed comparing one or both of these agents with oral drugs, immunocompromised patients with varicella should be hospitalized and treated with either vidarabine or acyclovir.

Herpes Zoster

The Immunologically Normal Host

Herpes zoster occurs in the immunologically normal host with increasing frequency with advancing age.[72] During an acute attack, most patients are troubled by pain at the site of involvement. In most patients this pain resolves with resolution of the cutaneous lesion. In patients 55 to 60 years old or older, the pain may persist as post-herpetic neuralgia for months after the disappearance of cutaneous lesions.[73] Dissemination of the virus to extradermatomal sites is rare in the nonimmunocompromised host. Occasionally patients may have neurologic complications, including encephalitis, meningitis, myelitis, or peripheral motor neuropathies.[74,75] The pathophysiology of these complications is incompletely established, although the virus has been isolated from the spinal cord of one immunologically normal patient with ascending myelitis.

The efficacy of intravenous acyclovir in the treatment of herpes zoster in the immunologically normal host has been investigated in two randomized placebo-controlled studies.[76,77] In the study in which virologic tests were performed, viral shedding ceased in a median of two days after initiation of treatment with acyclovir (1500 mg per square meter of body-surface area per day), as compared with five days after initiation of placebo. In addition, acyclovir accelerated the decrease in erythema, the cessation of new lesion formation, and healing. The median time to reduction of pain was two days in the acyclovir-treated group, as compared with five days in placebo recipients. In the second study, acyclovir (15 mg per kilogram per day) also accelerated healing according to several criteria. It decreased the persistence of pain from a median of 11 days to 4 days. The beneficial effect of acyclovir on pain was most demonstrable in patients over the age of 67 and in those who had been experiencing pain for three or fewer days before initiation of the drug. Neither study demonstrated an effect of acyclovir on the occurrence of post-herpetic neuralgia.

Antiviral therapy of the neurologic complications of herpes zoster has not yet been investigated in great detail. In one patient in whom ascending myelitis began two weeks after acute zoster infection, vidarabine therapy was associated with dramatic neurologic improvement.[78]

At present, antiviral therapy for acute herpes zoster in the immunologically normal host remains a subject of intense investigation. Although resolution of pain is hastened by intravenous acyclovir, this benefit does not appear to offset the inconvenience and expense of hospitalization for parenteral antiviral chemotherapy for the majority of patients. Further investigation may delineate subgroups of patients in whom this is reasonable, but it is likely that widespread application of antiviral chemotherapy in this setting will require demonstration of the efficacy of an effective outpatient regimen. Both oral acyclovir and intramuscular interferon alpha are under study, and investigations with oral bromovinyldeoxyuridine are contemplated.

The Immunocompromised Host

As in the normal host, herpes zoster in the immunocompromised host is predominantly a disease associated with morbidity rather than mortality. Patients may experience pain both acutely and after resolution of the cutaneous lesions. In addition, immunocompromised persons are at a higher risk for the development of disseminated zoster. This complication generally occurs between 2 and 11 days after the onset of dermatomal cutaneous lesions and is believed to represent blood-borne spread of the virus early during the reactivation period. Dissemination may involve only areas of skin remote from the initial dermatomal involvement, or it may involve any one or more of several organs, including the liver, lungs, central nervous system, or gastrointestinal tract. Although disseminated herpes zoster may be fatal, most patients eventually recover without sequelae. Prevention of dissemination has been one of the major goals for antiviral chemotherapy of herpes zoster in the immunocompromised host.

Two double-blind randomized studies comparing vidarabine with placebo in the treatment of immunocompromised patients with acute herpes zoster have been performed by the National Institute of Allergy and Infectious Diseases Collaborative Antiviral Study Group. The initial study was constructed with a crossover design because of ethical concerns about the morbidity and mortality of herpes zoster in the immunocompromised host.[79] In this study, patients were randomized to receive either placebo or vidarabine (10 mg per kilogram per day) for five days. During the second five-day period, they received the alternative study drug. Patients taking vidarabine initially had more rapid cessation of viral shedding and acceleration of healing of cutaneous lesions. Benefits were most apparent in patients with reticuloendothelial cancer who received vidarabine within six days of the initial appearance of cutaneous lesions. Because of the crossover design of the study, conclusions could not be reached about the effect of the drug on dissemination, post-herpetic neuralgia, or other long-term complications.

The low mortality rate in the initial study, coupled with the need to ascertain the effect of vidarabine on the long-term complications of herpes zoster, prompted a follow-up placebo-controlled study employing the same dose of drug for five days without subsequent crossover.[80] Patients were eligible for inclusion in the study only if the initial dermatomal lesions had been present for 72 hours or less. In this study, the local effects of the drug were once again apparent, but in addition, the drug decreased distal cutaneous dissemination from 24 to 8 per cent, and visceral dissemination from 19 to 5 per cent. Local pain resolved relatively rapidly in both drug and placebo groups, but in older patients, resolution of pain was accelerated by vidarabine. Post-herpetic neuralgia occurred in 45 per cent of both vidarabine and placebo recipients, but its duration was significantly shorter among vidarabine recipients.

The efficacy of interferon alpha has been studied in three randomized placebo-controlled studies.[81] In the third study, which used the highest dose of interferon alpha (5.1×10^5 U per kilogram per day), the drug slowed progression of disease in the primary dermatome and eliminated distal cutaneous spread. When the three studies were taken together, interferon could also be demonstrated to decrease the frequency of visceral dissemination and to hasten resolution of pain.

Intravenous acyclovir therapy of herpes zoster in the immunocompromised host has also been studied in both open and controlled studies.[82-84] In a controlled study, 94 patients were randomized to receive either placebo or acyclovir (1500 mg per square meter per day) for seven days.[84] Although efforts were made to enroll patients within three days of the onset of initial cutaneous lesions, patients with older lesions were included if new skin lesions were forming at the time of entry into the study. Acyclovir retarded the spread of cutaneous lesions in patients with either localized or disseminated cutaneous zoster at entry. In addition, the drug significantly reduced the frequency of development of visceral zoster. Effects of the drug on localized healing, pain, and viral shedding were relatively small but generally suggested benefit.

Thus, studies with vidarabine, acyclovir, and interferon alpha have demonstrated efficacy in the therapy of herpes zoster in the immunosuppressed host. Of the three drugs, only vidarabine is currently licensed by the Food and Drug Administration for this indication. No study has directly compared the agents in a controlled fashion in a single group of patients. Several benefits of therapy are apparent, although each of the drugs has some toxicity and all must be given parenterally. The ultimate role of these drugs in the therapy of zoster in the immunocompromised host has not yet been completely elucidated. Although the studies necessary to do this are under way, it would seem prudent to treat the most severely immunocompromised patients with herpes zoster — e.g., those with advanced Hodgkin's disease or lymphoreticular neoplasms — at an early stage of the disease (while lesions are still localized) with either vidarabine or acyclovir. The latter agent should be particularly suited to patients with renal insufficiency or bone-marrow suppression. As in the case of herpes zoster in the normal host, development of effective orally administered drugs that can be used on an outpatient basis will facilitate treatment of a much larger number of patients.

Epstein–Barr Virus

Epstein–Barr virus is the etiologic agent for all cases of heterophil-positive infectious mononucleosis and some cases of heterophil-negative mononucleosis. In addition, the virus has been associated with African Burkitt's lymphoma, nasopharyngeal carcinoma, and lymphoproliferative diseases associated with immunodeficiency disorders or with immunosuppression occurring after allograft transplantation.[85-91] Epstein–Barr virus is sensitive in vitro to several antiviral agents, including interferon alpha,[92-94] vidarabine,[95] and phosphonoacetic acid.[96-100] Although the virus lacks a virus-specified thymidine kinase, it is susceptible to acyclovir because of the exquisite sensitivity of the viral DNA polymerase to the drug.[14,101,102] Acyclovir prevents in vitro production of the virus by producer cell lines but has no effect on latent viral genomes.[103]

Although primary infection with Epstein–Barr virus may be associated with considerable morbidity, most cases are self-limited. Double-blind, placebo-controlled trials of oral acyclovir in Epstein–Barr virus mononucleosis are currently under way. Purtilo and his colleagues have outlined an X-linked syndrome in which an incompletely defined immunologic defect appears to enhance susceptibility to the virus.[87,104] Primary infection may result in death in these patients, due either to uncontrolled lymphoproliferation or to any one of several sequelae of disordered immunoregulation triggered by the primary infection. Two patients with this syndrome have been treated with intravenous acyclovir during primary Epstein–Barr virus infection. The drug had little apparent effect on progression of the disease.[105,106] At post-mortem examination, cells that were positive for Epstein–Barr nuclear antigen were widespread in both patients.

Spontaneous reactivation of Epstein–Barr virus occurs frequently both in normal and immunosuppressed hosts and is generally asymptomatic.[107] In one study that addressed the impact of the virus on renal-allograft recipients, 6 of 41 patients had episodes of fever and leukopenia associated temporally with virus reactivation.[108] In this same study, the effect of interferon alpha (3×10^6 units twice weekly for six weeks after transplantation) on Epstein–Barr virus excretion and serologic reactivity was examined. This regimen decreased the frequency of oropharyngeal excretion of the virus from 65 to 38 per cent of patients, but had no demonstrable effect on the frequency of rises in antibody titer to the virus or on symptoms apparently related to viral reactivation.

The role of Epstein–Barr virus in the pathogenesis of B-cell lymphoproliferative syndromes and lymphomas in the presence of immunosuppression is becoming increasingly apparent.[88-90] This relation has been best established in organ-allograft recipients, but recently a number of Epstein–Barr virus–associated B-cell lymphomas have been noted in patients with the acquired immunodeficiency syndrome.[91,109] It has been hypothesized that impaired cell-mediated immunity in these settings allows an increased opportunity for Epstein–Barr virus–induced polyclonal B-cell proliferation.[89,110,111] In time, a monoclonal B-cell lymphoma may develop. In the past, post-transplantation lymphoma has been treated with withdrawal of immunosuppression or with conventional combination chemotherapy. Neither approach has been particularly successful.

A potential role for antiviral chemotherapy has been suggested by a recently reported case of post-transplantation lymphoma in a 12-year-old boy.[110] In this child, acyclovir therapy had a dramatic effect in twice inducing remission of Epstein–Barr nuclear-antigen–positive polyclonal B-cell lymphoma. Immunosuppressive therapy was continued, and the tumor recurred a third time. On this occasion, the tumor was monoclonal and did not respond to acyclovir therapy. This experience, coupled with the observation that acyclovir is able to inhibit productive but not latent Epstein–Barr virus infection in vitro, has led to speculation that in the early polyclonal phase of the disease, intervention with acyclovir may be useful.

Cytomegalovirus

Cytomegalovirus is a major cause of congenital malformations and an important opportunistic pathogen in immunocompromised hosts.[112] In transplant recipients, it may cause interstitial pneumonitis, fever–leukopenia syndromes, hepatitis, glomerulopathy, retinopathy, and other disorders, and may enhance susceptibility to superinfection with fungi, protozoa, and bacteria.[113,114] It also causes a heterophil-negative mononucleosis syndrome in both immunocompetent and immunosuppressed hosts.[115,116]

No agent has shown clinical usefulness in the therapy of cytomegalovirus infection. Therapeutic trials in ongoing cytomegalovirus pneumonia have been carefully conducted in bone-marrow–transplant recipients in Seattle.[117,118] Treatment with vidarabine, alpha interferon, acyclovir, and combinations of vidarabine and alpha interferon or of acyclovir and alpha interferon have not altered the high mortality rate from this disease. In contrast to these results, Balfour et al. reported a double-blind, placebo-controlled trial of acyclovir in a heterogeneous group of 16 immunocompromised patients with a variety of cytomegalovirus syndromes.[119] Acyclovir-treated patients appeared to improve more rapidly, but larger numbers of patients with more homogeneous disorders will need to be studied before conclusions are drawn. An uncontrolled trial of high-dose vidarabine in patients with cytomegalovirus retinitis also suggested some benefit, with decreases in inflammation and urinary virus excretion; marked hematologic, gastrointestinal, and neurologic toxicity was also observed.[120] Thus, at present, no treatment can be recommended for serious cytomegalovirus syndromes. Several newer nucleoside derivatives — e.g., fluoroiodoaracytosine — show in vitro activity against cytomegalovirus and will require further study.

Use of alpha interferon as prophylaxis against cytomegalovirus syndromes in high-risk patients shows some promise. A double-blind, placebo-controlled trial in 41 renal-transplant recipients showed delayed shedding of cytomegalovirus and decreased viremia in those who received a six-week course of twice-weekly alpha interferon (3×10^6 U per dose).[121]

Another double-blind, placebo-controlled trial of interferon prophylaxis has recently been completed in renal-transplant recipients susceptible to cytomegalovirus reactivation infection. In patients receiving 102×10^6 U of interferon over 14 weeks, cytomegalovirus syndromes and superinfections were reduced.[122] Thus, interferon prophylaxis may be useful in high-risk patients susceptible to reactivation cytomegalovirus syndromes, whereas therapy for ongoing infections appears less promising. In patients susceptible to primary cytomegalovirus infections, other potential methods of prophylaxis — e.g., vaccines and hyperimmune globulin — are also under investigation. Initial results with cytomegalovirus immune globulin or plasma in bone-marrow recipients suggest that some prophylactic effects occur in seronegative patients not given granulocyte transfusions.[123,124]

Herpes Simplex Virus

Neonatal Infections

Herpes simplex virus infection of the newborn can be devastating, particularly when central-nervous-system involvement or other visceral dissemination occurs. The majority of such infections are secondary to herpes simplex Type 2 involvement, often unrecognized, in the mother. A multicenter, double-blind, placebo-controlled trial has demonstrated the efficacy of vidarabine treatment in neonatal herpes.[125] In this study, 56 infected newborns, 27 of whom had disseminated disease, were randomized to receive vidarabine (15 mg per kilogram of body weight per day) or placebo intravenously for 10 days. Vidarabine reduced mortality in infants with central-nervous-system or disseminated disease from 74 to 38 per cent. When these disease categories were separated, vidarabine reduced death rates from disseminated disease from 85 to 57 per cent and deaths from localized central-nervous-system disease from 50 to 10 per cent. Among survivors judged to be normal at one year, those with disseminated disease included 14 per cent of the vidarabine recipients and 8 per cent of the placebo recipients; those with central-nervous-system disease included 50 per cent of the vidarabine recipients and 17 per cent of the placebo recipients. Subsequent studies have suggested that newborns can tolerate higher doses of vidarabine than older patients, and that progression of localized skin involvement to central-nervous-system disease is reduced when doses of 30 mg per kilogram per day are employed (Whitley R: unpublished data).

The usefulness of acyclovir in neonatal herpes simplex virus infections has not been established. Current multicenter collaborative trials are comparing intravenous acyclovir with intravenous vidarabine. Until these studies are completed, vidarabine remains the drug of choice in this disorder.

Encephalitis

Initial double-blind, placebo-controlled, multicenter collaborative trials demonstrated the effectiveness of vidarabine in reducing the mortality from herpes simplex encephalitis.[126] Twenty-eight patients with herpes encephalitis confirmed at brain biopsy received either vidarabine (15 mg per kilogram per day) or placebo for 10 days. Mortality was reduced by vidarabine from 70 to 28 per cent at one month and to 44 per cent at six months, without notable drug toxicity.

Recently, the same multicenter collaborative group reported a follow-up study involving 132 patients considered on clinical grounds to have herpes simplex encephalitis.[127] This diagnosis was confirmed on brain biopsy in 75 patients (57 per cent), and all were treated with vidarabine, with a mortality of 39 per cent.

Analysis of combined data from the two vidarabine studies resulted in several additional observations. Fifty-four per cent (30 of 56) of vidarabine-treated survivors had normal central-nervous-system function at one year; this accounts for 32 per cent of all the vidarabine-treated patients (30 of 93). Age and level of consciousness at entry were important variables in determining outcome; younger patients (under age 30) with higher levels of consciousness did better. Biopsy was associated with a low rate of complications (2 per cent) and a high degree of sensitivity (4 per cent false-negative results). A variety of potentially treatable conditions could mimic the clinical presentation of herpes encephalitis, including cryptococcosis, tuberculosis, and bacterial abscess. These observations, plus the potential fluid-overload problems associated with vidarabine, point out the utility of early brain biopsy in diagnosis, in the absence of safer diagnostic tests.

No controlled trials of acyclovir in herpes encephalitis have been reported. Double-blind studies comparing vidarabine and acyclovir are under way in the United States, and similar trials comparing acyclovir and placebo are in progress in the United Kingdom. Until results from such trials are available, vidarabine remains the drug of choice for treatment of herpes simplex encephalitis.

Mucocutaneous Infection in the Immunosuppressed Host

Acyclovir has been studied extensively for both the prophylaxis and therapy of mucocutaneous herpes simplex virus infections in immunosuppressed hosts. Saral et al. reported a double-blind trial of intravenous prophylactic acyclovir in bone-marrow-transplant recipients seropositive for herpes simplex virus.[128] Patients received acyclovir (250 mg per square meter of body-surface area) or placebo every eight hours for 18 days, starting three days before transplantation. Culture-positive lesions developed in 7 of 10 placebo recipients but in none of 10 acyclovir recipients. Once acyclovir was discontinued, herpes infections developed in seven patients, five of whom were symptomatic, indicating no effect of acyclovir on latent virus.

The only other analogous prophylactic study in immunosuppressed hosts was performed by Cheeseman et al. in renal-transplant recipients given alpha interferon.[121] Patients received either intramuscular interferon (3×10^6 U) or placebo on the day of transplantation and then twice weekly, for a total of 15 doses. No appreciable effects of interferon were demonstrated on virus shedding or lesions.

Thus, acyclovir appears to be the drug of choice for prevention of herpes simplex infections in high-risk immunosuppressed patients when prophylaxis is indicated. Studies of prophylactic oral acyclovir in this setting are currently being conducted. Preliminary studies indicate that oral-acyclovir prophylaxis is also effective in preventing herpes simplex infections in recipients of bone-marrow transplants.[129] The indications for prophylactic acyclovir in the immunosuppressed host are few. The exception may be a patient with frequently recurrent, severe herpes who is undergoing a short but intense period of immunosuppression.[130] More generally useful is therapeutic acyclovir for ongoing herpes infections in the compromised host. A number of studies have addressed the utility of intravenous, topical, and oral acyclovir for the treatment of mucocutaneous herpesvirus infections among immunosuppressed patients.

A randomized double-blind trial of intravenous acyclovir for culture-proved herpes simplex virus infections after marrow transplantation was conducted at the University of Washington.[131] Patients received either intravenous acyclovir (750 mg per square meter per day) or placebo for seven days. Thirteen of 17 patients given acyclovir had therapeutic responses, as compared with 2 of 17 given placebo. Acyclovir-treated patients also had shorter durations of positive cultures and shorter times to resolution of lesions and pain. Again, no effect on latency was observed; 16 of the 17 acyclovir-treated patients had reactivated infection after termination of therapy.

Similar controlled treatment studies have been performed in heart-transplant recipients and other immunosuppressed patients. Some of the accumulated data have been incorporated into an expanded report of double-blind, placebo-controlled trials of intravenous acyclovir in 97 immunocompromised patients with mucocutaneous herpes simplex infection.[132] Acyclovir shortened periods of virus shedding, lesion pain, and times to scabbing and healing. Toxicity was limited to local venous irritation.

Uncontrolled trials of oral acyclovir in immunosuppressed patients with herpes simplex virus infection (200 mg every four hours while the patients were awake) have also been encouraging,[133] and true double-blind studies are currently being performed. Topical five per cent acyclovir ointment in polyethylene glycol has also been evaluated in a double-blind, placebo-controlled trial in 43 immunocompromised patients with progressive mucocutaneous herpes simplex infections.[134] The cessation of virus shedding and pain occurred more rapidly in the acyclovir-treated patients than in their placebo-treated counterparts, although the total time to healing was not different in the two groups.

Intravenous vidarabine has also been the subject of double-blind, placebo-controlled trials in progressive mucocutaneous herpes simplex infections in immunocompromised patients. The data from this trial are currently under analysis, though preliminary examination indicates beneficial effects of vidarabine (Whitley R: unpublished data.) Nevertheless, intravenous acyclovir is the current drug of choice for such patients. Clearly, not every immunosuppressed patient with herpes simplex requires this therapy. Patients will require individualization and those at highest risk whose lesions do not heal promptly without therapy should receive intravenous acyclovir. In time, we will learn whether oral acyclovir is equally beneficial, and by natural-history studies we will be able to determine who requires no treatment, who requires oral acyclovir, and who requires intravenous acyclovir.

Genital Herpes

The clinical importance of genital herpes in the United States has been amply documented, but until recently, no therapeutic or prophylactic agent has withstood careful and critical investigations.[135] A multitude of clinical trials studying various formulations of acyclovir have recently been reported or are in progress. Both topical and intravenous preparations are now licensed for initial episodes of genital herpes, and oral acyclovir looks promising, both in acute treatment and prophylaxis.

Acyclovir as a 5 per cent ointment in a polyethylene glycol base was evaluated in a double-blind, placebo-controlled trial among 77 patients with first episodes of genital herpes and 111 patients with recurrent episodes treated in Seattle or Atlanta.[136] Topical acyclovir or placebo was applied four times a day for seven days. In acyclovir-treated patients with first-episode primary genital herpes, the mean duration of viral shedding was reduced by acyclovir from 7.0 to 4.1 days, and the time to complete crusting from 10.5 to 7.1 days. Acyclovir also reduced viral shedding in men with recurrent herpes, but only by approximately one day. The time to crusting and healing appeared to be reduced in acyclovir-treated men with recurrent infections, though these differences were not statistically significant (P = 0.07 and 0.08, respectively.) Acyclovir did not facilitate healing in women with recurrent infection or delay recurrences in either sex. The Seattle group subsequently presented an expanded report of their own studies, including 111 patients with recurrent infections.[137] In addition to shortened time of virus shedding, slight beneficial effects were seen in pain reduction and healing in men. A second controlled trial in 88 patients with recurrent herpes genitalis demonstrated similar small effects of acyclovir —i.e., shortened virus shedding in men — but no other significant differences between acyclovir and placebo groups.[138] In this study, patients were treated within 48 hours of the onset of lesions, and ointments were administered six times a day.

The beneficial effects observed in first-episode primary genital herpes after topical acyclovir ointment are clear-cut. Although very slight effects may be seen in recurrent disease in men, we believe that use of present formulations of topical acyclovir in recurrent disease is unjustified. It is possible that other topical formulations — e.g., 5 per cent acyclovir in cream base — may be more effective, and that patient-initiated treatment at the time of prodrome or early lesions may yield better results. Nevertheless, at present the risks of enhancing the emergence of resistant organisms, together with the costs involved, do not justify treatment of recurrent genital infection.

Intravenous acyclovir exerts more dramatic effects on initial genital herpes than does the topical form. Thirty patients with a first attack severe enough to warrant hospital admission were studied at London's Middlesex Hospital in a randomized, double-blind, placebo-controlled trial.[139] Twenty had true primary infections. Patients received acyclovir (5 mg per kilogram) or placebo every eight hours, for 15 doses. Acyclovir shortened median healing times (from 15 to 9 days), duration of new lesion formation (2 to 0 days), vesicle persistence (5 to 2.5 days), duration of symptoms (8.8 to 6.3 days), and times of virus shedding (8.8 to 2 days.)

Oral acyclovir is under investigation in the treatment of both primary and recurrent genital herpes. Nilsen et al. conducted a double-blind, placebo-controlled trial in 31 patients with initial cases of genital herpes and 85 patients with recurrent disease.[140] Patients received oral acyclovir (200 mg) or placebo five times a day for five days. Among patients with initial episodes, none of the acyclovir recipients had new lesion formation, whereas 43 per cent of placebo recipients had new lesions. Times to crusting and healing, viral shedding, and duration of pain were also substantially shortened by oral acyclovir. In recurrent disease, acyclovir shortened viral shedding, healing time, and new lesion formation. Although the differences between acyclovir and placebo in median healing time were statistically significant, they were far smaller than those observed in initial episodes of the disease.

Bryson et al. conducted a similar trial of oral acyclovir in initial-episode genital herpes, with treatment continuing for 10 days rather than 5.[141] The periods before virus disappearance, lesion crusting, and lesion healing were shorter in acyclovir recipients than placebo recipients. The severity of clinical symptoms was markedly reduced by oral acyclovir, both in men and women. Subsequent recurrences were unaffected. Similar results have been presented in abstract form by other investigators, indicating that oral acyclovir will be a useful addition to the treatment of primary genital herpes.

Reichman et al. have reported two trials of oral acyclovir in recurrent genital herpes.[142,143] In one, treatment was begun by physicians within 48 hours of the onset of lesions, whereas in the other, therapy was initiated by patients at the onset of lesions. In both studies, the duration of virus shedding and times to crusting and healing were shortened in acyclovir recipients. Patient-initiated therapy resulted in the most rapid healing and cessation of viral shedding.

The question of long-term prophylaxis of frequently recurrent genital herpes by oral acyclovir has recently also been addressed.[143a] Thirty-five patients received oral acyclovir or placebo for 125 days. Significantly fewer recurrences were observed in acyclovir than in placebo recipients. Prolonged prophylaxis was well tolerated, but all patients had recurrences once acyclovir was discontinued.

It appears clear that when licensed, oral acyclovir will represent a major advance in the management of genital herpes. It will probably become the agent of choice for initial attacks of genital herpes, and it may well be useful when begun early in recurrent disease as well, particularly when patient-initiated therapy is begun at the first signs of recurrence. The use of oral prophylaxis should be limited to the few patients with frequent (e.g., monthly) severe recurrent attacks. Prophylactic courses of oral acyclovir should be relatively brief because of the theoretical possibilities of host-cell DNA damage and emergence of resistant viruses, and because the natural course of recurrent episodes may be to diminish with time.

Until oral acyclovir becomes licensed, acyclovir treatment of only initial-episode genital herpes is recommended. The intravenous route is recommended when hospitalization is required, and the topical preparation when hospitalization is not necessary.

Herpes Labialis (Febrilis)

Studies of orolabial herpes in the immunocompetent host have not yet shown substantial benefit from any treatment program. There is no currently available effective therapy for herpes fever blisters or cold sores. Neither vidarabine mono-phosphate cream nor acyclovir ointment has been found to be clinically effec-tive.[144-146] A double-blind, placebo-controlled trial of topical 5 per cent acyclovir in polyethylene glycol was carried out in 208 patients with recurrent herpes labialis.[145] Although virus titers were reduced in the group receiving acyclovir early (within eight hours after onset of lesions) four times a day, no clinical benefits were observed. In a subsequent study, 10 per cent acyclovir in polyethyl-ene glycol was begun in the prodromal or early erythema stages, and doses were applied every two hours.[147] No beneficial effects were observed. The effects of topical acyclovir cream and oral acyclovir are under study in cases of herpes labialis.

Interferon alpha has been evaluated as a prophylactic agent in herpes sim-plex—seropositive patients at high risk for reactivation after trigeminal-ganglion surgery.[147,148] In a double-blind study, patients were given placebo or 7×10^4 U of alpha interferon per kilogram for five days, beginning the day before sur-gery. Both herpes simplex shedding and herpes labialis were reduced in inter-feron recipients, but latent virus was not eliminated. Several trials of recombinant interferons in various forms of herpes infection are under way. Trials of other agents, including phosphonoformate and bromovinyldeoxyuridine, are also in progress.

Herpes Keratitis

The treatment of ocular herpesvirus infections is complex and has been reviewed in detail elsewhere.[149,150] A number of well-controlled trials have been conduct-ed, and three topical agents are now licensed for use in this country: idoxuridine, vidarabine, and trifluorothymidine. Because of better solubility, less viral resist-ance, less toxicity, and greater therapeutic efficacy, trifluorothymidine and vidar-abine are favored by many clinicians for the initial management of epithelial herpes infections of the eye.

| Summary

Guidelines for the prophylaxis or therapy of herpesvirus infections are shown in Table 1. Progress is so rapid in this area that frequent revisions of such guidelines will be necessary. Newer drugs or new formulations of older agents are constantly being developed. Combination therapies — e.g., interferon plus acyclovir — appear promising in laboratory models of herpesvirus infections[151,152] and will undoubtedly receive clinical investigation in the years ahead. The problem of dealing with latent virus infections still eludes us, and major breakthroughs will be necessary before we can discuss cure of recurrent infections. Nevertheless, important strides have been made in the past few years, and further progress is predictable in the years ahead.

TABLE 1.   Guidelines for the Management of Herpesvirus Infections.

Herpes Simplex

Encephalitis
Recommended — Vidarabine (intravenous), 15 mg/kg/day for
   10 days
Investigational — Acyclovir (intravenous)

Neonatal
Recommended — Vidarabine (intravenous), 30 mg/kg/day for
   10 days
Investigational — Acyclovir (intravenous)

Progressive mucocutaneous
Recommended — Acyclovir (intravenous), 15 mg/kg/day for 7 days
Alternative — Vidarabine (intravenous), 10 mg/kg/day for 10 days
Investigational — Acyclovir (oral)

Genital (primary)

   Severe
   Recommended — Acyclovir (intravenous), 15 mg/kg/day for
      5 days
   Investigational alternative — Acyclovir (oral)

   Moderate
   Recommended — Acyclovir (topical), 5% ointment for 7 days
   Investigational alternative — Acyclovir (oral)

Genital (recurrent)
Recommended — None
Investigational — Acyclovir (oral), interferons, phosphonoformate

Labial (primary or recurrent)
Recommended — None
Investigational — Acyclovir (oral or topical), phosphonoformate,
   bromovinyldeoxyuridine, fluoroiodoaracytosine, interferons

Prophylaxis, high-risk groups
Recommended in individualized situations — Acyclovir (intravenous or oral)
   (investigational)
Investigational — Interferon alpha

Keratitis
Recommended — Trifluorothymidine (topical), 1% for 7 to 21 days, or vidarabine
   (topical), 3% for 7 to 21 days
Alternative — Idoxuridine

TABLE 1. (continued)

Varicella Zoster

Chickenpox, high-risk patients
Prophylaxis
Recommended — Varicella zoster immune globulin (intramuscular), 1 vial per 10 kg
Investigational — Varicella zoster vaccine, transfer factor

Treatment
Recommended — Vidarabine (intravenous), 10 mg/kg/day for 5 days, or acyclovir
(intravenous), 15 mg/kg/day for 7 days
Investigational — Interferon alpha, acyclovir (oral), bromovinyldeoxyuridine

Herpes zoster
Immunocompetent patients
Investigational — Acyclovir (oral or intravenous), interferons

Immunosuppressed patients
Recommended — Vidarabine (intravenous), 10 mg/kg/day for 5 days, or acyclovir
(intravenous), 1500 mg/m^2/day for 7 days
Investigational — Interferons

Cytomegalovirus

Prophylaxis, high-risk patients
Investigational — Interferon alpha, cytomegalovirus immune globulin,
cytomegalovirus vaccine

Treatment
Recommended — None
Investigational — Interferons, fluoroiodoaracytosine

Epstein–Barr Virus

Prophylaxis, high-risk patients
Investigational — Interferons, acyclovir (oral)

Treatment
Investigational — acyclovir (intravenous or oral)

References

1. Hirsch MS, Swartz MN. Antiviral agents. N Engl J Med 1980; 302:903-7, 949-53.
2. Shipman C Jr, Smith SH, Carlson RH, Drach JC. Antiviral activity of arabinosyladenine and arabinosylhypoxanthine in herpes simplex virus-infected KB cells: selective inhibition of viral deoxyribonucleic acid synthesis in synchronized suspension
   cultures. Antimicrob Agents Chemother 1976; 9:120-7.

3. Müller WEG. Mechanisms of action and pharmacology: chemical agents. In: Galasso GJ, Merigan TC, Buchanan RA, eds. Antiviral agents and viral diseases of man. New York: Raven Press 1979:77-149.

4. Whitley R, Alford C, Hess F, Buchanan R. Vidarabine: a preliminary review of its pharmacological properties and therapeutic use. Drugs 1980; 20:267-82.

5. Ross AH, Julia A, Balakrishnan C. Toxicity of adenine arabinoside in humans. J Infect Dis 1976; 133: Suppl:A192-8.

6. Sacks SL, Smith JL, Pollard RB, et al. Toxicity of vidarabine. JAMA 1979; 241:28-9.

7. Friedman HM, Grasela T. Adenine arabinoside and allopurinol — possible adverse drug interaction. N Engl J Med 1981; 304:423.

8. Ramos E, Timmons RF, Schimpff SC. Inappropriate antidiuretic hormone following adenine arabinoside administration. Antimicrob Agents Chemother 1979; 15:142-4.

9. Elion GB. Mechanism of action and selectivity of acyclovir. Am J Med 1982; 73(1A):7-13.

10. St. Clair MH, Furman PA, Lubbers CM, Elion GB. Inhibition of cellular α and virally induced deoxyribonucleic acid polymerases by the triphosphate of acyclovir. Antimicrob Agents Chemother 1980; 18:741-5.

11. Allaudeen HS, Descamps J, Sehgal RK. Mode of action of acyclovir triphosphate on herpesviral and cellular DNA polymerases. Antiviral Res 1982; 2:123-33.

12. Schaeffer HJ. Acyclovir chemistry and spectrum of activity. Am J Med 1982; 73(1A):4-6.

13. McGuirt PV, Furman PA. Acyclovir inhibition of viral DNA chain elongation in herpes simplex virus-infected cells. Am J Med 1982; 73(1A):67-71.

14. Datta AK, Colby BM, Shaw JE, Pagano JS. Acyclovir inhibition of Epstein–Barr virus replication. Proc Natl Acad Sci USA 1980; 77:5163-6.

15. Tyms AS, Scamans EM, Naim HM. The in vitro activity of Acyclovir and related compounds against cytomegalovirus infections. J Antimicrob Chemother 1981; 8:65-72.

16. Coen DM, Schaffer PA. Two distinct loci confer resistance to acycloguanosine in herpes simplex type 1. Proc Natl Acad Sci USA 1980; 77:2265-9.

17. Schnipper LE, Crumpacker CS. Resistance of herpes simplex virus to acycloguanosine: role of viral thymidine kinase and DNA polymerase loci. Proc Natl Acad Sci USA 1980; 77:2270-3.

18. Burns WH, Saral R, Santos GW, et al. Isolation and characterisation of resistant herpes simplex virus after acyclovir therapy. Lancet 1982; 1:421-4.

19. Crumpacker CS, Schnipper LE, Marlowe SI, Kowalsky PN, Hershey BJ, Levin MJ. Resistance to antiviral drugs of herpes simplex virus isolated from a patient treated with acyclovir. N Engl J Med 1982; 306:343-6.

20. Sibrack CD, Gutman LT, Wilfert CM, et al. Pathogenicity of acyclovir-resistant herpes simplex virus type 1 from an immunodeficient child. J Infect Dis 1982; 146:673-82.

21. Field HJ, Darby G. Pathogenicity in mice of strains of herpes simplex virus which are resistant to acyclovir in vitro and in vivo. Antimicrob Agents Chemother 1980; 17:209-16.

22. Darby G, Field HJ, Salisbury SA. Altered substrate specificity of herpes simplex virus thymidine kinase confers acyclovir-resistance. Nature 1981; 289:81-3.

23. Field HJ, Larder BA, Darby G. Isolation and characterization of acyclovir-resistant strains of herpes simplex virus. Am J Med 1982; 73(1A):369-71.

24. Laskin OL, Longstreth JA, Saral R, de Miranda P, Keeney R, Lietman PS. Pharmacokinetics and tolerance of acyclovir, a new anti-herpesvirus agent, in humans. Antimicrob Agents Chemother 1982; 21:393-8.

25. Whitley RJ, Blum MR, Barton N, de Miranda P. Pharmacokinetics of acyclovir in humans following intravenous administration: a model for the development of parenteral antivirals. Am J Med 1982; 73(1A):165-71.

26. Van Dyke RB, Connor JD, Wyborny C, Hintz M, Keeney RE. Pharmacokinetics of orally administered acyclovir in patients with herpes progenitalis. Am J Med 1982; 73(1A):172-5.

27. Laskin OL, Longstreth JA, Whelton A, et al. Acyclovir kinetics in end-stage renal failure. Clin Pharmacol Ther 1982; 31:594-601.

28. Peterslund NA, Black PFT, Tauris P. Impaired renal function after bolus injections of acyclovir. Lancet 1983; 1:243-4.

29. Steele RW, Marmer DJ, Keeney RE. Comparative in vitro immunotoxicology of acyclovir and other antiviral agents. Infect Immun 1980; 28:957-62.

30. McGuffin RW, Shiota FM, Meyers JD. Lack of toxicity of acyclovir to granulocyte progenitor cells in vitro. Antimicrob Agents Chemother 1980; 18:471-3.

31. Parker LM, Lipton JM, Binder N, Crawford EL, Kudisch M, Levin MJ. Effect of acyclovir and interferon on human hematopoietic progenitor cells. Antimicrob Agents Chemother 1981; 21:146-50.

32. Stewart WE II. The interferon system. 2d ed. New York: Springer-Verlag, 1982.

33. Baron S, Dianzani F, Stanton GJ. The interferon system: a review to 1982. Texas Rep Biol Med 1981-82; 41.

34. Ho M. Recent advances in the study of interferon. Pharmacol Rev 1982; 34:119-29.

35. Jordan GW, Fried RP, Merigan TC. Administration of human leukocyte interferon in herpes zoster. I. Safety, circulating antiviral activity, and host responses to infection. J Infect Dis 1974; 130:56-62.

36. Pollard RB, Merigan TC. Experience with clinical applications of interferon and interferon inducers. Pharmacol Ther 1978; 2:783-811.

37. Hirsch MS, Tolkoff-Rubin NE, Kelly AP, Rubin RH. Pharmacokinetics of human and recombinant alpha interferons in patients with chronic renal failure who are undergoing hemodialysis. J Infect Dis 1983; 148:335.

38. Ingimarsson S, Cantell K, Strander H. Side effects of long-term treatment with human leukocyte interferon. J Infect Dis 1979; 140:560-3.

39. Smedley H, Katrak M, Sikora K, Wheeler T. Neurological effects of recombinant human interferon. Br Med J 1983; 286:262-4.

40. Gutterman JU, Fine S, Quesada J, et al. Recombinant leucocyte A interferon: pharmocokinetics, single dose tolerance, and biologic effects in cancer patients. Ann Intern Med 1982; 96:549-56.

41. Horning SJ, Levine JF, Miller RA, Rosenberg SA, Merigan TC. Clinical and immunologic effects of recombinant leukocyte A interferon in eight patients with advanced cancer. JAMA 1982; 247:1718-22.

42. Helgstrand E, Eriksson B, Johansson NG, et al. Trisodium phosphonoformate, a new antiviral compound. Science 1978; 201:819-21.

43. Wallin J, Lernestedt JO, Lycke E. Therapeutic efficacy of trisodium phosphonoformate in treatment of recurrent herpes labialis. In: Nahmias AJ, Dowdle WR,

Schinazi RF, eds. The human herpesviruses: an interdisciplinary perspective. New York: Elsevier Press, 1981:681.

44. De Clercq E, Descamps J, Verhelst G, et al. Comparative efficacy of antiherpes drugs against different strains of herpes simplex virus. J Infect Dis 1980; 141:563-74.

45. De Clercq E. Comparative efficacy of antiherpes drugs in different cell lines. Antimicrob Agents Chemother 1982; 21:661-3.

46. Allaudeen HS, Kozarich JW, Bertino JR, De Clercq E. On the mechanism of selective inhibition of herpesvirus replication by (E)-5-(2-bromovinyl)-2'-deoxyuridine. Proc Natl Acad Sci USA 1981; 78:2698-702.

47. De Clercq E, Zhang Z-X, Sim IS. Treatment of experimental herpes simplex virus encephalitis with (E)-5-(2-bromovinyl)-2'-deoxyuridine in mice. Antimicrob Agents Chemother 1982; 22:421-5.

48. de Clercq E, Degreef H, Wildiers J, et al. Oral (E)-5-(2-bromovinyl)-2'-deoxyuridine in severe herpes zoster. Br Med J 1980; 281:1178.

49. Lopez C, Watanabe KA, Fox JJ. 2'-Fluoro-5-iodo-aracytosine, a potent and selective anti-herpesvirus agent. Antimicrob Agents Chemother 1980; 17:803-6.

50. Fox JJ, Watanabe KA, Lopez C, Philips FS, Leyland-Jones B. Chemistry and potent antiviral activity of 2'-fluoro-5-substituted-arabinosyl-pyrimidine-nucleosides. In: Shiota H, Cheng Y-C, Prusoff WH, eds. Herpesvirus: clinical, pharmacological and basic aspects. Amsterdam: Excerpta Medica, 1982:135-47.

51. Meyers JD. Congenital varicella in term infants: risk considered. J Infect Dis 1974; 129:215-7.

52. Dolin R, Reichman RC, Mazur MH, Whitley RJ. Herpes zoster-varicella infections in immunosuppressed patients. Ann Intern Med 1978; 89:375-88.

53. Triebwasser JH, Harris RE, Bryant RE, Rhoades ER. Varicella pneumonia in adults: report of seven cases and a review of literature. Medicine (Baltimore) 1967; 46:409-23.

54. Mazur M, Dolin R. Herpes zoster at the NIH: a 20 year experience. Am J Med 1978; 65:738-44.

55. Merselis JG Jr, Kaye D, Hook EW. Disseminated herpes zoster: a report of 17 cases. Arch Intern Med 1964; 113:679-86.

56. Gephart JF, Lerner AM. Comparison of the effects of arabinosyladenine, arabinosylhypoxanthine, and arabinosyladenine 5'-monophosphate against herpes simplex virus, varicella-zoster virus and cytomegalovirus with their effects on cellular deoxyribonucleic acid synthesis. Antimicrob Agents Chemother 1981; 19:170-8.

57. Biron KK, Elion GB. In vitro susceptibility of varicella-zoster virus to acyclovir. Antimicrob Agents Chemother 1980; 18:443-7.

58. De Clercq E, Descamps J, Ogata M, Shigeta S. In vitro susceptibility of varicella zoster virus to E-5-(2-bromovinyl)-2'-deoxyuridine and related compounds. Antimicrob Agents Chemother 1982; 21:33-8.

59. Iltis JP, Lin T-S, Prusoff WH, Rapp F. Effect of 5-iodo-5' amino-2'5'-dideoxyuridine on varicella zoster virus in vitro. Antimicrob Agents Chemother 1979; 16:92-7.

60. Shigeta S, Yokota T, Iwabuchi T, et al. Comparative efficacy of antiherpes drugs against various strains of varicella-zoster virus. J Infect Dis 1982; 147:576-84.

61. Machida H, Kuninaka A, Yoshino H. Inhibitory effects of antiherpesviral thymidine analogs against varicella-zoster virus. Antimicrob Agents Chemother 1982; 21:358-61.

62. Takahashi M, Otsuka T, Okuno Y, Asano Y, Yazaki T, Isomura S. Live vaccine used to prevent the spread of varicella in children in hospital. Lancet 1974; 2:1288-90.

63. Asano Y, Nakayama H, Yazaki T, et al. Protection against varicella in family contacts by immediate inoculation with live varicella vaccine. Pediatrics 1977; 59:3-7.

64. Brunell PA, Ross A, Miller LH, Kuo B. Prevention of varicella by zoster immune globulin. N Engl J Med 1969; 280:1191-4.

65. Zaia JA, Levin MJ, Preblud SR, et al. Evaluation of varicella-zoster immune globulin: protection of immunosuppressed children after household exposure to varicella. J Infect Dis 1983; 147:737-43.

66. Balfour HH Jr, Groth KE, McCullough J, et al. Prevention or modification of varicella using zoster immune plasma. Am J Dis Child 1977; 131:693-6.

67. Orenstein WA, Heymann DL, Ellis RJ, et al. Prophylaxis of varicella in high-risk children: dose-response effect of zoster immune globulin. J Pediatr 1981; 98:368-73.

68. Whitley R, Hilty M, Haynes R, et al. Vidarabine therapy of varicella in immunosuppressed patients. J Pediatr 1982; 101:125-31.

69. Prober CG, Kirk LE, Keeney RE. Acyclovir therapy of chickenpox in immunosuppressed children — a collaborative study. J Pediatr 1982; 101:622-5.

70. Arvin AM, Feldman S, Merigan TC. Human leucocyte interferon in the treatment of varicella in children with cancer: a preliminary controlled trial. Antimicrob Agents Chemother 1978; 13:605-7.

71. Arvin AM, Kushner JH, Feldman S, Baehner RL, Hammond D, Merigan TC. Human leukocyte interferon for the treatment of varicella in children with cancer. N Engl J Med 1982; 306:761-5.

72. Hope-Simpson RE. The nature of herpes zoster: a long-term study and a new hypothesis. Proc R Soc Med 1965; 58:9-20.

73. Burgoon CF Jr, Burgoon JS, Baldridge GD. The natural history of herpes zoster. JAMA 1957; 164:265-9.

74. Dolin R, Reichman RC, Mazur MH, Whitley RJ. Herpes zoster-varicella infections in immunosuppressed patients. Ann Intern Med 1978; 89:375-88.

75. Jemsek J, Greenberg SB, Taber L, Harvey D, Gershon A, Couch RB. Herpes zoster-associated encephalitis: clinicopathologic report of 12 cases and review of the literature. Medicine (Baltimore) 1983; 62:81-97.

76. Peterslund NA, Seyer-Hansen K, Ipsen J, Esmann V, Schonheyder H, Juhl H. Acyclovir in herpes zoster. Lancet 1981; 2:827-30.

77. Bean B, Braun C, Balfour HH Jr. Acyclovir therapy for acute herpes zoster. Lancet 1982; 2:118-21.

78. Corston RN, Logsdail S, Godwin-Austen RB. Herpes-zoster myelitis treated successfully with vidarabine. Br Med J 1981; 283:698-9.

79. Whitley RJ, Ch'ien LT, Dolin R, et al. Adenine arabinoside therapy of herpes zoster in the immunosuppressed: NIAID Collaborative Antiviral Study. N Engl J Med 1976; 294:1193-9.

80. Whitley RJ, Soong S-J, Dolin R, et al. Early vidarabine therapy to control the complications of herpes zoster in immunosuppressed patients. N Engl J Med 1982; 307:971-5.

81. Merigan TC, Rand KH, Pollard RB, Abdallah PS, Jordan GW, Fried RP. Human leukocyte interferon for the treatment of herpes zoster in patients with cancer. N Engl J Med 1978; 298:981-7.

82. Spector SA, Hintz M, Wyborny L, Connor JD, Keeney RE, Liao S. Treatment of herpes virus infections in immunocompromised patients with acyclovir by continuous intravenous infusion. Am J Med 1982; 73(1A):275-80.

83. Serota FT, Starr SE, Bryan CK, Kock PA, Plotkin SA, August CS. Acyclovir treatment of herpes zoster infections: use in children undergoing bone marrow transplantation. JAMA 1982; 247:2132-5.

84. Balfour HH Jr, Bean B, Laskin OL, et al. Acyclovir halts progression of herpes zoster in immunocompromised patients. N Engl J Med 1983; 308:1448-53.

85. Henle W, Henle G, Ho H-C, et al. Antibodies of Epstein–Barr virus in nasopharyngeal carcinoma, other head and neck neoplasms, and control groups. JNCI 1970; 44:225-31.

86. Epstein MA, Achong BA, Barr YM. Virus particles in cultured lymphoblasts from Burkitt's lymphoma. Lancet 1964; 1:702-3.

87. Purtilo DT. Pathogenesis and phenotypes of an X-linked recessive lymphoproliferative syndrome. Lancet 1976; 2:882-5.

88. Hanto DW, Frizzera G, Gajl-Peczalska J, et al. The Epstein–Barr virus (EBV) in the pathogenesis of posttransplant lymphoma. Transplant Proc 1981; 13:756-60.

89. Hanto DW, Frizzera G, Purtilo DT, et al. Clinical spectrum of lymphoproliferative disorders in renal transplant recipients and evidence for the role of Epstein–Barr virus. Cancer Res 1981; 41:4253-61.

90. Klein G, Purtilo DT. Summary: symposium on Epstein–Barr virus-induced lymphoproliferative diseases in immunodeficient patients. Cancer Res 1981; 41:4302-4.

91. Ziegler JL, Drew WL, Miner RC, et al. Outbreak of Burkitt's-like lymphoma in homosexual men. Lancet 1982; 2:631-3.

92. Adams A, Strander H, Cantell K. Sensitivity of the Epstein–Barr virus transformed human lymphoid cell lines to interferon. J Gen Virol 1975; 28:207-17.

93. Thorley-Lawson DA. The transformation of adult but not newborn lymphocytes by Epstein Barr virus and phytohemagglutinin is inhibited by interferon: the early suppression by T cells of Epstein Barr infection is mediated by interferon. J Immunol 1981; 126:829-33.

94. Garner JG, Hirsch MS, Schooley RT. IFN-alpha inhibition of B-cell transformation by Epstein-Barr virus. 22nd Interscience Conference on Antimicrobial Agents and Chemotherapy. American Society for Microbiology. Miami Beach, Fla. Oct. 4-6, 1982.

95. Coker-Vann M, Dolin R. Effect of adenine arabinoside on Epstein–Barr virus in vitro. J Infect Dis 1977; 135:447-53.

96. Thorley-Lawson D, Strominger JL. Transformation of human lymphocytes by Epstein–Barr virus is inhibited by phosphonoacetic acid. Nature 1976; 263:332-4.

97. Nyormoi O, Thorley-Lawson DA, Elkington J, Strominger JL. Differential effect of phosphonoacetic acid on the expression of Epstein–Barr viral antigens and virus production. Proc Natl Acad Sci USA 1976; 73: 1745-8.

98. Summers WC, Klein G. Inhibition of Epstein–Barr virus DNA synthesis and late gene expression by phosphonoacetic acid. J Virol 1976; 18:151-5.

99. Rickinson AB, Epstein MA. Sensitivity of the transforming and replicative functions of Epstein–Barr virus to inhibition by phosphonoacetate. J Gen Virol 1978; 40:409-20.

100. Thorley-Lawson DA, Strominger JL. Reversible inhibition by phosphonoacetic acid of human B lymphocyte transformation by Epstein–Barr virus. Virology. 1978; 86:423-31.

101. Colby BM, Shaw JE, Elion GB, Pagano JS. Effect of acyclovir [9-(2-hydroxyethoxy-methyl)guanine] on Epstein–Barr virus DNA replication. J Virol 1980; 34: 560-8.

102. Colby BM, Shaw JE, Datta AK, Pagano JS. Replication of Epstein–Barr virus DNA in lymphoblastoid cells treated for extended periods with acyclovir. Am J Med 1982; 73(1A):77-81.

103. Pagano JS, Datta AK. Perspectives on interactions of acyclovir with Epstein–Barr and other herpes viruses. Am J Med 1982; 73(1A):18-26.

104. Sullivan JL, Byron JS, Brewster FE, Baker SM, Ochs HS. X-linked lymphoprolifera-tive syndrome: natural history of the immunodeficiency. J Clin Invest 1983; 71:1765-78.

105. Sullivan JL, Byron KS, Brewster FE, Sakamoto K, Shaw JE, Pagano JS. Treatment of life-threatening Epstein–Barr virus infections with acyclovir. Am J Med 1982; 73(1A):262-6.

106. Sullivan JL, Baker JN, Byron KS, Brewster FE, Mulder C. Failure of acyclovir to inhibit polyclonal Epstein-Barr virus induced lymphoproliferation. Fed Proc 1983; 42:458.

107. Chang RS, Lewis JP, Abildgaard CF. Prevalence of oropharyngeal excreters of leuko-cyte-transforming agents among a human population. N Engl J Med 1973; 289:1325-9.

108. Chesseman SH, Henle W, Rubin RH, et al. Epstein-Barr virus infection in renal transplant recipients: effects of antithymocyte globulin and interferon. Ann Intern Med 1980; 93:39-42.

109. Diffuse, undifferentiated non-Hodgkins lymphoma among homosexual males — United States. MMWR 1982; 31:277-9.

110. Hanto DW, Frizzera G, Gajl-Peczalska KJ, et al. Epstein–Barr virus-induced B-cell lymphoma after renal transplantation: acyclovir therapy and transition from poly-clonal to monoclonal B-cell proliferation. N Engl J Med 1982; 306:913-8.

111. Frizzera G, Hanto DW, Gajl-Peczalska KJ, et al. Polymorphic diffuse B-cell hyper-plasias and lymphomas in renal transplant recipients. Cancer Res 1981; 41:4262-79.

112. Ho M. Cytomegalovirus: biology and infection. New York: Plenum, 1982.

113. Glenn J. Cytomegalovirus infections following renal transplantation. Rev Infect Dis 1981; 3:1151-78.

114. Schooley RT, Hirsch MS, Colvin RB, et al. Association of herpesgroup virus infec-tions with T-lymphocyte-subset alterations, glomerulopathy, and opportunistic in-fections following renal transplantation. N Engl J Med 1983; 308:307-13.

115. Lang DJ, Hanshaw JB. Cytomegalovirus infection and the postperfusion syndrome: recognition of primary infections in four patients. N Engl J Med 1969; 280:1145-9.

116. Hirsch MS. Herpesgroup virus infections in the compromised host. In: Rubin RH, Young LS, eds. Clinical approach to infection in the immunosuppressed host. New York: Plenum, 1981:389-415.

117. Meyers JD, McGuffin RW, Neiman PE, Singer JW, Thomas ED. Toxicity and efficacy of human leukocyte interferon for treatment of cytomegalovirus pneumonia after marrow transplantation. J Infect Dis 1980; 141:555-62.

118. Meyers JD, McGuffin RW, Bryson YJ, Cantell K, Thomas ED. Treatment of cyto-megalovirus pneumonia after marrow transplant with combined vidarabine and hu-man leukocyte interferon. J Infect Dis 1982; 146:80-4.

119. Balfour HH Jr, Bean B, Mitchell CD, Sachs GW, Boen JR, Edelman CK. Acyclovir in immunocompromised patients with cytomegalovirus disease: a controlled trial at one institution. Am J Med 1982; 73(1A):241-8.

120. Pollard RB, Egbert PR, Gallagher JG, Merigan TC. Cytomegalovirus retinitis in immunosuppressed hosts. I. Natural history and effects of treatment with adenine arabinoside. Ann Intern Med 1980; 93:655-64.

121. Cheeseman SH, Rubin RH, Stewart JA, et al. Controlled clinical trial of prophylactic human-leukocyte interferon in renal transplantation: effects on cytomegalovirus and herpes simplex virus infections. N Engl J Med 1979; 300:1345-9.

122. Hirsch MS, Schooley RT, Cosimi AB, et al. Effects of interferon-alpha on cytomegalovirus reactivation syndromes in renal-transplant recipients. N Engl J Med 1983; 308:1489-93.

123. Winston DJ, Pollard RB, Ho WG, et al. Cytomegalovirus immune plasma in bone marrow transplant recipients. Ann Intern Med 1982; 97:11-8.

124. Meyers JD, Leszczynski J, Zaia JA, et al. Prevention of cytomegalovirus infection by cytomegalovirus immune globulin after marrow transplantation. Ann Intern Med 1983; 98:442-6.

125. Whitley RJ, Nahmias AJ, Soong S-J, et al. Vidarabine therapy of neonatal herpes simplex virus infection. Pediatrics 1980; 66:495-501.

126. Whitley RJ, Soon S, Dolin R, et al. Adenine arabinoside therapy of biopsy-proved herpes simplex encephalitis: National Institute of Allergy and Infectious Diseases Collaborative Antiviral Study. N Engl J Med 1977; 297:289-94.

127. Whitley RJ, Soong S-J, Hirsch MS, et al. Herpes simplex encephalitis: vidarabine therapy and diagnostic problems. N Engl J Med 1981; 304:313-8.

128. Saral R, Burns WH, Laskin OL, Santos GW, Lietman PS. Acyclovir prophylaxis of herpes-simplex-virus infections: a randomized, double-blind controlled trial in bone-marrow-transplant recipients. N Engl J Med 1981; 305:63-7.

129. Wade JC, Newton B, Flournoy H, Meyers JD. Oral acyclovir prophylaxis of herpes simplex virus infections after marrow transplant. Presented at the 22d Interscience Conference on Antimicrobial Agents and Chemotherapy, Miami Beach, Fla., October 4-6, 1982.

130. Burns WH, Saral R. Chemotherapy of herpes simplex virus infections. In: Ennis F, ed. Immune response of humans to viruses: recent developments. New York: Academic Press. (in press).

131. Wade JC, Newton B, McLaren C, Flournoy N, Keeney RE, Meyers JD. Intravenous acyclovir to treat mucocutaneous herpes simplex virus infection after marrow transplantation: a double-blind trial. Ann Intern Med 1982; 96:265-9.

132. Meyers JD, Wade JC, Mitchell CD, et al. Multicenter collaborative trial of intravenous acyclovir for treatment of mucocutaneous herpes simplex virus infection in the immunocompromised host. Am J Med 1982; 73(1A):229-35.

133. Straus SE, Smith HA, Brickman C, de Miranda P, McLaren C, Keeney RE. Acyclovir for chronic mucocutaneous herpes simplex virus infection in immunosuppressed patients. Ann Intern Med 1982; 96:270-7.

134. Whitley R, Barton N, Collins E, Whelchel J, Diethelm AG. Mucocutaneous herpes simplex virus infections in immunocompromised patients: a model for evaluation of topical antiviral agents. Am J Med 1982; 73(1A):236-40.

135. Guinan ME. Therapy for symptomatic genital herpes simplex virus infection: a review. Rev Infect Dis 1982; 4: Suppl:S819-28.

136. Corey L, Nahmias AJ, Guinan ME, Benedetti JK, Critchlow CW, Holmes KK. A trial of topical acyclovir in genital herpes simplex virus infections. N Engl J Med 1982; 306:1313-9.

137. Corey L, Benedetti JK, Critchlow CW, et al. Double-blind controlled trial of topical acyclovir in genital herpes simplex virus infections. Am J Med 1982; 73(1A):326-34.

138. Reichman RC, Badger GJ, Guinan ME, et al. Topically administered acyclovir in the treatment of recurrent herpes simplex genitalis: a controlled trial. J Infect Dis 1983; 147:336-40.

139. Mindel A, Adler MW, Sutherland S, Fiddian AP. Intravenous acyclovir treatment for primary genital herpes. Lancet 1982; 1:697-700.

140. Nilsen AE, Aasen T, Halsos AM, et al. Efficacy of oral acyclovir in the treatment of initial and recurrent genital herpes. Lancet 1982; 2:571-3.

141. Bryson YJ, Dillon M, Lovett M, et al. Treatment of first episodes of genital herpes simplex virus infection with oral acyclovir: a randomized double-blind controlled trial in normal subjects. N Engl J Med 1982; 308:916-21.

142. Reichman RC, Ginsberg M, Barrett-Connor E, et al. Controlled trial of oral acyclovir in the therapy of recurrent herpes simplex genitalis: a preliminary report. Am J Med 1982; 73(1A):338-41.

143. Mertz GJ, Reichman R, Dolin R, et al. Double blind placebo controlled trial of oral acyclovir for first episode genital herpes. Presented at the 22d Interscience Conference on Antimicrobial Agents and Chemotherapy, Miami Beach, Fla., October 4-6, 1982.

143a. Strauss SE, Seidlin M, Takiff HE. Suppression of recurrent genital herpes with oral acyclovir. Clin Res 1983; 31:543A.

144. Spruance SL, Crumpacker CS, Haines H, et al. Ineffectiveness of topical adenine arabinoside 5'-monophosphate in the treatment of recurrent herpes simplex labialis. N Engl J Med 1979; 300:1180-4.

145. Spruance SL, Schnipper LE, Overall JC Jr, et al. Treatment of herpes simplex labialis with topical acyclovir in polyethylene glycol. J Infect Dis 1982; 146:85-90.

146. Spruance SL, Crumpacker CS, Schnipper LE, et al. Topical 10% acyclovir in polyethylene glycol for herpes simplex labialis: results of treatment begun in the prodrome and erythema stages. Presented at the 22d Interscience Conference on Antimicrobial Agents and Chemotherapy. Miami Beach, Fla., October 4-6, 1982.

147. Pazin GJ, Armstrong JA, Lam MT, Tarr GC, Janetta PJ, Ho M. Prevention of reactivated herpes simplex infection by human leukocyte interferon after operation on the trigeminal root. N Engl J Med 1979; 301:225-30.

148. Haverkos HW, Pazin GJ, Armstrong JA, Ho M. Follow-up of interferon treatment of herpes simplex. N Engl J Med 1980; 303:699.

149. Kaufman HE. Local therapy of herpes simplex virus ocular infections. In: Nahmias AJ, Dowdle WR, Shinazi RF, eds. The human herpesviruses: an interdisciplinary perspective. New York: Elsevier Press, 1981:466-77.

150. Pavan-Langston D. Herpetic diseases. In: Smulin G, Thoft R. The cornea: scientific foundations and clinical practice. Boston: Little, Brown, 1982:178-95.

151. Hammer SM, Kaplan JC, Lowe BP, Hirsch MS. Alpha interferon and acyclovir treatment of herpes simplex virus in lymphoid cell cultures. Antimicrob Agents Chemother 1982; 21:634-40.

152. Levin MJ, Leary PL. Inhibition of human herpesviruses by combinations of acyclovir and human leukocyte interferon. Infect Immun 1981; 32: 995-9.

Correspondence

Treatment of Herpesvirus Infections*

To the Editor:

A recent article (Oct. 20 and 27 issues) describes various therapies for managing several herpesvirus infections.† In the discussion of vidarabine, the article states that the use of a more soluble analogue, vidarabine monophosphate, in herpes simplex encephalitis was curtailed because of an apparent lack of efficacy or because of increased toxicity in collaborative trials.

In the final analysis of the vidarabine monophosphate limb of the multi-center clinical study sponsored by the National Institute of Allergy and Infectious Diseases, the following conclusions were reached by the Collaborative Antiviral Study Group and the manufacturer, Warner–Lambert: Patients with herpes simplex encephalitis who received vidarabine monophosphate did not benefit from the treatment but did not have evidence of toxicity. It was considered likely that the inability to benefit from the treatment was directly related to increased risk factors, the age of the patient, and the level of consciousness at the time of initiation of therapy.

Vidarabine monophosphate continues to be used both intramuscularly and topically in studies of other herpesvirus infections, including varicella zoster and genital herpes.

RICHARD J. WHITLEY, M.D.
University of Alabama in Birmingham
School of Medicine
Birmingham, AL 35294

To the Editor:

In their review of the treatment of herpesvirus infections, Drs. Hirsch and Schooley state that the toxicity of acyclovir has been minimal. However, there have been recent reports of neuropsychiatric symptoms associated with acyclovir therapy, including delirium,[1-3] tremors,[1,3,4] and transient hemiparesthesias.[1] In the most recent study, of six patients who had received high doses of acyclovir (mean dosage, >2000 mg per square meter of body-surface area per day), all had diffuse slowing on their electroencephalograms, and five had increased levels of myelin basic protein suggestive of a demyelinating process.[1] However, a cause-and-effect relationship between acyclovir and these symptoms has not been clearly established, and further study is needed. When immunocompromised patients receiving acyclovir begin to have neuropsychiatric symptoms, other causes must also be considered, including high-dose corticosteroids, herpes encephalitis,

*Originally published on March 8, 1984 (310:654-655).

†Hirsch MS, Schooley RT. Treatment of herpesvirus infections. N Engl J Med 1983; 309:963-70, 1034-9.

other central-nervous-system infections, vidarabine,[5] necrotizing leukoencephalopathy,[6] and central-nervous-system neoplasms.

JAMES L. LEVENSON, M.D.
Medical College of Virginia
Richmond, VA 23298-0001

1. Wade JC, Meyers JD. Neurologic symptoms associated with parenteral acyclovir treatment after marrow transplantation. Ann Intern Med 1983; 98:921-5.
2. Saral R, Burns WH, Laskin OL, Santos GW, Lietman PS. Acyclovir prophylaxis of herpes-simplex-virus infections: a randomized, double-blind, controlled trial in bone-marrow-transplant recipients. N Engl J Med 1981; 305:63-7.
3. Meyers JD, Wade JC, Mitchell CD, et al. Multicenter collaborative trial of intravenous acyclovir for treatment of mucocutaneous herpes simplex virus infection in the immunocompromised host. Am J Med 1982; 73: Suppl 1A:229-35.
4. Straus SE, Smith HA, Brickman C, et al. Acyclovir for chronic mucocutaneous herpes simplex virus infection in immunosuppressed patients. Ann Intern Med 1982; 96:270-7.
5. Sacks SL, Smith JL, Pollard RB, et al. Toxicity of vidarabine. JAMA 1979; 241:28-9.
6. Gangji D, Reaman GH, Cohen SR, Bleyer WA, Poplack DG. Leukoencephalopathy and elevated levels of myelin basic protein in the cerebrospinal fluid of patients with acute lymphoblastic leukemia. N Engl J Med 1980; 303:19-21.

To the Editor:

In the review by Hirsch and Schooley the discussion of vidarabine is confusing. The reader is led to believe that the half-life of vidarabine may be three to four hours. In fact, the half-life of this agent cannot be determined accurately because in most cases the drug cannot be detected in plasma at all. Its arabinosyl nucleoside metabolites, most notably arabinosyl hypoxanthine, account for the majority of measurable drug. These metabolites, rather than vidarabine, have an estimated half-time of disappearance of three to four hours,[1] with cerebrospinal-fluid levels of one third to one half those in serum.[2]

Suppression of erythrocyte levels of *S*-adenosylhomocysteine hydrolase activity is seen during and for several weeks after withdrawal of vidarabine therapy.[3] Inactivation of this enzyme may interrupt *S*-adenosylmethionine-dependent methylation pathways, which might help to explain the mechanisms of action and toxicity of this agent. Although mechanisms and toxicity are discussed, the methylation pathways have been entirely ignored in this review.

One further point: The toxicity of vidarabine, although largely reversible,[4] can occasionally progress to long-term sequelae and even death[5,6] — an issue that should not have been forgotten, especially in a review article containing information that a clinician may wish to use at the bedside.

STEPHEN L. SACKS, M.D.
University of British Columbia
Vancouver, BC V6T 1W5, Canada

1. Le Page GA, Khaliq A, Gottlieb JA. Studies of 9-β-D-arabinofuranosyladenine in man. Drug Metab Dispos 1973; 1:756-9.
2. Whitley R, Alford C, Hess F, Buchanan R. Vidarabine: a preliminary review of its pharmacological properties and therapeutic use. Drugs 1980; 20:267-82.
3. Sacks SL, Merigan TC, Kaminska J, Fox IH. Inactivation of S-adenosylhomocysteine hydrolase during adenine arabinoside therapy. J Clin Invest 1982; 69:226-30.
4. Sacks SL, Scullard GH, Pollard RB, Gregory PB, Robinson WS, Merigan TC. Antiviral treatment of chronic hepatitis B virus infection: pharmacokinetics and side effects of interferon and adenine arabinoside alone and in combination. Antimicrob Agents Chemother 1982; 21:93-100.
5. Van Etta L, Brown J, Mastri A, Wilson T. Fatal vidarabine toxicity in a patient with normal renal function. JAMA 1981; 246:1703-5.
6. Marker SC, Howard RJ, Groth KE, Mastri AR, Simmons RL, Balfour HH Jr. A trial of vidarabine for cytomegalovirus infection in renal transplant patients. Arch Intern Med 1980; 140:1441-4.

To the Editor:

I found the recent review on the drug therapy of herpesvirus infections by Hirsch and Schooley to be extremely informative and well written. In Table 1 of the article, the dosage of intravenous acyclovir for treatment of progressive mucocutaneous herpesvirus infections in immunocompromised patients is given as 15 mg per kilogram of body weight daily for seven days. This regimen is approximately 20 per cent lower than the daily dose (750 mg per square meter of body-surface area) that was used in the properly controlled trials showing efficacy and safety.[1-3] Assuming that the normal adult has a surface area of 1.73 m^2 and weighs 70 kg, the correct conversion from square meters to milligrams per kilogram is about 18.5 mg per kilogram daily (6.2 mg per kilogram every eight hours). In these and other trials,[1-6] the toxicity of acyclovir was minimal, and no serious adverse effects attributable to acyclovir were demonstrated at this dose administered as a one-hour infusion. Since it is not known whether the efficacy of intravenous acyclovir at a dosage of 5 mg per kilogram every eight hours is equivalent to its efficacy at a dosage of 250 mg per square meter every eight hours, and since acyclovir can be given with relative safety at the higher dosage, I would like to know why Drs. Hirsch and Schooley, as well as the package insert, recommend a lower dose than that used in the double-blind, placebo-controlled trials.

OSCAR L. LASKIN, M.D.
Cornell University Medical College
New York, NY 10021

1. Meyers JD, Wade JC, Mitchell CD, et al. Multicenter collaborative trial of intravenous acyclovir for treatment of mucocutaneous herpes simplex virus infection in the immunocompromised host. Am J Med 1982; 73: Suppl 1A:229-35.
2. Mitchell CD, Bean B, Gentry SR, Groth KE, Boen JR, Balfour HH Jr. Acyclovir therapy for mucocutaneous herpes simplex infections in immunocompromised patients. Lancet 1981; 1:1389-92.

3. Wade JC, Newton B, McLaren C, Flournoy N, Keeney RE, Meyers JD. Intravenous acyclovir to treat mucocutaneous herpes simplex virus infection after marrow transplantation: a double blind trial. Ann Intern Med 1982; 96:265-9.
4. Keeney RE, Kirk LE, Bridgen D. Acyclovir tolerance in humans. Am J Med 1982; 73: Suppl 1A:176-81.
5. Laskin OL. Clinical pharmacokinetics of acyclovir. Clin Pharmacokinet 1983; 8:187-201.
6. Laskin OL, Saral R, Burns WH, Angulopulos CM, Lietman PS. Acyclovir concentrations and tolerance during repetitive administration for 18 days. Am J Med 1982; 73: Suppl 1A:221-4.

The above letters were referred to the authors of the article in question, who offer the following reply:

To the Editor:

We thank Dr. Whitley for providing an updated analysis of the role of vidarabine monophosphate in herpes encephalitis, and Dr. Levenson for a current summary of acyclovir's possible neurotoxicity. The paper by Wade and Meyers cited by Dr. Levenson was published after submission of our manuscript. We agree that none of the publications demonstrates a causal relationship between acyclovir and the neuropsychiatric findings observed and that further study is needed, particularly in patients not receiving other potentially neurotoxic agents.

We regret that Dr. Sacks has misinterpreted our comments concerning vidarabine. We state that vidarabine is readily deaminated in vivo to arabinosyl hypoxanthine, which has a half-life of three to four hours. Space considerations did not permit us to discuss all the postulated mechanisms of action and toxicity, and thus, we were forced to omit mention of Dr. Sacks' paper on methylation pathways. We agree that vidarabine may have neurotoxicity and that this is usually, but not always, reversible. This point is clearly made in our article, as is the corollary that vidarabine should be used cautiously in patients with preexisting neurologic, hepatic, or renal dysfunction, or in those receiving allopurinol.

Dr. Laskin is correct in his discussion of the differences between the recommended acyclovir dose of 15 mg per kilogram for mucocutaneous herpes and that used in several studies (750 mg per square meter). Other studies using lower intravenous doses or even oral acyclovir have also shown efficacy in progressive herpesvirus infections in immunosuppressed subjects (King D: personal communication). For these reasons, we and the manufacturer are confident that the doses of 15 mg per kilogram and 750 mg per square meter are equally appropriate for this indication.

MARTIN S. HIRSCH, M.D. AND ROBERT T. SCHOOLEY, M.D.
Massachusetts General Hospital
Boston, MA 02114

Current Status of Benzodiazepines
(In Two Parts)

David J. Greenblatt, M.D.,

Richard I. Shader, M.D.,

and Darrell R. Abernathy, M.D., Ph.D.

W HEN the pharmacologic and clinical properties of the benzodiazepine sedative–anxiolytics were last reviewed comprehensively in 1973 and 1974,[1-3] their use in clinical practice was very extensive and increasing.[4-6] It was pointed out that a continuation of the yearly rate of increase would lead to the total tranquilization of America by the turn of the century.[7] During the mid-1970s, however, concern emerged among both prescribers and users of these medications about this continuously increasing use. Articles in scientific publications and the lay press suggested some apparently dramatic consequences and hazards of tranquilizer use.[8-12] Although the validity of most such reports was never confirmed, the overall result was a reversal of the trend, and by the end of the decade benzodiazepine use was decreasing. Meanwhile, the continuing scientific interest in the basic and clinical pharmacologic properties of these drugs has greatly expanded our knowledge about them.

Neuropharmacology of the Benzodiazepines

In 1977, two research groups independently reported the existence of brain fractions having a high and specific affinity for compounds of the benzodiazepine class.[13-15] These sites, termed benzodiazepine receptors, have been found in both animal and human brains. Although benzodiazepine-binding sites are also found in other organs, their density is highest in the central nervous system, particularly in cortical and limbic-forebrain areas. Furthermore, the pharmacologic profile or specificity of the peripheral benzodiazepine-binding sites is different from that of the brain "receptors" and does not correlate with the behavioral properties of these drugs. The binding of benzodiazepines to their brain receptors is of very high

From the Division of Clinical Pharmacology, Departments of Psychiatry and Medicine, Tufts University School of Medicine and New England Medical Center Hospital, Boston.

Supported in part by grants (MH-34223 and AM-MH-32050) from the U.S. Public Health Service and by a Research Fellowship from the Charles A. King Trust of Boston.

Originally published in two parts on August 11, 1983 (309:354-358) and August 18, 1983 (309:410-416).

affinity and is stereospecific and saturable. The affinity of a given benzodiazepine for such receptor sites approximately parallels its pharmacologic potency both in animals and in human beings. Binding of a benzodiazepine to its specific receptor site is postulated to be the initial step in a sequence of events that eventually leads to pharmacodynamic activity. The net effect of the interaction of benzodiazepines with their receptors is to enhance the inhibitory neuronal properties of the neurotransmitter gamma-aminobutyric acid (GABA). Thus, benzodiazepine receptors appear to enhance GABA-mediated chloride conductance allosterically across the neuronal membrane.[16,17]

Since their initial recognition and description, benzodiazepine receptors have been the subject of hundreds of papers in the scientific literature.[16-18] The rapid emergence of new scientific data has emphasized the complexity of this neuropharmacologic phenomenon. The presence of an endogenous receptor suggests that an endogenous neurotransmitter or ligand may exist, but none has yet been conclusively identified. Evidence for multiple benzodiazepine-receptor subtypes has emerged, and specific actions of benzodiazepines may be mediated by different populations of receptors. Certain non-benzodiazepines also bind to the specific receptor site. Some such compounds have at least some of the same pharmacologic properties as benzodiazepines, whereas others have no agonist activity and act as benzodiazepine-receptor antagonists.[19-22] A number of antagonists have been described, and some produce a behavioral syndrome that is consistent with fear or anxiety when they are administered to animals.[22]

Attempts to correlate alterations in pharmacodynamic sensitivity to benzodiazepines — such as may occur in aging human or animal populations[23] or as a consequence of prolonged exposure to benzodiazepines[24,25] — with corresponding changes in the number, density, or affinity of benzodiazepine receptors have so far yielded inconsistent results. Despite this complex and sometimes baffling information, research on benzodiazepine receptors represents a major advance in understanding the mechanism of action of this class of compounds.

Pharmacokinetics of Benzodiazepines

Behavioral and neuroreceptor studies of the benzodiazepines have clearly established large quantitative differences in the potency of the various derivatives, but qualitative differences among them are at best subtle. In experimental models, all currently available benzodiazepines are anxiolytic, sedative–hypnotic, and anticonvulsant, in ascending order of dose and brain concentration. Similarly, it is difficult to find consistent scientific validation of differences among drugs in approved clinical indications, which, for example, suggest that some benzodiazepines are primarily anxiolytic, whereas others are primarily hypnotic (Table 1). This lack of evidence greatly complicates the task for practicing physicians, who must choose from among an increasing number of marketed benzodiazepines, each promoted as having unique clinical properties and for each of which a specifically approved clinical indication may be based on incomplete or selectively

TABLE 1. Characteristics of Benzodiazepines Used in the United States.

Administered Drug (Year Introduced)	Approved Indications	Rate of Appearance after Oral Dose	Active Substances in Blood *	Overall Rate of Elimination
Chlordiazepoxide (1960)	Anxiety Alcohol withdrawal Preoperative sedation	Intermediate	Chlordiazepoxide Desmethylchlordiaze- poxide Demoxepam Desmethyldiazepam	Slow
Diazepam (1961)	Anxiety Alcohol withdrawal Muscle spasm Preoperative sedation Status epilepticus	Rapid	Diazepam Desmethyldiazepam	Slow
Oxazepam (1963)	Anxiety Anxiety–depression Alcohol withdrawal	Intermediate to slow	Oxazepam	Intermediate to rapid
Flurazepam (1970)	Insomnia	Rapid to intermediate	Hydroxyethyl flurazepam [Flurazepam aldehyde] Desalkylflurazepam	Slow
Clorazepate (1972)	Anxiety Seizure disorders Alcohol withdrawal	Rapid	Desmethyldiazepam	Slow

*Brackets indicate compounds of minor quantitative importance.

TABLE 1. (continued)

Administered Drug (Year Introduced)	Approved Indications	Rate of Appearance after Oral Dose	Active Substances in Blood *	Overall Rate of Elimination
Clonazepam (1974)	Seizure disorders	Intermediate	Clonazepam	Intermediate
Lorazepam (1977)	Anxiety Anxiety–depression Preoperative sedation	Intermediate	Lorazepam	Intermediate
Prazepam (1977)	Anxiety	Slow	Desmethyldiazepam	Slow
Temazepam (1981)	Insomnia	Intermediate to slow	Temazepam	Intermediate
Alprazolam (1981)	Anxiety Anxiety–depression	Intermediate	Alprazolam	Intermediate
Halazepam (1981)	Anxiety	Intermediate to slow	[Halazepam] Desmethyldiazepam	Slow
Triazolam (1983)	Insomnia	Intermediate	Triazolam	Rapid

obtained scientific data. Some cost-conscious hospital formulary committees have, not surprisingly, concluded that clinical differences among benzodiazepines are not meaningful and that all needs can be adequately met if one or possibly two benzodiazepines are made available. In some hospitals, only chlordiazepoxide is listed in the formulary, since it can be inexpensively obtained from generic sources.

This approach appears rational at some levels, but it has been resisted by many physicians in both primary care and specialty practices who contend that important differences in clinical action do exist among various benzodiazepines despite their neuropharmacologic similarities.[26] Advances in understanding of the kinetic properties of the benzodiazepines have at least partly corroborated and explained these clinical observations.[27-30]

Determinants of Activity after Single Doses

The time of onset, intensity, and duration of clinical action after single doses of benzodiazepines are of great importance to physicians using the drugs for short-term and intermittent treatment of anxiety, for the therapy of sleep disorders, as anesthetic-induction agents or premedicants before surgical or diagnostic procedures, in the short-term treatment of seizure disorders, and in the treatment of severe agitation or panic.

The capacity of drugs to traverse the blood–brain barrier by means of a passive diffusion process depends in part on their intrinsic lipid solubility at physiologic pH. Increasing lipophilicity is associated with more rapid diffusion across such membranes. Benzodiazepines differ in relative lipid solubility, but all consist of highly lipophilic molecules that rapidly cross the blood–brain barrier and enter brain tissue after single intravenous injections.[31] The onset of clinical sedative–anxiolytic activity of all benzodiazepines injected intravenously is rapid, ranging from a single circulation time (15 to 30 seconds) to no more than a few minutes, depending on the size of the dose, the particular pharmacologic response, and the patient's sensitivity. The onset of action of such relatively less lipophilic benzodiazepines as lorazepam and chlordiazepoxide may be slightly slower than that of the highly lipophilic derivatives such as diazepam, desmethyl-diazepam, and midazolam, but this is not a consistent finding. The duration of action, on the other hand, differs considerably among drugs. The more lipophilic benzodiazepines have a shorter duration of clinical activity after a single intra-venous dose than do the less lipid-soluble derivatives, apparently because increasing lipophilicity increases the extent of drug distribution into peripheral sites, principally adipose tissue. This in turn leads to the rapid egress of the drug out of blood and brain into these inactive storage sites, thereby diminishing or terminating its effects on the central nervous system. For drugs that are less lipophilic, "effective" brain concentrations may persist longer because of reduced peripheral distribution. Thus, the dependence of the duration of activity on drug distribution rather than on the rate of elimination explains the apparent paradox that benzodiazepines with a long half-life of elimination, such as diazepam, may have a shorter duration of action than derivatives with a short half-life, such as lorazepam, when given in single doses.

The onset of action after single oral doses of benzodiazepines is limited by the rate of absorption from the gastrointestinal tract into the circulation rather than by the much more rapid passage from blood into brain. The large differences among benzodiazepines in their rate of gastrointestinal absorption are partly attributable to the characteristics of the pharmaceutical formulation (such as particle size), but they are primarily determined by intrinsic physicochemical properties. Diazepam and desmethyldiazepam (administered as its precursor clorazepate dipotassium) are the two most rapidly absorbed benzodiazepines; they rapidly attain peak concentrations in the blood and have a correspondingly rapid onset of clinical sedative–anxiolytic effects. At the other extreme is another desmethyldiazepam precursor, prazepam; it is slowly transformed into the active substance desmethyldiazepam, which therefore appears in the blood slowly. Other benzodiazepines fall between these extremes (Table 1). Differences in absorption rates have predictable clinical consequences. The pharmacologic effects of diazepam and clorazepate are perceived to be of rapid onset after single oral doses. This property may be desirable for patients who perceive the prompt onset of effects as being therapeutically beneficial, but less desirable in other patients, who experience such onset as an unwelcome feeling of drowsiness, excessive relaxation, or loss of control.

A slowly absorbed drug such as prazepam, on the other hand, reaches the peripheral blood gradually and has a slower onset of clinical action. This may or may not be therapeutically beneficial, depending on the expectations or needs of an individual patient. Thus, differences among benzodiazepines in rates of absorption may greatly influence their clinical profile of efficacy or toxicity when they are administered in a single dose for the treatment of anxiety or insomnia.[32-34]

The slow absorption of intramuscular chlordiazepoxide was first described[35] in 1974 and has been confirmed in several subsequent studies.[36-38] In contrast, the absorption of lorazepam after intramuscular injection is rapid, reliable, and complete.[39,40] Early studies of intramuscular diazepam suggested that the rate and completeness of absorption may be variable and unpredictable,[41,42] but the site of injection is of critical importance.[42] The likelihood of rapid and complete drug absorption is increased when diazepam is injected into the deltoid-muscle area because of the higher blood flow to the deltoid muscles relative to the gluteal or vastus lateralis sites.[43] Although chlordiazepoxide is more hydrophilic at physiologic pH than either diazepam or lorazepam, it is poorly absorbed even after injection into the deltoid muscle. This may be because of the higher absolute concentrations of chlordiazepoxide present in the injection vehicle (50 mg per milliliter) as compared with the concentrations of lorazepam or diazepam (2 and 5 mg per milliliter, respectively), which increases the likelihood of local precipitation.

Drug Effects during Multiple Dosage

Clinical effects of benzodiazepines during and after repeated dosage are partly related to the rate and extent of drug accumulation, which in turn are determined by the elimination half-life and metabolic clearance of the administered
drug or its principal active metabolite or both. When the half-life is long,
accumulation is slow and extensive (Fig. 1). Conversely, drugs with short half-
lives attain the steady state rapidly, and the extent of accumulation is minimal.
Intermediate values can be anticipated for drugs with half-lives that fall between
these two extremes (Table 1). The steady-state condition is reached when the
average rate of drug intake equals its rate of removal by metabolic clearance.
When treatment has been in progress for at least four to five times as long as the
elimination half-life, the accumulation process will be more than 90 per cent
complete.

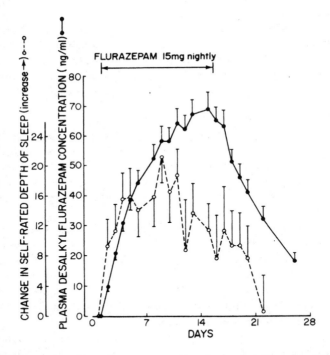

Figure 1. Plasma Desalkylflurazepam Concentrations and Morning Self-Ratings of Depth
(Soundness) of Sleep (Relative to Pre-Drug Base Line) during and after 15 Consecutive Nights of
Flurazepam Administration (15 mg) in a Series of 18 Volunteers.[44]

Each point is the mean (±S.E.) for all subjects at the corresponding time. Plasma concentrations
rose progressively during the course of treatment, but self-ratings of sleep soundness did not increase
in a parallel fashion after the ninth day. After treatment was terminated, self-ratings returned to
base line gradually but more rapidly than the decline in plasma concentrations.

These principles have been repeatedly confirmed in human pharmacokinetic studies of benzodiazepines[27-30] and have led to speculation about the clinical risks and benefits of accumulation versus nonaccumulation of benzodiazepines. Much of this conjecture is incompletely validated, but a number of clinical phenomena are consistent with the pharmacokinetic profile of benzodiazepines during and after repeated doses.

The day-by-day buildup of active substances in the blood and brain as a result of repeated doses of benzodiazepines with long half-lives raises concern that the degree of drowsiness, sedation, memory impairment, and impairment of intellectual and psychomotor performance may increase correspondingly.[45,46] This is clearly relevant to benzodiazepine users who routinely engage in potentially dangerous tasks, such as operating an automobile, or whose occupations demand unimpaired intellectual function. Excessive drug accumulation causing drowsiness, mental confusion, and motor incoordination leading to ataxia and falling is of particular concern with respect to elderly or chronically ill patients, especially those in nursing homes or other institutional settings. These concerns are logical, and some well-controlled studies comparing benzodiazepine hypnotic agents with long versus short half-lives indicate that there is more frequent drowsiness and sedation with the drugs with long half-lives, possibly because of greater drug accumulation.[47-50]

However, most studies of sedation, drowsiness, and impairment of performance among long-term users of benzodiazepines with long half-lives reveal minimal if any detectable impairment and no consistent differences between agents with long versus short half-lives.[51] When they occur, such effects usually develop early in the course of therapy and then increase no further or even wane, despite continued drug use and continued drug accumulation.[44,51-54] Analogous phenomena are observed in experimental models.[55] The divergence between sedative effects and drug concentrations in the plasma or brain during prolonged benzodiazepine exposure is operationally described as "adaptation" or "tolerance" (Fig. 1) and explains why long-term use of benzodiazepines with long half-lives, such as diazepam, clorazepate, or flurazepam, has not produced the epidemic of drug-induced obtundation that one would predict on the basis of plasma concentrations alone.

Since benzodiazepines cure neither anxiety nor insomnia, symptom recurrence can be anticipated after discontinuation of the drug. The rate of drug disappearance from blood and brain and the "uncovering" of the benzodiazepine receptor after termination of long-term treatment will correspond to the drug's elimination half-life, which in turn will influence the time course and intensity of symptom recurrence. The consequences of differences in half-life are most convincingly demonstrated in comparisons of the recurrence of insomnia after discontinuation of hypnotic agents with long versus short half-lives. When treatment with a drug with a short half-life, such as triazolam, is terminated, insomnia recurs rapidly, and in some cases there is a transient period of "rebound" sleep disturbance.[49,56-61] When a drug with a long half-life, such as flurazepam, is discontinued, insomnia recurs gradually over a period of days, with minimal if any withdrawal or rebound phenomenon.[44,62] The time course of disappearance of adverse drug effects will have a similar profile. If long-term therapy has caused sedation or performance impairment, the effect will persist longer after discontinuation of benzodiazepines with long half-lives than after those with short ones.[63]

Clinical Implications of Benzodiazepine Oxidation versus Conjugation

Hepatic biotransformation accounts for essentially all benzodiazepine clearance or elimination by the human organism. The two principal pathways involve either hepatic microsomal oxidation (N-dealkylation or aliphatic hydroxylation) or glucuronide conjugation. These two pathways are differently controlled and differently influenced by factors altering the capacity for drug biotransformation. Oxidation is "susceptible," since it can be impaired by certain population characteristics (such as old age), disease states (such as hepatic cirrhosis), or the coadministration of other drugs that can impair oxidizing capacity (such as cimetidine, estrogens, disulfiram, or isoniazid). Conjugation, on the other hand, is "nonsusceptible," being far less impaired, if at all, by the same factors.[64,65] These well-established pharmacokinetic and metabolic facts have led to the logical hypothesis that conjugated benzodiazepines may be safer and more appropriate than oxidized benzodiazepines for such groups as the elderly, patients with cirrhosis, and persons receiving other drugs that impair oxidation. However, these speculations are incompletely validated in clinical studies. Coadministration of cimetidine to a patient being treated with diazepam will increase steady-state plasma concentrations of diazepam and its major metabolite, desmethyldiazepam, in a manner consistent with the impaired oxidative clearance of these two compounds.[66] This could be clinically important if the increase in blood concentrations were sufficient to cause sedation or to increase anxiolytic effects, but such consequences have not been documented. The therapeutic index of benzodiazepines in general is high, and the increase in blood concentrations may be partly or completely offset by tolerance.[54]

Clinical Use of Benzodiazepines

Anxiety

Since 1977, several new benzodiazepines have been marketed in the United States for the treatment of anxiety syndromes[67-71] (Table 1). These drugs may offer some subtle clinical options. Prazepam, for example, may cause less drowsiness after single doses than do comparable doses of other benzodiazepines because of the slow appearance of desmethyldiazepam in the blood.[72] Some clinical studies suggest a reduced incidence of sedation during treatment with lorazepam and alprazolam — benzodiazepines that have an intermediate half-life — possibly because the extent of drug accumulation is reduced; however, this is not a consistent finding.[69,70] In general, the newer benzodiazepine anxiolytics appear clinically similar or equivalent in both efficacy and toxicity to such standard older ones as diazepam during intermediate-term treatment of ambulatory patients with neurotic anxiety. This interchangeability is partly predictable, since many benzodiazepine derivatives are biotransformed into the same final metabolic product, desmethyldiazepam.[27] Chlordiazepoxide and diazepam both have desmethyldiazepam as a major metabolite; halazepam is rapidly transformed into desmethyldiazepam shortly after reaching the systemic circulation[73]; prazepam and clorazepate are essentially completely transformed into this metabolite even before reaching systemic blood (Table 1). Because of the long elimination half-life of desmethyldiazepam, any benzodiazepine biotransformed into this compound will be an effective anxiolytic with the overall profile of a benzodiazepine with a long half-life.

Controlled clinical trials evaluating new benzodiazepine anxiolytics are generally of four weeks' duration or less, and drug efficacy has been repeatedly and consistently established.[2,74,75] However, many anxious patients who use benzodiazepines take the drugs for periods of months or years. Concern regarding the continued efficacy and possible hazards of benzodiazepines during long-term treatment has led the Food and Drug Administration to mandate caution against anxiolytic treatment of more than four months' duration. Because of the difficult methodologic and logistic problems of long-term studies of anxiolytic drugs, little controlled evidence has been available to support or refute this position. Recent studies are reassuring, however, in that they have demonstrated continued anxiolytic benefit for periods of up to six months, with recurrence of symptoms approximately to the pretreatment base-line level after medications are discontinued.[76] Among long-term users of benzodiazepines, symptom recurrence has been observed in groups in which placebo has been substituted but not in control groups that have continued to take their usual dose of medication.[77]

Further controlled studies of these critical issues are needed, but an individualized common-sense approach can increase the likelihood of benefit and decrease the risks associated with anxiolytic pharmacotherapy.[78,79] Situational anxiety that is not disproportionately intense may improve performance and stimulate adaptive and coping behavior; such anxiety is generally nonpathologic and probably better left untreated. Pathologic anxiety, on the other hand, is maladaptive and impairs rather than improves functioning in occupation and family. Pathologic anxiety typically includes some combination of the following: apprehension (e.g., worrying, rumination), vigilance, hyperresponsiveness and autonomic arousal, and motor tension. When symptoms last more than one month and are not distinguished by a pattern of panic attacks and avoidance behavior on the one hand or of obsessive-compulsive thinking and ritualistic behavior on the other, or both, a diagnosis of generalized anxiety disorder is usually warranted.[80]

Anxiolytic medications are but one option available to patients with maladaptive anxiety. Decisions about which patients are candidates for medication and the role of anxiolytic therapy in the overall treatment plan are matters for individually tailored clinical judgment. When drug therapy is undertaken, it is not necessarily possible to predict how long it will be needed. Physicians should be committed to close monitoring of patients, particularly early in the course of therapy. Periodic attempts to discontinue or withdraw the drug should help establish whether treatment continues to be necessary and, if so, whether it is optimally effective. These are also matters of clinical judgment, since a role for monitoring plasma concentrations of benzodiazepines is not clearly established. For some patients with chronic anxiety, long-term anxiolytic pharmacotherapy will be necessary and appropriate in much the same way that insulin is needed for diabetics, salicylates for patients with rheumatoid arthritis, or diuretics for patients with hypertension. Such chronically anxious patients are seldom physiologically addicted to benzodiazepines, nor should they be considered drug abusers. Although benzodiazepines do not cure their anxiety, the medications can restore some degree of functionality and render life bearable for a person who might otherwise be incapacitated.

Anxiety Associated with Medical Disease

In patients with anxiety associated with gastrointestinal disorders or with cardiovascular disease such as hypertension or arteriosclerotic heart disease, benzodiazepines are effective in alleviating the anxiety component of the disorder but have no effect on the underlying disease process. Many controlled studies have involved lorazepam as the active agent,[69] but other benzodiazepines should be similarly effective. Anxiety associated with medical disease should be clearly distinguished from anxiety-like symptoms caused by such disorders as pheochromocytoma, hypothyroidism, hypoxia, or hypoglycemia. Treatment of the underlying medical cause in such conditions should alleviate the symptoms of anxiety.

Depression and Mixed-Anxiety Depression

Controlled studies of benzodiazepines in the treatment of depressive disorders have yielded conflicting results, which are partly attributable to the nonspecificity of the term "depression," which refers to a heterogeneous group of diseases or syndromes.[81] Highly variable effects of benzodiazepines in depression may reflect inaccuracy of diagnosis or heterogeneity of treatment groups.

True endogenous or autonomous depression (major affective disorder[80]), occurring cyclically and alternating with either periods of normal mood (unipolar depression) or episodes of mania (bipolar depression), clearly responds best to treatment with heterocyclic antidepressants, monoamine oxidase inhibitors, lithium, or electroshock. Many depressed patients also have agitation, anxiety, or sleep-onset insomnia as a component of the disease. Adjunctive therapy with benzodiazepines may alleviate some of these concurrent symptoms but is generally of little benefit for the underlying depressive disorder. Depressive symptoms, as opposed to true depressive disease, may occur in otherwise healthy persons who experience a loss. Depending on the importance of the lost object or person, the resulting reactive or situational depression can vary in severity from simple sadness to true grief and mourning. Such persons may experience anxiety, agitation, or difficulty falling asleep that may be helped by short-term treatment with benzodiazepines; however, benzodiazepines are not a substitute for the time and emotional work needed to adjust to the loss. Finally, many patients who are primarily anxious also have feelings of depression, inadequacy, or demoralization as a part of the anxiety syndrome. The efficacy of benzodiazepines in such neurotic or anxious depressions is determined by the extent to which anxiety as such contributes to overall debility. Preliminary studies with the new triazolobenzo-diazepine, alprazolam, suggest that this drug may provide more specific efficacy in the treatment of endogenous depression than has previously been reported with other benzodiazepine derivatives.[82,83] These observations require further confirmation in controlled studies.

Panic Disorders

Patients suffering from recurrent panic attacks (panic disorder) commonly have secondary anxiety syndromes due to anticipation of these attacks.[84,85] Typical avoidance behavior may also develop when patients avoid situations in which an attack, if it occurred, would be particularly embarrassing or debilitating. Controlled trials generally demonstrate that tricyclic antidepressants and monoamine oxidase inhibitors are effective in reducing the frequency and severity of panic attacks as such.[86,87] Benzodiazepines are useful in alleviating anticipatory anxiety but have no important influence on the underlying panic disorder. Preliminary studies suggest that alprazolam may also have a specific anti-panic effect.[88,89] If this effect is replicated and confirmed in controlled studies, the use of alprazolam would constitute another important therapeutic alternative.

Sleep Disorders

Scientific data on the comparative efficacy and toxicity of benzodiazepine hypnotics after single doses and during repeated use are available from sleep-laboratory studies and from controlled clinical trials. Results from these two research settings are not always consistent with each other; but some generalizations can be made. Benzodiazepine derivatives are of well-established efficacy in the short-term or intermediate-term treatment of insomnia that is unrelated to identifiable medical or psychiatric disease. In a manner analogous to the treatment of anxiety with anxiolytic medications, the use of hypnotic drugs to treat insomnia constitutes but one management option in the overall clinical approach to patients with insomnia. Deciding which patients are candidates for hypnotic medications must be a matter for individualized clinical judgment. Most patients with insomnia do not require long-term treatment, and the hazards of well-monitored therapy of limited duration with hypnotic drugs appear to be small.[90]

Three benzodiazepines are indicated specifically for the treatment of insomnia (Table 1),[91-95] but this by no means precludes the use of other "anxiolytic" benzodiazepines, such as diazepam, lorazepam, or alprazolam, for this indication.[69,96,97] Most patients with insomnia report difficulty falling asleep, and the absorption rate of the benzodiazepine is a critical determinant of its efficacy in sleep-latency insomnia. Of the three available hypnotics, flurazepam (through its active metabolites) is absorbed most rapidly,[98] triazolam has an intermediate rate,[99] and temazepam is slowly absorbed.[100] These rates of absorption approximately parallel the relative clinical efficacy of the drugs in sleep-latency insomnia. The efficacy of a slowly absorbed drug such as temazepam may be improved by administration one to two hours before bedtime rather than just before retiring. Since the absorption of any benzodiazepine may be slowed if it is given with food, hypnotics should be given on an empty stomach, if possible.

Whether residual effects of hypnotics persist into the daytime hours depends partly on how much active substance remains in the blood and brain after drug removal by distribution and clearance has proceeded overnight.[101,102] Drugs that are rapidly eliminated by biotransformation (such as triazolam) and those that are rapidly and extensively distributed to peripheral tissues (such as diazepam) probably have the least likelihood of producing residual sequelae. For any given drug, the probability of daytime effects increases when higher doses are administered.

The consequences of accumulation as compared with nonaccumulation during repeated dosage with hypnotics were discussed above. Accumulation of compounds with long half-lives increases the likelihood of continued efficacy during repeated dosage and minimizes the probability that rebound insomnia will occur upon discontinuation of the drug.[60] The likelihood of daytime drowsiness and impairment of performance is also increased but is partly offset by clinical adaptation or tolerance.[45-49,103] Nonaccumulating hypnotics with short half-lives have a reduced likelihood of adverse daytime sequelae. Although it was previously disputed,[104] evidence from many laboratories now indicates an increased probability of transient rebound insomnia after discontinuation of hypnotics with short half-lives.[48,56-61,105-108]

Musculoskeletal Disorders

Only diazepam is specifically approved for the treatment of muscle spasm or musculoskeletal disorders. It is extensively prescribed for this purpose[109] and is also used to treat spasticity associated with spinal-cord injuries. High doses of diazepam have been reported to be effective against muscle spasm associated with tetanus or the stiff-man syndrome.[110,111]

The extensive clinical use of diazepam in the treatment of musculoskeletal disorders is not well supported by controlled studies that verify its efficacy.

Diazepam is not consistently more effective in the treatment of such common problems as low back pain than are conventional measures, such as analgesics, rest, and local application of heat. Furthermore, it seems unlikely that usual or even high therapeutic doses of diazepam would be sufficient to achieve the very high drug concentrations in brain-stem tissue that are necessary to produce clinically important objective relaxation of peripheral skeletal musculature.[112] The efficacy of diazepam in these disorders probably results from its sedative and anxiolytic effects, since patients with muscle spasm and low back pain commonly experience considerable anxiety or agitation, which may exacerbate pain and spasm. It also seems likely that appropriate doses of any benzodiazepine would have an efficacy similar to that of diazepam in the treatment of musculoskeletal disorders.

Seizure Disorders

Intravenous diazepam remains one of several drugs of choice for the treatment of repetitive grand mal seizures,[113] although in some cases its duration of action is short because of rapid and extensive distribution in peripheral tissues. Recent studies suggest that lorazepam has an efficacy similar to that of diazepam.[114] The onset of activity of lorazepam may be slightly slower than that of diazepam, but lorazepam's action may last considerably longer because the extent of its peripheral distribution is more limited.[31] Lorazepam, therefore, may provide a useful option for the treatment of status epilepticus. Some data suggest a possible adjunctive role for oral benzodiazepine in the long-term prevention of grand mal seizures,[115,116] but benzodiazepines are generally less effective than phenytoin or phenobarbital. The use of clonazepam for certain seizure disorders in childhood has been limited by a relatively high incidence of side effects and by the apparent development of tolerance,[117] but it remains one of several drugs of choice for some types of seizures.

Withdrawal from Alcohol

The reduction of morbidity and mortality associated with the alcohol-withdrawal syndrome by early and aggressive treatment with appropriate sedative–hypnotic agents appears to be reasonably well established. Benzodiazepine derivatives are now used almost exclusively in most medical centers for this indication because of their efficacy as well as their relatively low incidence of cardiovascular and respiratory depression.[118,119] Clinical success appears equally likely with any benzodiazepine derivative, provided the approach to therapy is appropriate. Guidelines for the use of diazepam in this syndrome can now be based on well-controlled objective data.[120] Single 20-mg intravenous or oral doses can be administered on an hourly basis until the desired degree of symptom reduction or sedation is achieved. At that point, no more diazepam is administered, since the slow elimination of diazepam and its metabolite will produce a carry-over effect. Clinically equivalent doses of other benzodiazepines can also be used, although for drugs with a shorter half-life, such as oxazepam or lorazepam, subsequent maintenance doses may be needed after the titration end point is reached, because of the more rapid elimination of the active compounds. In all cases, benzodiazepine therapy constitutes only a component of the overall treatment program, which must also include supportive care and follow-up. [121,122]

Anesthesia and Surgery

Benzodiazepine derivatives continue to be widely used as preoperative medications before surgical or endoscopic procedures and as induction agents before the initiation of inhalational anesthesia. Administration of benzodiazepine premedicants by intramuscular injection is becoming less common, since injections may be painful and do not necessarily lead to more reliable absorption than oral administration. Benzodiazepines administered orally are completely absorbed and produce sedative, anxiolytic, and anterograde amnestic effects that are dose dependent for any given drug. [123] The onset of action depends on the gastrointestinal absorption rate and is most rapid for drugs such as diazepam. The duration of action, on the other hand, is determined by drug distribution and is shortest for such extensively distributed drugs as diazepam, regardless of the route of administration. [31,124,125] Preliminary studies of the sublingual administration of benzodiazepines such as lorazepam indicate that absorption from this site is complete and comparable in rate to that of oral administration. [40]

Benzodiazepines are a logical choice as induction agents before general anesthesia, since they carry a low risk of cardiovascular and respiratory depression as compared with barbiturates. However, the physicochemical properties of induction agents must allow for second-to-second titration of the state of consciousness, which in turn requires sufficient lipid solubility to allow rapid equilibration between blood and brain. All benzodiazepines are lipophilic, but lorazepam is not sufficiently so to allow the needed titration. [126] Diazepam is considerably more lipophilic and is successfully used as an induction agent. The most promising benzodiazepine for this indication is midazolam, which is even more lipid soluble at physiologic pH than diazepam. Midazolam allows titration of consciousness similar to that possible with thiopental but without the concurrent hazards of cardiopulmonary depression. [127,128] Midazolam has been marketed as an induction agent in Europe and is under clinical study in the United States.

Adverse Reactions, Side Effects, and Hazards

Sedation and Impairment of Performance

Excessive depression of the central nervous system is the most common side effect associated with benzodiazepine treatment. Specific manifestations in any given clinical or experimental setting depend on the sensitivity of the individual subject or patient as well as the approach to evaluation or testing. Commonly reported effects include a reduced level of consciousness (drowsiness, excessive somnolence), impairment of intellectual function, reduced motor coordination, and impairment of memory and recall.[50,129,130] When such effects complicate long-term treatment, they usually occur early in the course of therapy and wane over time because of adaptation or tolerance or after a reduction of dosage.[131] The potential hazards of drowsiness or impaired performance for an individual patient should be jointly evaluated by the patient and physician as they assess the risks and benefits of therapy. It is extremely difficult to interpret the clinical importance of studies of benzodiazepine effects on performance in laboratory settings. Many of these studies are of the most rigorous scientific quality, yet all share the limitation that the relation of laboratory to real-life performance can never be determined with certainty.[50,129,130] Even the most seemingly realistic laboratory tasks, such as simulated or controlled driving,[132-136] lack the stimulus to vigilance associated with actual automobile operation and the potentially lethal consequences of error. It is also difficult to interpret epidemiologic studies that document, for example, an increased frequency of automobile accidents among users of benzodiazepines.[137,138] Such studies suggest but certainly do not prove that benzodiazepines cause automobile accidents, since the association of road accidents with drug use could be due to the emotional disorders for which the medications are being taken as much as to the effect of the drugs themselves.[139]

Abuse, Addiction, and Dependence

Sensationalistic and terrifying depictions of benzodiazepine abuse and addiction have been a popular and recurrent subject of reports in the lay media. These reports usually assert or suggest the existence of a national epidemic of tranquilizer addiction, attributable to a pharmaceutical industry that encourages drug use for profit and to a medical profession that overprescribes tranquilizers as a substitute for more appropriate remedies for anxiety and insomnia.[12] Media sources commonly support their position with poorly validated and unreliable data bases, such as the Drug Abuse Warning Network.[140,141] Whenever this problem has been evaluated in systematic scientific studies, the results have not confirmed the implications of journalistic reports.[8,9] Such studies indicate that prescribing and clinical use of benzodiazepines generally reflect the symptoms for which pharmacotherapy is appropriate.[109,142-145] The majority of patients taking benzodiazepines appear to derive clinical benefit from them, even when the drugs are taken for prolonged periods. Evidence of drug abuse or excessive escalation of dosage is generally lacking,[109] and there is no consistent evidence that pharmacotherapy of anxiety impairs patients' incentive to seek more definitive solutions.[146] When drugs are discontinued, most people experience a recurrence or recrudescence of symptoms that are consistent with the original condition for which the drugs were taken.[76,77,147,148]

True physiologic addiction to benzodiazepines may nonetheless occur.[11,149] It is most commonly reported with high dosages but has also been documented with usual therapeutic dosages.[150-160] Since physiologic dependence is more likely to occur with longer drug exposure, minimizing the duration of continuous treatment as described in guidelines for anxiolytic therapy should allow many problems to be avoided. Patients should be counseled that discontinuation of benzodiazepine treatment after long-term use almost certainly will lead to the occurrence of symptoms, but that this does not suggest addiction. Symptoms that recur or recrudesce will qualitatively resemble those of the pretreatment emotional state and will gradually reappear over a period of weeks after discontinuation of therapy. Withdrawal symptoms appear more rapidly, reach a peak, and then wane over time. Symptoms consistent with withdrawal usually have an autonomic character and may include tremulousness, sweating, sensitivity to light and sound, difficulty in sleeping, abdominal discomfort, and systolic hypertension. Serious withdrawal syndromes such as seizures or psychosis, although well documented, are fortunately rare. Symptom recurrence or withdrawal or both appear to have a more rapid onset after discontinuation of benzodiazepines with short as opposed to long half-lives. The impact of drug discontinuation can be logically minimized by tapering rather than abruptly discontinuing treatment; this is particularly important for benzodiazepines with short half-lives. Unpleasant autonomic symptoms can be treated by coadministering a beta-adrenergic blocker such as propranolol.[159,160]

In contrast to patients who use benzodiazepines for appropriate therapeutic indications are substance-abusing populations, which commonly include benzodiazepines among the chemicals they abuse.[161-163] In controlled studies, benzodiazepines have been found to be less strongly reinforcing than barbiturates,[164,165] but the extensive therapeutic use of benzodiazepines has inevitably led to their appearance on the street. Heavy drug users may ingest huge amounts of benzodiazepines; it is not uncommon for them to take several hundred milligrams of diazepam or its equivalent per day.[162,163] Such patients may require detoxification or drug-substitution treatment in much the same way as would persons who abuse or are addicted to opiates or alcohol. The recent discovery of benzodiazepine-receptor antagonists, capable of immediately and transiently reversing the interaction of a benzodiazepine with its receptor, offers a promising approach to understanding the biologic mechanisms and clinical consequences of benzodiazepine addiction.[19,20,166,167]

Interaction with Alcohol

More than 100 scientific papers have appeared on the subject of the pharmacokinetic and clinical consequences of coadministration of benzodiazepines with ethanol.[168] The results of such studies are critically dependent on the particular methodologic design used, and a well-controlled study can be found to support almost any hypothesis. In general, the coadministration of single doses of benzodiazepines with single doses of alcohol causes a small pharmacokinetic interaction if any at all,[169] but it causes greater depression of the central nervous system than either given alone.[168] This is a valid response to the frequent questions of patients about the hazards of combining alcohol and benzodiazepines. Evidence for supra-additive or "knockout drop" effects of alcohol–benzodiazepine coadministration is lacking.

Benzodiazepine Overdosage

Probably the least controversial aspect of the pharmacology of benzodiazepines is their tremendous index of safety. The replacement of barbiturates by benzodiazepines as the primary agents for the treatment of anxiety and insomnia has greatly reduced the morbidity and mortality associated with overdosage of sedative–hypnotic drugs. When taken alone, massive quantities of benzodiazepines can be ingested with little or no hazard of prolonged or serious central-nervous-system depression. This conclusion has been repeatedly confirmed by a number of independent investigations that have included objective validation by measurement of plasma concentrations of the drug.[170-176] Fatal overdosage with a benzodiazepine taken alone is almost unheard of. Not surprisingly, many drug overdosages involve mixtures of benzodiazepines and drugs of other classes. The hazards of such drug mixtures can be considerably greater than those associated with benzodiazepines alone, depending on the coingested drug.

Although therapy of benzodiazepine overdosage beyond the usual supportive measures is usually not necessary, it is of interest that reversal of benzodiazepine-induced depression of the central nervous system by physostigmine has been reported on several occasions.[177] Should specific benzodiazepine antagonists become clinically available, such agents may be of value in the diagnosis and reversal of benzodiazepine intoxication.[178,179]

We are indebted to Marcia Divoll, Jerold S. Harmatz, Hermann R. Ochs, Rainer M. Arendt, Ann Locniskar, and Lawrence J. Moschitto for collaboration and assistance, and to Anthony Kales, Steven M. Paul, Leo E. Hollister, Edward M. Sellers, Markku Linnoila, Karl Rickels, Sidney Wolfe, Thomas R. Browne, and John W. Dundee for kindly providing reference materials, critical comments, and suggestions for the improvement of this manuscript.

| References

1. Garattini S, Mussini E, Randall LO, eds. The benzodiazepines. New York: Raven Press, 1973.
2. Greenblatt DJ, Shader RI. Benzodiazepines in clinical practice. New York: Raven Press, 1974.
3. *Idem.* Benzodiazepines. N Engl J Med 1974; 291:1011-5, 1239-43.
4. Parry HJ, Balter MB, Mellinger GD, Cisin IH, Manheimer DI. National patterns of psychotherapeutic drug use. Arch Gen Psychiatry 1973; 28:769-83.
5. Blackwell B. Psychotropic drugs in use today: the role of diazepam in medical practice. JAMA 1973; 225:1637-41.

6. Rucker TD. Drug use: data, sources, and limitations. JAMA 1974; 230:888-90.
7. Benzodiazepines: use, overuse, misuse, abuse? Lancet 1973; 1:1101-2.
8. Cole JO, Haskell DS, Orzack MH. Problems with the benzodiazepines: an assessment of the available evidence. McLean Hosp J 1981; 6:46-74.
9. Rickels K. Are benzodiazepines overused and abused? Br J Clin Pharmacol 1981; 11: Suppl:71s-83s.
10. Lasagna L. The Halcion story: trial by media. Lancet 1980; 1:815-6.
11. Marks J. The benzodiazepines: use, overuse, misuse, abuse. Lancaster, England: MTP Press, 1978.
12. Bargmann E, Wolfe SM, Levin J, et al. Stopping Valium. Washington, D.C., Public Citizen's Health Research Group, 1982.
13. Squires RF, Braestrup C. Benzodiazepine receptors in rat brain. Nature 1977; 266:732-4.
14. Braestrup C, Albrechtsen R, Squires RF. High densities of benzodiazepine receptors in human cortical areas. Nature 1977; 269:702-4.
15. Möhler H, Okada T. Benzodiazepine receptor: demonstration in the central nervous system. Science 1977; 198:849-51.
16. Tallman JF, Paul SM, Skolnick P, Gallager DW. Receptors for the age of anxiety: pharmacology of the benzodiazepines. Science 1980; 207:274-81.
17. Skolnick P, Paul SM. Benzodiazepine receptors in the central nervous system. Int Rev Neurobiol 1982; 23:103-40.
18. Müller WE. The benzodiazepine receptor: an update. Pharmacology 1981; 22:153-61.
19. Hunkeler W, Möhler H, Pieri L, et al. Selective antagonists of benzodiazepines. Nature 1981; 290:514-6.
20. Lukas SE, Griffiths RR. Precipitated withdrawal by a benzodiazepine receptor antagonist (Ro 15-1788) after 7 days of diazepam. Science 1982; 217:1161-3.
21. Darragh A, Lambe R, Kenny M, Brick I, Taaffe W, O'Boyle C. Ro 15-1788 antagonises the central effects of diazepam in man without altering diazepam bioavailability. Br J Clin Pharmacol 1982; 14:677-82.
22. Ninan PT, Insel TM, Cohen RM, Cook JM, Skolnick P, Paul SM. Benzodiazepine receptor–mediated experimental "anxiety" in primates. Science 1982; 218:1332-4.
23. Tsang CC, Speeg KV Jr, Wilkinson GR. Aging and benzodiazepine binding in the rat cerebral cortex. Life Sci 1982; 30:343-6.
24. Rosenberg HC, Chiu TH. Decreased ^{3}H-diazepam binding is a specific response to chronic benzodiazepine treatment. Life Sci 1979; 24:803-8.
25. Braestrup C, Nielsen M, Squires RF. No changes in rat benzodiazepine receptors after withdrawal from continuous treatment with lorazepam and diazepam. Life Sci 1979; 24:347-50.
26. Baskin I, Esdale A. Is chlordiazepoxide the rational choice among benzodiazepines? Pharmacotherapy 1982; 2:110-9.
27. Greenblatt DJ, Divoll M, Abernethy DR, Ochs HR, Shader RI. Benzodiazepine kinetics: implications for therapeutics and pharmacogeriatrics. Drug Metab Rev 1983; 14:251-92.
28. Klotz U, Kangas L, Kanto J. Clinical pharmacokinetics of benzodiazepines. Prog Pharmacol 1980; 3(3):1-72.

29. Greenblatt DJ, Shader RI, Divoll M, Harmatz JS. Benzodiazepines: a summary of pharmacokinetic properties. Br J Clin Pharmacol 1981; 11: Suppl:11s-6s.

30. Breimer DD, Jochemsen R, von Albert HH. Pharmacokinetics of benzodiazepines: short-acting versus long-acting. Arzneimittelforsch 1980; 30:875-81.

31. Arendt RM, Greenblatt DJ, deJong RH, et al. In vitro correlates of benzodiazepine CSF uptake, pharmacodynamic action, and peripheral distribution. J Pharmacol Exp Ther (in press).

32. Bliding Å. Effects of different rates of absorption of two benzodiazepines on subjective and objective parameters. Eur J Clin Pharmacol 1974; 7:201-11.

33. Greenblatt DJ, Shader RI, Harmatz JS, Franke K, Koch-Weser J. Absorption rate, blood concentrations, and early response to oral chlordiazepoxide. Am J Psychiatry 1977; 134:559-62.

34. Shader RI, Georgotas A, Greenblatt DJ, Harmatz JS, Allen MD. Impaired absorption of desmethyldiazepam from clorazepate by magnesium aluminum hydroxide. Clin Pharmacol Ther 1978; 24:308-15.

35. Greenblatt DJ, Shader RI, Koch-Weser J, Franke J. Slow absorption of intramuscular chlordiazepoxide. N Engl J Med 1974; 291:1116-8.

36. Greenblatt DJ, Shader RI, MacLeod SM, Sellers EM, Franke K, Giles HG. Absorption of oral and intramuscular chlordiazepoxide. Eur J Clin Pharmacol 1978; 13:267-74.

37. Perry PJ, Wilding DC, Fowler RC, Hepler CD, Caputo JF. Absorption of oral and intramuscular chlordiazepoxide by alcoholics. Clin Pharmacol Ther 1978; 23:535-41.

38. Morgan DD, Robinson JD, Mendenhall CL. Clinical pharmacokinetics of chlordiazepoxide in patients with alcoholic hepatitis. Eur J Clin Pharmacol 1981; 19:279-85.

39. Greenblatt DJ, Shader RI, Franke K, et al. Pharmacokinetics and bioavailability of intravenous, intramuscular, and oral lorazepam in humans. J Pharmaceut Sci 1979; 68:57-63.

40. Greenblatt DJ, Divoll M, Harmatz JS, Shader RI. Pharmacokinetic comparison of sublingual lorazepam with intravenous, intramuscular, and oral lorazepam. J Pharmaceut Sci 1982; 71:248-52.

41. Korttila K, Linnoila M. Absorption and sedative effects of diazepam after oral administration and intramuscular administration into vastus lateralis muscle and the deltoid muscle. Br J Anaesth 1975; 47:857-62.

42. Greenblatt DJ, Koch-Weser J. Intramuscular injection of drugs. N Engl J Med 1976; 295:542-6.

43. Divoll M, Greenblatt DJ, Ochs HR, Shader RI. Absolute bioavailability of oral and intramuscular diazepam: effect of age and sex. Anesth Analg (Cleve) 1983; 62: 1-8.

44. Greenblatt DJ, Divoll M, Harmatz JS, MacLaughlin DS, Shader RI. Kinetics and clinical effects of flurazepam in young and elderly noninsomniacs. Clin Pharmacol Ther 1981; 30:475-86.

45. Solomon F, White CC, Parron DL, Mendelson WB. Sleeping pills, insomnia and medical practice. N Engl J Med 1979; 300:803-8.

46. Church MW, Johnson LC. Mood and performance of poor sleepers during repeated use of flurazepam. Psychopharmacology 1979; 61:309-16.

47. Ogura C, Nakazawa K, Majima K, et al. Residual effects of hypnotics: triazolam, flurazepam, and nitrazepam. Psychopharmacology 1980; 68:61-5.

48. Oswald I. The why and how of hypnotic drugs. Br Med J 1979; 1:1167-8.

49. Oswald I, Adam K, Borrow S, Idzikowski C. The effects of two hypnotics on sleep, subjective feelings and skilled performance. In: Passouant P, Oswald I, eds. Pharmacology of the states of alertness. Oxford: Pergamon Press, 1979:51-63.

50. Carskadon MA, Seidel WF, Greenblatt DJ, Dement WC. Daytime carryover of triazolam and flurazepam in elderly insomniacs. Sleep 1982; 5:361-71.

51. Johnson LC, Chernik DA. Sedative-hypnotics and human performance. Psychopharmacology 1982; 76:101-13.

52. Ghoneim MM, Mewaldt SP, Berie JL, Hinrichs JV. Memory and performance effects of single and 3-week administration of diazepam. Psychopharmacology 1981; 73:147-51.

53. Palva ES, Linnoila M, Saario I, Mattila MJ. Acute and subacute effects of diazepam on psychomotor skills: interaction with alcohol. Acta Pharmacol Toxicol (Copenh) 1979; 45:257-64.

54. Ochs HR, Greenblatt DJ, Eckardt B, Harmatz JS, Shader RI. Repeated diazepam dosing in cirrhotic patients: cumulation and sedation. Clin Pharmacol Ther 1983; 33:471-6.

55. Margules DL, Stein L. Increase of "antianxiety" activity and tolerance of behavioral depression during chronic administration of oxazepam. Psychopharmacologia 1968; 13:74-80.

56. Kales A, Soldatos CR, Bixler EO, Kales JD. Rebound insomnia and rebound anxiety: a review. Pharmacology 1983; 26:121-37.

57. Kales A, Scharf MB, Kales JD. Rebound insomnia: a new clinical syndrome. Science 1978; 201:1039-41.

58. Kales A, Scharf MB, Kales JD, Soldatos CR. Rebound insomnia: a potential hazard following withdrawal of certain benzodiazepines. JAMA 1979; 241:1692-5.

59. Vogel GW, Barker K, Gibbons P, Thurmond A. A comparison of the effects of flurazepam 30 mg and triazolam 0.5 mg on the sleep of insomniacs. Psychopharmacology 1976; 47:81-6.

60. Kales A, Bixler EO, Kales JD, Scharf MB. Comparative effectiveness of nine hypnotic drugs: sleep laboratory studies. J Clin Pharmacol 1977; 17:207-13.

61. Monti JM, Debellis J, Gratadoux E, Alterwain P, Altier H, D'Angelo L. Sleep laboratory study of the effects of midazolam in insomniac patients. Eur J Clin Pharmacol 1982; 21:479-84.

62. Kales A, Bixler EO, Soldatos CR, Vela-Bueno A, Jacoby J, Kales JD. Quazepam and flurazepam: long-term use and extended withdrawal. Clin Pharmacol Ther 1982; 32:782-8.

63. Salzman C, Shader RI, Greenblatt DJ, Harmatz JS. Long *v.* short half-life benzodiazepines in the elderly: kinetics and clinical effects of diazepam and oxazepam. Arch Gen Psychiatry 1983; 40:293-7.

64. Greenblatt DJ. Clinical pharmacokinetics of oxazepam and lorazepam. Clin Pharmacokinet 1981; 6:89-105.

65. Greenblatt DJ, Sellers EM, Shader RI. Drug disposition in old age. N Engl J Med 1982; 306:1081-8.

66. Klotz U, Reimann I. Elevation of steady-state diazepam levels by cimetidine. Clin Pharmacol Ther 1981; 30:513-7.

67. Greenblatt DJ, Shader RI. Prazepam and lorazepam, two new benzodiazepines. N Engl J Med 1978; 299:1342-4.

68. Fann WE, Pitts WM, Wheless JC. Pharmacology, efficacy, and adverse effects of halazepam, a new benzodiazepine. Pharmacotherapy 1982; 2:72-8.

69. Ameer B, Greenblatt DJ. Lorazepam: a review of its clinical pharmacological properties and therapeutic uses. Drugs 1981; 21:161-200.

70. Cohn JB. Multicenter double-blind efficacy and safety study comparing alprazolam, diazepam and placebo in clinically anxious patients. J Clin Psychiatry 1981; 42:347-51.

71. Fawcett JA, Kravitz HM. Alprazolam: pharmacokinetics, clinical efficacy, and mechanism of action. Pharmacotherapy 1982; 2:243-53.

72. Allen MD, Greenblatt DJ, Harmatz JS, Shader RI. Desmethyldiazepam kinetics in the elderly after oral prazepam. Clin Pharmacol Ther 1980; 28:196-202.

73. Greenblatt DJ, Locniskar A, Shader RI. Halazepam, another precursor of desmethyldiazepam. Lancet 1982; 1:1358-9.

74. Rickels K. Use of antianxiety agents in anxious outpatients. Psychopharmacology 1978; 58:1-17.

75. Greenblatt DJ, Shader RI. Pharmacotherapy of anxiety with benzodiazepines and β-adrenergic blockers. In: Lipton MA, DiMascio A, Killam KF, eds. Psychopharmacology: a generation of progress. New York: Raven Press, 1978:1381-90.

76. Fabre LF, McLendon DM, Stephens AG. Comparison of the therapeutic effect, tolerance and safety of ketazolam and diazepam administered for six months to outpatients with chronic anxiety neurosis. J Int Med Res 1981; 9:191-8.

77. Bowden CL, Fisher JG. Safety and efficacy of long-term diazepam therapy. South Med J 1980; 73:1581-4.

78. Sellers EM. Clinical pharmacology and therapeutics of benzodiazepines. Can Med Assoc J 1978; 118:1533-8.

79. Rosenbaum JF. The drug treatment of anxiety. N Engl J Med 1982; 306:401-4.

80. Diagnostic and statistical manual of mental disorders. 3d ed. Washington, D.C.: American Psychiatric Association, 1980.

81. Schatzberg AF, Cole JO. Benzodiazepines in depressive disorders. Arch Gen Psychiatry 1978; 35:1359-65.

82. Fabre LF, McLendon DM. A double-blind study comparing the efficacy and safety of alprazolam with imipramine and placebo in primary depression. Curr Ther Res 1980; 27:474-82.

83. Rickels K, Cohen D, Csanalosi I, Harris H, Koepke H, Werblowsky J. Alprazolam and imipramine in depressed outpatients: a controlled study. Curr Ther Res 1982; 32:157-64.

84. Klein DG. Anxiety reconceptualized. In: Klein DF, Rabkin JG, eds. Anxiety: new research and changing concepts. New York: Raven Press, 1981:235-62.

85. Sheehan DV. Panic attacks and phobias. N Engl J Med 1982; 307:156-8.

86. Zitrin CM, Klein DF, Woerner MG. Treatment of agoraphobia with group exposure in vivo and imipramine. Arch Gen Psychiatry 1980; 37:63-72.

87. *Idem.* Behavior therapy, supportive psychotherapy, imipramine, and phobias. Arch Gen Psychiatry 1978; 35:307-16.

88. Shader RI, Goodman M, Gever J. Panic disorders: current perspectives. J Clin Psychopharmacol 1982; 2: Suppl:2S-10S.

89. Chouinard G, Annable L, Fontaine R, Solyom L. Alprazolam in the treatment of generalized anxiety and panic disorders: a double-blind placebo-controlled study. Psychopharmacology 1982; 77:229-33.

90. Clift AD. Factors leading to dependence on hypnotic drugs. Br Med J 1972; 3: 614-7.

91. Greenblatt DJ, Shader RI, Koch-Weser J. Flurazepam hydrochloride. Clin Pharmacol Ther 1975; 17:1-14.

92. Kales A, Bixler EO, Scharf M, Kales JD. Sleep laboratory studies of flurazepam: a model for evaluating hypnotic drugs. Clin Pharmacol Ther 1976; 19:576-83.

93. Pakes GE, Brogden RN, Heel RC, Speight TM, Avery GS. Triazolam: a review of its pharmacological properties and therapeutic efficacy in patients with insomnia. Drugs 1981; 22:81-110.

94. Mitler MM. Evaluation of temazepam as a hypnotic. Pharmacotherapy 1981; 1:3-11.

95. Bixler EO, Kales A, Soldatos CR, Scharf MB, Kales JD. Effectiveness of temazepam with short-, intermediate-, and long-term use: sleep laboratory evaluation. J Clin Pharmacol 1978; 18:110-8.

96. Roth T, Hartse KM, Saab PG, Piccione PM, Kramer M. The effects of flurazepam, lorazepam, and triazolam on sleep and memory. Psychopharmacology 1980; 70:231-7.

97. Bonnet MH, Kramer M, Roth T. A dose response study of the hypnotic effectiveness of alprazolam and diazepam in normal subjects. Psychopharmacology 1981; 75:258-61.

98. Greenblatt DJ, Divoll M, Abernethy DR, Shader RI. Benzodiazepine hypnotics: kinetic and therapeutic options. Sleep 1982; 5: Suppl:S18-S27.

99. Greenblatt DJ, Divoll M, Abernethy DR, Moschitto LJ, Smith RB, Shader RI. Reduced clearance of triazolam in old age: relation to antipyrine oxidizing capacity. Br J Clin Pharmacol 1983; 15:303-9.

100. Divoll M, Greenblatt DJ, Harmatz JS, Shader RI. Effect of age and gender on disposition of temazepam. J Pharm Sci 1981; 70:1104-7.

101. Nicholson AN. The use of short- and long-acting hypnotics in clinical medicine. Br J Clin Pharmacol 1981; 11: Suppl 1:61s-9s.

102. Roth T, Zorick F, Sicklesteel J, Stepanski E. Effects of benzodiazepines on sleep and wakefulness. Br J Clin Pharmacol 1981; 11: Suppl 1:31s-5s.

103. Salkind MR, Silverstone T. A clinical and psychometric evaluation of flurazepam. Br J Clin Pharmacol 1975; 2:223-6.

104. Nicholson AN. Hypnotics: rebound insomnia and residual sequelae. Br J Clin Pharmacol 1980; 9:223-5.

105. Adam K, Adamson L, Březinová V, Hunter WM, Oswald I. Nitrazepam: lastingly effective but trouble on withdrawal. Br Med J 1976; 1:1558-60.

106. Oswald I, French C, Adam K, Gilham J. Benzodiazepine hypnotics remain effective for 24 weeks. Br Med J 1982; 284:860-3.

107. Kales A, Soldatos CR, Bixler EO, Goff PJ, Vela-Bueno A. Midazolam: dose-response studies of effectiveness and rebound insomnia. Pharmacology 1983; 26:138-49.

108. Linnoila M, Viukari M, Lamminsivu U, Auvinen J. Efficacy and side effects of lorazepam, oxazepam, and temazepam as sleeping aids in psychogeriatric inpatients. Int Pharmacopsychiatry 1980; 15:129-35.

109. Hollister LE, Conley FK, Britt RH, Shuer L. Long-term use of diazepam. JAMA 1981; 246:1568-70.

110. Dasta JF, Brier KL, Kidwell GA, Schonfeld SA, Couri D. Diazepam infusion in tetanus: correlation of drug levels with effect. South Med J 1981; 74:278-80.

111. Ochs HR, Greenblatt DJ, Lauven PM, Stoeckel H, Rommelsheim K. Kinetics of high-dose I.V. diazepam. Br J Anaesth 1982; 54:849-52.

112. Lossius R, Dietrichson P, Lunde PKM. Effect of diazepam and desmethyl-diazepam in spasticity and rigidity: a quantitative study of reflexes and plasma concentrations. Acta Neurol Scand 1980; 61:378-83.

113. Browne TR, Penry JK. Benzodiazepines in the treatment of epilepsy: a review. Epilepsia 1973; 14:277-310.

114. Walker JE, Homan RW, Vasko MR, Crawford IL, Bell RD, Tasker WG. Lorazepam in status epilepticus. Ann Neurol 1979; 6:207-13.

115. Wilensky AJ, Ojemann LM, Temkin NR, Troupin AS, Dodrill CB. Clorazepate and phenobarbital as antiepileptic drugs: a double-blind study. Neurology (NY) 1981; 31:1271-6.

116. Troupin AS, Friel P, Wilensky AJ, Moretti-Ojemann L, Levy RH, Feigl P. Evaluation of clorazepate (Tranxene®) as an anticonvulsant — a pilot study. Neurology 1979; 29:458-66.

117. Browne TR. Clonazepam. N Engl J Med 1978; 299:812-6.

118. Thompson WL, Johnson AD, Maddrey WL, et al. Diazepam and paraldehyde for treatment of severe delirium tremens: a controlled trial. Ann Intern Med 1975; 82:175-80.

119. Sellers EM, Kalant H. Alcohol intoxication and withdrawal. N Engl J Med 1976; 294:757-62.

120. Sellers EM, Naranjo CA, Harrison M, Devenyi P, Roach C. Simplifying treatment of alcohol withdrawal: diazepam loading. Clin Pharmacol Ther 1982; 31:268. abstract.

121. Naranjo CA, Chater K, Iversen P, Roach C, Sykora K, Sellers EM. Importance of nonpharmacologic factors in the treatment of acute alcohol withdrawal. Clin Pharmacol Ther 1982; 31:254-5. abstract.

122. Shaw JM, Kolesar GS, Sellers EM, Kaplan HL, Sandor P. Development of optimal treatment tactics for alcohol withdrawal. I. Assessment and effectiveness of supportive care. J Clin Psychopharmacol 1981; 1:382-9.

123. Kanto J. Benzodiazepines as oral premedicants. Br J Anaesth 1981; 53:1179-87.

124. Kothary SP, Brown ACD, Pandit UA, Samra SK, Pandit SK. Time course of antirecall effect of diazepam and lorazepam following oral administration. Anesthesiology 1981; 55:641-4.

125. George KA, Dundee JW. Relative amnesic actions of diazepam, flunitrazepam and lorazepam in man. Br J Clin Pharmacol 1977; 4:45-50.

126. Conner JT, Katz RL, Bellville JW, Graham C, Pagano R, Dorey F. Diazepam and lorazepam for intravenous surgical premedication. J Clin Pharmacol 1978; 18:285-92.

127. Reves JG, Vinik R, Hirschfield AM, Holcomb C, Strong S. Midazolam compared with thiopentone as a hypnotic component in balanced anaesthesia: a randomized, double-blind study. Can Anaesth Soc J 1979; 26:42-9.

128. Sarnquist FH, Mathers WD, Brock-Utne J, Carr B, Canup C, Brown CR. A bioassay of a water-soluble benzodiazepine against sodium thiopental. Anesthesiology 1980; 52:149-53.

129. McNair DM. Antianxiety drugs and human performance. Arch Gen Psychiatry 1973; 29:611-7.
130. Wittenborn JR. Effects of benzodiazepines on psychomotor performance. Br J Clin Pharmacol 1979; 7: Suppl 1:61s-7s.
131. Greenblatt DJ, Allen MD, Shader RI. Toxicity of high-dose flurazepam in the elderly. Clin Pharmacol Ther 1977; 21:355-61.
132. Seppala T, Linnoila M, Mattila MJ. Drugs, alcohol and driving. Drugs 1979; 17:389-408.
133. de Gier 't Hart BJ, Nelemans FA, Bergman H. Psychomotor performance and real driving performance of outpatients receiving diazepam. Psychopharmacology 1981; 73:340-4.
134. Palva ES, Linnoila M, Routledge P, Seppälä T. Actions and interactions of diazepam and alcohol on psychomotor skills in young and middle-aged subjects. Acta Pharmacol Toxicol 1982; 50:363-9.
135. O'Hanlon JF, Haak TW, Blaauw GJ, Riemersma JBJ. Diazepam impairs lateral position control in highway driving. Science 1982; 217:79-82.
136. Betts TA, Birtle J. Effect of two hypnotic drugs on actual driving performance next morning. Br Med J 1982; 285:852.
137. Skegg DCG, Richards SM, Doll R. Minor tranquillisers and road accidents. Br Med J 1979; 1:917-9.
138. Honkanen R, Ertama L, Linnoila M, et al. Role of drugs in traffic accidents. Br Med J 1980; 281:1309-12.
139. Silverstone T. Drugs and driving. Br J Clin Pharmacol 1974; 1:451-4.
140. Ungerleider JT, Lundberg GD, Sunshine I, Walberg CB. The Drug Abuse Warning Network (DAWN) Program: toxicologic verification of 1,008 emergency room 'mentions.' Arch Gen Psychiatry 1980; 37:106-9.
141. Idem. DAWN: Drug Abuse Warning Network or Data About Worthless Numbers? J Anal Toxicol 1980; 4:269-71.
142. Manheimer DI, Davidson ST, Balter MB, Mellinger GD, Cisin IH, Parry HJ. Popular attitudes and beliefs about tranquilizers. Am J Psychiatry 1973; 130:1246-53.
143. Uhlenhuth EH, Balter MB, Lipman RS. Minor tranquilizers: clinical correlates of use in an urban population. Arch Gen Psychiatry 1978; 35:650-5.
144. Mellinger GD, Balter MB, Manheimer DI, Cisin IH, Parry HJ. Psychic distress, life crisis, and use of psychotherapeutic medications: national household survey data. Arch Gen Psychiatry 1978; 35:1045-52.
145. Hesbacher P, Stepansky P, Stepansky W, Rickels K. Psychotropic drug use in family practice. Pharmakopsychiatr Neuropsychopharmakol 1976; 9:50-60.
146. Balmer R, Battegay R, von Marschall R. Long-term treatment with diazepam: investigation of consumption habits and the interaction between psychotherapy and psychopharmacology: a prospective study. Int Pharmacopsychiatry 1981; 16:221-34.
147. Rickels K, Case WG, Diamond L. Relapse after short-term drug therapy in neurotic outpatients. Int Pharmacopsychiatry 1980; 15:186-92.
148. Lapierre YD, Tremblay A, Gagnon A, Monpremier P, Berliss H, Oyewumi LK. A therapeutic and discontinuation study of clobazam and diazepam in anxiety neurosis. J Clin Psychiatry 1982; 43:372-4.
149. Greenblatt DJ, Shader RI. Dependence, tolerance, and addiction to benzodiazepines: clinical and pharmacokinetic considerations. Drug Metab Rev 1978; 8:13-28.

150. Winokur A, Rickels K, Greenblatt DJ, Snyder PJ, Schatz NJ. Withdrawal reaction from long-term, low-dosage administration of diazepam: a double-blind, placebo-controlled case study. Arch Gen Psychiatry 1980; 37:101-5.

151. Hallstrom C, Lader M. Benzodiazepine withdrawal phenomena. Int Pharmacopsychiatry 1981; 16:235-44.

152. Petursson H, Lader MH. Withdrawal from long-term benzodiazepine treatment. Br Med J 1981; 283:643-5.

153. Preskorn SH, Denner LJ. Benzodiazepines and withdrawal psychosis: report of three cases. JAMA 1977; 237:36-8.

154. Fruensgaard K. Withdrawal psychosis: a study of 30 consecutive cases. Acta Psychiatr Scand 1976; 53:105-18.

155. Khan A, Joyce P, Jones AV. Benzodiazepine withdrawal syndromes. NZ Med J 1980; 92:94-6.

156. de la Fuente JR, Rosenbaum AH, Martin HR, Niven RG. Lorazepam-related withdrawal seizures. Mayo Clin Proc 1980; 55:190-2.

157. Pevnick JS, Jasinski DR, Haertzen CA. Abrupt withdrawal from therapeutically administered diazepam: report of a case. Arch Gen Psychiatry 1978; 35:995-8.

158. Mellor CS, Jain VK. Diazepam withdrawal syndrome: its prolonged and changing nature. Can Med Assoc J 1982; 127:1093-6.

159. Tyrer P, Rutherford D, Huggett T. Benzodiazepine withdrawal symptoms and propranolol. Lancet 1981; 1:520-2.

160. Abernethy DR, Greenblatt DJ, Shader RI. Treatment of diazepam withdrawal syndrome with propranolol. Ann Intern Med 1981; 94:354-5.

161. Tennant FS Jr. Outpatient treatment and outcome of prescription drug abuse. Arch Intern Med 1979; 139:154-6.

162. Stitzer ML, Griffiths RR, McLellan AT, Grabowski J, Hawthorne JW. Diazepam use among methadone maintenance patients: patterns and dosages. Drug Alcohol Depend 1981; 8:189-99.

163. Woody GE, O'Brien CP, Greenstein R. Misuse and abuse of diazepam: an increasingly common medical problem. Int J Addict 1975; 10:843-8.

164. Griffiths RR, Bigelow G, Liebson I. Human drug self-administration: double-blind comparison of pentobarbital, diazepam, chlorpromazine and placebo. J Pharmacol Exp Ther 1979; 210:301-10.

165. Griffiths RR, Bigelow GE, Liebson I, Kaliszak JE. Drug preference in humans: double-blind choice comparison of pentobarbital, diazepam and placebo. J Pharmacol Exp Ther 1980; 215:649-61.

166. Cumin R, Bonetti EP, Scherschlicht R, Haefely WE. Use of the specific benzodiazepine antagonist, Ro 15-1788, in studies of physiological dependence on benzodiazepines. Experientia 1982; 38:833-4.

167. McNicholas LF, Martin WR. The effect of a benzodiazepine antagonist, Ro 15-1788, in diazepam dependent rats. Life Sci 1982; 31:731-7.

168. Sellers EM, Busto U. Benzodiazepines and ethanol: assessment of the effects and consequences of psychotropic drug interactions. J Clin Pharmacol 1982; 22:249-62.

169. Sellers EM, Holloway MR. Drug kinetics and alcohol ingestion. Clin Pharmacokinet 1978; 3:440-52.

170. Greenblatt DJ, Allen MD, Noel BJ, Shader RI. Acute overdosage with benzodiazepine derivatives. Clin Pharmacol Ther 1977; 21:497-514.

171. Finkle BS, McCloskey KL, Goodman LS. Diazepam and drug-associated deaths: a survey in the United States and Canada. JAMA 1979; 242:429-34.

172. Jatlow P, Dobular K, Bailey D. Serum diazepam concentrations in overdose: their significance. Am J Clin Pathol 1979; 72:571-7.

173. Busto U, Kaplan HL, Sellers EM. Benzodiazepine-associated emergencies in Toronto. Am J Psychiatry 1980; 137:224-7.

174. Greenblatt DJ, Woo E, Allen MD, Orsulak PJ, Shader RI. Rapid recovery from massive diazepam overdose. JAMA 1978; 240:1872-4.

175. Allen MD, Greenblatt DJ, LaCasse Y, Shader RI. Pharmacokinetic study of lorazepam overdosage. Am J Psychiatry 1980; 137:1414-5.

176. Divoll M, Greenblatt DJ, Lacasse Y, Shader RI. Benzodiazepine over-dosage: plasma concentrations and clinical outcome. Psychopharmacology 1981; 73:381-3.

177. Avant GR, Speeg KV Jr, Freemon FR, Schenker S, Berman ML. Physostigmine reversal of diazepam-induced hypnosis: a study in human volunteers. Ann Intern Med 1979; 91:53-5.

178. Darragh A, Lambe R, Scully M, Brick I, O'Boyle C, Downie WW. Investigation in man of the efficacy of a benzodiazepine antagonist, Ro 15-1788. Lancet 1981; 2:8-10.

179. Mendelson WB, Cain M, Cook JM, Paul SM, Skolnick P. A benzodiazepine receptor antagonist decreases sleep and reverses the hypnotic actions of flurazepam. Science 1983; 219:414-6.

| Correspondence

Benzodiazepines*

To the Editor:

We were surprised to note that paradoxical effects of benzodiazepines are not mentioned by Greenblatt and colleagues (Aug. 11 and 18 issues).[1] These adverse reactions, including hyperactivity and irritability, were first described, for chlordiazepoxide, by Ingram and Timbury.[2] Since then, other paradoxical reactions, such as paradoxical excitement,[3] hostile behavior,[4] verbal and physical aggression,[5] symptoms of delirium,[6] rage reaction,[7] increased anxiety or panic,[8] and increased seizure frequency,[3] have been reported. Several benzodiazepines, including chlordiazepoxide,[2] diazepam,[3,6] clonazepam,[3] triazolam,[5] lorazepam,[6] clorazepate,[7] temazepam,[8] and clobazam[9] have been associated with such reactions.

Unlike common side effects (drowsiness and ataxia), which are related to a more intense expression of the desired pharmacologic effects of benzodiazepines, paradoxical reactions appear to be related to personal or environmental factors.[4] It is extremely difficult to interpret the clinical importance of the paradoxical effects of benzodiazepines, but their incidence seems to be low.

JEAN-LUC FOUILLADIEU, M.D., JEROME D'ENFERT, M.F.,
CHRISTIAN CONSEILLER, M.D.
Hopital Cochin
75014, Paris, France

*Originally published on February 16, 1984 (310:464-466).

1. Greenblatt DJ, Shader RI, Abernethy DR. Drug therapy: current status of benzodiazepines. N Engl J Med 1983; 309:354-58, 410-16.
2. Ingram IM, Timbury GC. Side effects of librium. Lancet 1960; 2:766.
3. Brown TR, Feldman RG. Clinical experience with benzodiazepines in neurological disorders. In: Priest RG, Filho UV, Amrein R, Skreta M, eds. Benzodiazepines today and tomorrow. Lancaster, Pa.: MTP, 1980:113-22.
4. Tranquillizers causing aggression. Br Med J 1975; 1:113-4.
5. van der Kroef C. Reactions to triazolam. Lancet 1979; 2:526.
6. Ong BY, Pickering BG, Palahniuk RJ, Cumming M. Lorazepam and diazepam as adjuncts to epidural anesthesia for caesarean section. Can Anaesth Soc J 1982; 29:31-4.
7. Karch FE. Rage reaction associated with clorazepate dipotassium. Ann Intern Med 1979; 91:61-2.
8. Heel RC, Brogden RN, Speight TM, Avery GS. Temazepam: a review of its pharmacological properties and therapeutic efficacy as an hypnotic. Drugs 1981; 21:321-40.
9. Brogden RN, Heel RC, Speight TM, Avery GS. Clobazam: a review of its pharmacological properties and therapeutic use in anxiety. Drugs 1980; 20:161-78.

To the Editor:

In the excellent review of benzodiazepines by Greenblatt et al., mention is made of the use of diazepam and lorazepam for status epilepticus and of diazepam for possible adjunctive maintenance treatment of generalized tonic-clonic seizures. I believe it should be added, however, that the benzodiazepines are increasingly being employed in the treatment of a variety of seizure disorders. Specifically, diazepam has been advocated as an adjunctive anticonvulsant for absence seizures[1] and is also used routinely for treatment of akinetic and myoclonic seizures.[2,3] Nitrazepam (not yet available in the United States but extensively prescribed in Europe and elsewhere) has also been used as a principal treatment of childhood myoclonic epilepsy, either as the drug of choice[4] or as an alternative treatment when clonazepam, diazepam, or valproic acid cannot be used.[5]

In short, the efficacy of benzodiazepines may be limited in the maintenance pharmacotherapy of generalized tonic-clonic seizures, but as a class of drugs they are of undoubted value in the treatment of certain other seizure types; indeed, Calne[4] has emphasized that the myoclonic and akinetic epilepsies "are commonly refractory to any treatment other than benzodiazepines."[4] It seems that such considerations merit at least some mention.

ROBERT HAUSNER, M.D.
Mount Zion Hospital and Medical Center
San Francisco, CA 94120

1. Penry JK. Medical treatment of convulsive disorders. In: Chase TN, ed. The nervous system. Vol. 2. The clinical neurosciences. New York: Raven Press, 1975:267-75.
2. Wilder BJ, Ramsay RE. Antiepileptic drugs: epilepsy and its treatment. In: Davis FA, ed. Neurological reviews. Minneapolis: American Academy of Neurology, 1976:53-71.

3. Dodson WE. Pharmacology and therapeutics of epilepsy in childhood. In: Klawans HL, ed. Clinical neuropharmacology. Vol. 4. New York: Raven Press, 1979:1-29.
4. Calne DB. Therapeutics in neurology. Oxford: Blackwell, 1975:163-89.
5. Eadie MJ, Tyrer JH. Neurological clinical pharmacology. Sydney: ADIS Press, 1980:163-229.

To the Editor:

Is the reference by Greenblatt et al. to hypothyroidism as a cause of anxiety a semantic error? Do they not mean hyperthyroidism? Hypothyroidism may cause various mental syndromes, including apathy, depression, and psychosis, but because of the reduced autonomic arousal with underactivity of the thyroid gland, anxiety does not occur.

Their view that the alcohol-withdrawal syndrome should be aggressively treated with appropriate sedative-hypnotic agents needs to be tempered with the awareness that benzodiazepines may precipitate irreversible acute hepatic coma in an alcoholic with cirrhosis and impaired liver function.[1] Benzodiazepines share with alcohol a common metabolic pathway of degradation.[2] Hepatic cellular damage by alcohol has been demonstrated to be related to anoxic changes in the liver cell because ethanol is preferentially oxidized, with consequent insufficient oxygen availability for vital hepatic cellular function.[3] In fact, no alcoholic with the withdrawal syndrome should be detoxicated with benzodiazepines until serum ammonia and blood urea nitrogen levels indicate that hepatic urea synthesis is proceeding normally and that the risk of acute hepatic failure through the use of benzodiazepines is unlikely.

THEODORE PEARLMAN, M.D.
Suite 717 Medical Towers
6608 Fannin
Houston, TX 77030

1. Pearlman T. Diagnostic pitfalls and therapeutic hazards encountered in treating alcoholism. J St Joseph Hosp 1982; 17:154-5.
2. Torrielli MV, Gabriel L, Dianzani MU. Ethanol-induced hepatotoxicity: experimental observations on the role of lipid peroxidation. J Pathol 1978; 126:11-25.
3. Israel Y, Kalent H, Khanna JM. Ethanol metabolism, oxygen availability, and alcohol-induced liver damage. J Adv Exp Med Biol 1976; 85:343.

To the Editor:

The suggestion of Greenblatt and colleagues that the symptoms patients experience after discontinuation of long-term benzodiazepine use do not indicate addiction seems questionable. I work in a clinic that treats a sizable number of patients with regular daily doses of diazepam. Over 50 per cent of this group have been taking diazepam for more than five years. It is difficult for clinicians to be certain whether this treatment is necessary to provide relief for an unremitting anxiety disorder or to prevent withdrawal symptoms. It is clear, however, that the majority of these patients are physiologically or psychologically dependent on diazepam and that cessation of medication leads to withdrawal symptoms or rebound anxiety more severe than the symptoms for which the drug was initially prescribed.

DAVID HASKELL, M.D.
68 Amory St.
Brookline, MA 02146

To the Editor:

Greenblatt et al. are surprisingly cavalier about the long-term use of benzodiazepines, overstating the benefits and minimizing the risks. The addictive potential of benzodiazepines, even when taken in therapeutic doses, is well established.[1,2] Confirming this, a double-blind study published at the same time as Greenblatt's review found withdrawal symptoms in 43 per cent of patients who had taken benzodiazepines for eight months or more when the drugs were suddenly withdrawn.[3]

Equally distressing is the absence of placebo-controlled studies demonstrating the long-term efficacy of benzodiazepines. Placebo-substitution studies, although quite useful for measuring adverse reactions such as withdrawal, cannot be used as evidence of long-term efficacy, because symptoms of withdrawal from benzodiazepines can mimic anxiety, so that patients going through drug withdrawal are mistakenly believed to be having a recurrence of their original symptoms.[4] In the absence of well-designed studies of efficacy showing a continued benefit in comparison to that seen in a placebo group, long-term use of a drug with a known addictive potential strikes us as poor medical practice.

Even as medical evidence mounts on the risk of addiction in long-term benzodiazepine users, while evidence of a long-term benefit is wanting, prescription of benzodiazepines for months or years continues at a stunning rate. A 1979 survey found that 2.2 per cent of Americans between 18 and 79 years of age had used antianxiety agents daily for four months or more.[5] (This figure may have changed since 1979 but is unlikely to have fallen dramatically.) On the basis of July 1983 population estimates, this means that approximately 3.5 million Americans are receiving from their physicians a treatment with risks that are real and benefits that are dubious at best.

Studies of the safety and efficacy of long-term use of benzodiazepines are not at all reassuring. Benzodiazepine prescribers and users alike should look at the evidence and then think again about long-term use.

EVE BARGMANN, M.D. AND SIDNEY M. WOLFE, M.D.
Public Citizen Health Research Group
Washington, DC 20036

1. Petursson H, Lader MH. Withdrawal from long-term benzodiazepine treatment. Br Med J 1981; 283:643-5.

2. Tyrer P, Rutherford D, Huggett T. Benzodiazepine withdrawal symptoms and propranolol. Lancet 1981; 1:520-2.

3. Rickels K, Case WG, Downing RW, Winokur A. Long-term diazepam therapy and clinical outcome. JAMA 1983; 250:767-71.

4. Maletzky BM, Klotter J. Addiction to diazepam. Int J Addict 1976; 11:95-115.

5. Mellinger GD, Balter MB. Prevalence and patterns of use of psychotherapeutic drugs: results from a 1979 national survey of American adults. In: Tognoni G, Bellantuono C, Lader M, eds. Epidemiologic impact of psychotropic drugs. New York: Elsevier/North Holland, 1981:117-35.

The above letters were referred to the authors of the article in question, who offer the following reply:

To the Editor:

Space constraints precluded our discussing every pharmacologic effect ever attributed to benzodiazepines. The "paradoxical" reactions described by Dr. Fouilladieu and associates are interesting but clearly unusual; furthermore, such reactions are not always established as causally related to drug therapy. Anger and hostility are not necessarily "paradoxical" effects of benzodiazepines but may represent behavior released by anxiolytic therapy under some circumstances in some patients.[1] Likewise, Dr. Hausner's observations on the antiseizure effects of benzodiazepines are of interest, but we caution against concluding that benzodiazepines are effective for a specific type of seizure disorder until the benefits are clearly established in controlled trials.

Dr. Pearlman correctly points out a typographical error in our paper: among medical conditions that can produce secondary anxiety, we meant to include hyperthyroidism, not hypothyroidism. We agree that sedative-hypnotic therapy carries risk in alcoholics with the withdrawal syndrome and impaired hepatic function, but the severe stress of untreated withdrawal may be equally or more hazardous in such patients. In the absence of controlled clinical data defining the risks and benefits of sedative-hypnotic therapy in this patient group, we recommend carefully titrated and monitored use of benzodiazepines in low doses to control withdrawal symptoms.

We reviewed in some depth (and will not reiterate here) the scientific evidence on benzodiazepine abuse and dependence and suggested practical guidelines to minimize the likelihood of problems. Our conclusions on the relative benefits and risks of benzodiazepine therapy are consistent with those of other investigators and scientists.[2-4] We find the stern warnings by Dr. Haskell and by Drs. Bargmann and Wolfe against long-term use of benzodiazepine, to be ironically misplaced. They make no mention of the current epidemic of truly lethal drug addiction — cigarette smoking.

DAVID J. GREENBLATT, M.D. AND RICHARD I. SHADER, M.D.
Tufts–New England Medical Center
Boston, MA 02111

1. Salzman C, Kochansky GE, Shader RI, Porrino LJ, Harmatz JS, Swett CP Jr. Chlordiazepoxide-induced hostility in a small group setting. Arch Gen Psychiatry 1974; 31:401-5.
2. Rickels K, Case WG, Downing RW, Winokur A. Long-term diazepam therapy and clinical outcome. JAMA 1983; 250:767-71.
3. Owen RT, Tyrer P. Benzodiazepine dependence: a review of the evidence. Drugs 1983; 25:385-98.
4. Lader M. Dependence on benzodiazepines. J Clin Psychiatry 1983; 44:121-7.

Pindolol: A New β-Adrenoceptor Antagonist with Partial Agonist Activity

William H. Frishman, M.D.

PINDOLOL (Visken) is a β-adrenoceptor antagonist that was released in November 1982 for clinical use in the United States (Fig. 1). After propranolol, metoprolol, nadolol, atenolol, and timolol, it is the sixth orally active β-blocker to be approved by the Food and Drug Administration for the treatment of systemic hypertension. The drug has been marketed widely outside the United States since 1969 for hypertension, angina pectoris, and arrhythmias.

Despite the therapeutic similarity of the β-blocking drugs, some differences in their pharmacodynamic and pharmacokinetic properties may be clinically important.[1] The β-blockers are usually classified according to the presence or absence of β_1-adrenergic selectivity, intrinsic sympathomimetic activity (partial agonist activity), and membrane-stabilizing properties.[1] Differences in potency, metabolism, half-life, lipophilicity, and protein binding are also recognized.[1] Pindolol, like propranolol, is a nonselective β-blocker with a relatively short plasma half-life.[1] However, pindolol differs from other β-blocking drugs currently available in the United States, because of its partial agonist activity.

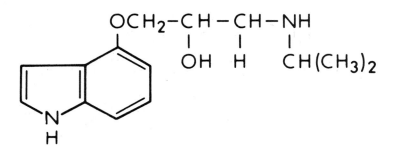

Figure 1. Molecular Structure of Pindolol.

From the Department of Medicine, Albert Einstein College of Medicine, Bronx, N.Y.
Supported in part by a grant (HL-00653-3) from the National Institutes of Health.
Originally published on April 21, 1983 (308:940-944).

Intrinsic Sympathomimetic Activity (Partial Agonist Activity)

Certain β-adrenoceptor blockers (acebutolol, alprenolol, oxprenolol, and pindolol) possess partial agonist activity.[2] These drugs cause a slight to moderate activation of the β-receptor,[1,3] in addition to preventing the access of natural or synthetic catecholamines to the receptor sites (Fig. 2). Dichloroisoproterenol, the first β-adrenoceptor blocking drug, exerted such marked partial agonist activity that it caused tachycardia in patients and was unsuitable for clinical use.[4] However, compounds with less partial agonist activity, such as pindolol, are effective β-blocking drugs.[5]

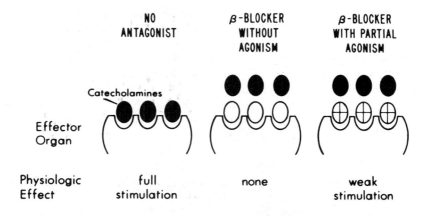

Figure 2. *Physiologic Effects of β-Adrenergic Blocking Drugs with and without Partial Agonist Activity, in the Presence of Circulating Catecholamines.*

When circulating catecholamines (●) combine with β-adrenergic receptors, they produce a full physiologic response. When these receptors are occupied by a β-blocker lacking partial agonist activity (○), no physiologic effects from catecholamine stimulation can occur. A β-blocking drug with partial agonist activity (⊕) also blocks the binding of catecholamines to β-adrenergic receptors, but in addition the drug causes a relatively weak stimulation of the receptor.

A quantitative assessment of the partial agonist activity in a β-blocker can be made in animals whose resting sympathetic tone has been abolished by adrenalectomy and pretreatment with reserpine or syringoserpine.[6,7] If in such animals a β-blocker increases the heart rate or force of myocardial contraction, the drug has partial agonist activity.[7] The increases in heart rate and contractility are mediated through β-adrenergic stimulation since they can be antagonized by propranolol.[7] The partial agonist effects of β-adrenoceptor blocking drugs differ from those of such agonists as epinephrine and isoproterenol in that the maximum pharmacologic effect is less, although the affinity for the receptor is high.[1,3] In laboratory animals pindolol has up to 50 per cent of the agonist activity of isoproterenol[3];

however, this activity is probably lower in human beings.[8] Unlike the relative selectivity of atenolol and metoprolol for β_1-adrenoceptors, which is attenuated as higher therapeutic doses are used,[1,9,10] the partial agonist activity of pindolol is not lost when higher doses are given.[11] The partial agonist effect of pindolol appears with low doses and has a flat dose–response curve, since the effect on the resting heart rate remains unchanged within a wide range of therapeutic doses.[11,12]

The evaluation of the partial agonist activity of β-blockers administered to human beings is complicated by the necessity to study the intact subject. However, the presence, extent, and clinical relevance of partial agonist activity can be assessed if equivalent pharmacologic doses of β-blocking drugs with and without this property are compared. Drugs with partial agonist activity, such as pindolol, cause less slowing of the resting heart rate than drugs without this activity, such as propranolol, atenolol, or metoprolol.[13-16] On the other hand, the increments in heart rate with exercise[13,15] or isoproterenol are decreased similarly by both types of β-blockers. An explanation for these findings is that the relative importance of the partial agonist effect of pindolol, as compared with its β-blocking action, is greatest when sympathetic tone is low[16] and therefore is appreciated only in resting subjects.[16] Since the drug's chronotropic effect is weak relative to endogenous catecholamines, the net effect of pindolol in resting subjects is not, however, a positive chronotropic action but either no change in heart rate or a smaller decrease than that caused by β-blockers lacking partial agonist activity. During exercise, when sympathetic activity is high, the β-blocking effect of pindolol predominates over its partial agonist activity. Thus, all β-blockers, with or without partial agonist activity, are equally effective in reducing the increases in heart rate and blood pressure that occur with exercise[16] — a finding that has been verified in many clinical studies.[11,13,17]

Studies in animals and human beings suggest that β-blockers with partial agonist activity may cause less depression of left ventricular function[18-20] and intracardiac conduction[21] than drugs lacking this property. Unlike propranolol and metoprolol, pindolol has been shown to reduce resistance in the femoral vascular bed of dogs[3] and to lower the total peripheral vascular resistance of patients with hypertension at rest and during exercise.[22-24] These effects on resistance appear to be mediated through peripheral β_2-receptor stimulation.[25] In other animal studies, drugs with partial agonist activity were found to have a relaxing effect on bronchial smooth muscle, although much less than that observed with isoproterenol.[3] Pindolol does not produce airways obstruction in normal subjects and appears to be better tolerated than propranolol in patients with bronchospasm.[26-28] Despite these reports, it is still not clear whether partial agonist activity actually has a beneficial role in patients with myocardial dysfunction, atrioventricular conduction disease, peripheral vascular disease, or bronchial asthma who require treatment with β-blocking drugs.[16,18,21,27-29]

Abrupt discontinuation of long-term pindolol therapy in patients with hypertension may be associated with fewer withdrawal reactions than sudden cessation of propranolol or metoprolol.[30,31] However, the clinical importance of this observation for patients with ischemic heart disease who are withdrawn from long-term pindolol treatment has not been determined.

Clinical Effectiveness

It has been postulated that partial agonist activity may detract from the beneficial actions of β-adrenergic blockade and clinical effectiveness.[1,16] However, in the treatment of patients with hypertension,[5,15] angina pectoris,[5,13,32] or arrhythmias,[28,33,34] pindolol appears to be as efficacious as β-blockers lacking this property. When given orally to normal subjects, pindolol is six to eight times more potent per milligram than propranolol in inhibiting isoproterenol-induced tachycardia.[1]

Hypertension

The various β-adrenoceptor blocking drugs appear to have comparable effectiveness in hypertension.[5,35] The mechanisms for the antihypertensive effects of β-blocking agents are not known. In most patients with hypertension, lowering of the blood pressure by long-term administration of β-blockers without partial agonist activity results from a reduction of cardiac output, largely mediated by blockade of β-receptors in the myocardium, sinoatrial node, and possibly the capacitance vessels.[2,36] The ability of the β-blockers to reduce plasma renin activity may also contribute to their antihypertensive effects in certain patients.[2,36] Other antihypertensive mechanisms, such as the resetting of peripheral baroreceptors or the attenuation of sympathetic outflow from the central nervous system, are hypothesized but remain unproved.[2,36] Pindolol has a variable effect on plasma renin activity[37] and causes a lesser decrement in cardiac output than metoprolol or propranolol, with similar reductions in blood pressure.[23,24] The antihypertensive effect of pindolol thus appears to derive more from a reduction in peripheral vascular resistance.[24] Whether this effect of pindolol on peripheral vascular resistance in hypertension is related to direct stimulation of peripheral β_2-receptors[25] or to other actions of the drug needs further clarification.

Despite the concern that partial agonist activity may impose a therapeutic ceiling on the antihypertensive effect of pindolol, numerous comparative studies have failed to demonstrate any difference in efficacy between β-blocking drugs with partial agonist activity and those without it.[14,15,38] Increasing the dose of pindolol within the recommended therapeutic range increases its effectiveness.[15]

The effectiveness of pindolol in hypertension has been established in numerous placebo-controlled trials.[15] Its antihypertensive action appears to be quantitatively similar to that of propranolol, thiazides, methyldopa, and chlorthalidone.[15] When administered two or three times daily to patients with hypertension, pindolol reduces both systolic and diastolic blood pressure by about 15 per cent.[15]

The drug is equally effective in the supine and standing positions; postural hypotension has rarely been observed.[15] The dose–response curve for pindolol in hypertension is relatively flat, with the maximal effect on blood pressure usually occurring by the first week of treatment with a dose of 15 to 20 mg a day.[15] As compared with other available β-blockers, pindolol, in effective β-blocking doses, is usually associated with a smaller reduction in resting cardiac output and heart rate.[23,38] When lowering the blood pressure, pindolol has a variable effect on plasma renin activity,[37] and blood pressure appears to be reduced equally well in patients with low, normal, or elevated renin levels before treatment.[37,38] Adjustment of the dosage to achieve an optimal antihypertensive effect may require a few weeks.[15] When therapy with pindolol is discontinued, the blood pressure tends to return gradually to pretreatment levels.[15] Drug tolerance does not appear to develop with long-term use.[15,38]

As is true of other β-blockers used to treat hypertension, there are differences among patients in the response of blood pressure to pindolol. The drug is more effective when combined with a diuretic, which may permit reduction of the dose of pindolol.[15,38] The addition of methyldopa, hydralazine, and guanethidine to pindolol enhances the reduction of blood pressure.[15,38] The drug appears to be safe and effective for the treatment of hypertension in patients with renal dysfunction.[39] Like the dosage of any other antihypertensive drug, the dosage of pindolol may have to be reduced in most patients undergoing hemodialysis. Despite its fairly short plasma half-life, pindolol has a relatively long duration of pharmacologic action.[40] It has been given once daily in the treatment of hypertension,[41,42] but further clinical study is needed to substantiate the efficacy of this regimen.

Ischemic Heart Disease

Like other β-blockers, pindolol can be expected to protect the heart from the deleterious effects of excessive adrenergic stimulation during exercise, excitement, or stress. By blocking catecholamine-induced increments in heart rate, in the velocity and extent of myocardial contraction, and in blood pressure, pindolol generally reduces the oxygen requirements of the heart at any given level of activity.[2] This pharmacologic effect makes it a useful agent for the long-term treatment of patients with stable angina pectoris.

In a placebo-controlled clinical study of 52 patients with classic angina pectoris, pindolol (10 to 40 mg per day in four divided doses) reduced angina attacks and nitroglycerin consumption, and increased exercise tolerance at least as effectively as propranolol (40 to 160 mg per day in four divided doses).[13] Both drugs effectively blunted the increments in blood pressure and heart rate occurring with exercise.[13] However, unlike propranolol, pindolol did not reduce the resting heart rate.[13] Although both β-blocking drugs are effective in patients with angina pectoris of effort, in patients with angina pectoris at rest, propranolol, by lowering the resting heart rate, appears to have a distinct advantage over pindolol.[16] Pindolol is used in many countries for the treatment of angina pectoris with effort, but this indication has not been approved as yet in the United States. In contrast to metoprolol, propranolol, and timolol, the use of pindolol has not been reported in any major trials in survivors of acute myocardial infarction, and the drug is not approved for use as prophylactic treatment for reducing the incidence of reinfarction and death in survivors of acute myocardial infarction.

Arrhythmias

Like other β-blockers, pindolol has antiarrhythmic properties that stem from its ability to antagonize the effects of catecholamines on cardiac automaticity.[2] It has been suggested that partial agonist activity in a β-blocker may partially negate the antiarrhythmic efficacy of β-blockade. However, pindolol has been shown to be as effective as propranolol for treatment of supraventricular tachyarrhythmias[28,33] and efficacious for treatment of ventricular tachyarrhythmias.[34] Like other β-blockers, pindolol has been shown to be effective in arrhythmias associated with thyrotoxicosis.[43] The relative safety of pindolol in patients with arrhythmias who have associated conduction abnormalities has not been demonstrated. The drug is not yet approved for the treatment of arrhythmia in the United States.

| Pharmacokinetics

Pindolol is rapidly and nearly completely (95 per cent) absorbed after oral ingestion. Absorption is not influenced by the presence of food.[40,44] The drug is detectable in the blood within half an hour, and peak plasma drug levels occur in one to two hours.[40,44] Pindolol undergoes little metabolism during its first pass through the liver, and its oral bioavailability is about 90 per cent.[40,44] Any increase in the daily dose within the therapeutic range can be expected to result in a proportional increase in the amount of drug in the body (linear pharmacokinetics).[40,44] There is a fourfold variation in plasma drug levels among patients after a single dose.[40,44] Interpatient variation decreases to twofold after multiple doses.[44] Pindolol is only 40 per cent bound to plasma proteins[40]; its volume of distribution in healthy subjects is about 2 liters per kilogram of body weight.[40] The drug crosses the placenta and is excreted in milk in measurable amounts. Pindolol is lipophilic and rapidly enters the central nervous system.

Sixty per cent of an oral dose of pindolol is metabolized in the liver, and the other 40 per cent is excreted unchanged in the urine.[40,44] No active metabolites are formed. The plasma concentration of pindolol declines monoexponentially after oral administration, and in patients with normal renal function the plasma half-life is three to four hours.[44] The half-life of pindolol is not altered by long-term administration or by moderate renal dysfunction.[40,44,45] In elderly patients with hypertension and normal renal function, the half-life is more variable and averages about seven hours.[44]

Gas chromatographic methods for determining plasma levels of pindolol are available.[46] As with all β-blockers, such measurements have little to offer as therapeutic guides, except for assessing compliance.[1] Pharmacodynamic characteristics and clinical response should be used as guides in determining the optimal dosage for each patient.

Clinical Use

The only indication approved for pindolol in the United States is the treatment of hypertension. Pindolol is available in tablets containing 5 or 10 mg. The standard wholesale costs are $0.14 for the 5-mg tablet and $0.21 for the 10-mg tablet. The initial dosage is 10 mg twice daily alone or in combination with a thiazide diuretic. Many patients will respond to 5 mg three times daily.[15] The antihypertensive response is usually seen within the first week of treatment.[15,38] If a satisfactory response does not occur within two to three weeks, the dose may be increased by 10 mg at intervals of two to three weeks, up to a maximum of 60 mg per day. The most useful drug combinations are with diuretics or vasodilating drugs, such as hydralazine or prazosin.[15,38]

Caution should be exercised when pindolol is given to patients with impaired hepatic function, since plasma drug levels may increase substantially in this situation.[40,44] The pharmacokinetics of pindolol are not greatly altered by renal impairment, and unlike atenolol and nadolol, which are predominantly excreted unchanged by the kidney, pindolol can be used safely in patients with renal dysfunction.

Despite the evidence that abrupt withdrawal of pindolol may be better tolerated by patients than the withdrawal of other β-blockers,[30] it is recommended that pindolol not be abruptly withdrawn and that patients receiving the drug be cautioned against interrupting therapy on their own. If the drug needs to be discontinued, it should be withdrawn cautiously over one to two weeks.[47] The safety of pindolol during pregnancy and lactation and its effectiveness and safety in children have not been established.

In certain clinical situation (cardiac failure, heart block, and bronchial asthma), preservation of adequate sympathetic-nervous-system stimulation may be necessary to maintain vital function. Although a β-blocker with partial agonist activity does not eliminate sympathetic stimulation entirely, there is no controlled evidence to show that pindolol is safer than other β-blockers in these conditions or less likely to cause them. Pindolol may be given cautiously with digitalis and diuretics to a patient with compensated congestive heart failure. The drug should not be administered or should be used with extreme caution in patients with bronchospastic disease.

When therapy is changed to pindolol from moderate daily doses of atenolol, metoprolol, nadolol, propranolol, or timolol, the recommended starting dose is 10 mg, given twice daily. Further dosage adjustments will depend on "titrating" for optimal clinical response.

Side Effects and Precautions

Any serious side effects of pindolol are related to its β-adrenergic blocking activity and are similar to those described with other β-adrenergic blocking drugs.[48-50] The occurrence of unwanted depression of myocardial function and cardiac electrical activity by pindolol and other β-blockers used in therapeutic doses is related to the dependence of these functions on adrenergic stimulation in individual patients. Similarly, pindolol can interfere with ventilatory functions in patients who are dependent on adrenergic stimulation of β_2-receptors.

Most of the less serious side effects reported with pindolol are similar in type and frequency to those reported with propranolol. They include a low incidence of dizziness, vivid dreams, fatigue, weakness, headache, muscle cramps, and nausea.[48-50] There is no evidence to date to suggest that pindolol can cause a general oculomucocutaneous syndrome like that caused by practolol.[48] An average increase of 1.4 kg in body weight has been described with pindolol — a larger increase than reported with either propranolol or placebo.[48] The weight gain appears to be unrelated to the blood-pressure response and is not associated with an increase in heart failure, although edema has been found to be more prevalent with pindolol than with placebo treatment.[48] Minor persistent elevations in serum transaminases have been described in 7 per cent of patients during pindolol treatment, but progressive elevations were not observed. Moreover, hepatic injury related to pindolol treatment has not been reported after 10 years of clinical use outside the United States.[50] Like all other β-blockers, pindolol can mask some clinical signs of hypoglycemia or hyperthyroidism, and the package insert advises that the drug be used with caution in diabetes. Treatment of pindolol overdosage should follow that described for other β-blockers.[51] Pindolol, like all other systemically active β-blockers, has an enormous margin of safety in patients who do not depend on functioning β-adrenoceptors.

References

1. Frishman WH. β-Adrenoceptor antagonists: new drugs and new indications. N Engl J Med 1981; 305:500-6.
2. Frishman W, Silverman R. Clinical pharmacology of the new beta-adrenergic blocking drugs. 2. Physiologic and metabolic effects. Am Heart J 1979; 97:797-807.
3. Clark BJ, Menninger K, Bertholet A. Pindolol — the pharmacology of a partial agonist. Br J Clin Pharmacol 1982; 13: Suppl 2:149s-58s.
4. Glover WE, Greenfield ADM, Shanks RG. Effects of dichloroisoprenaline on the peripheral vascular responses to adrenaline in man. Br J Pharmacol Chemother 1962; 19:235-44.
5. Frishman W, Silverman R. Clinical pharmacology of the new beta-adrenergic blocking drugs. 3. Comparative clinical experiences and new therapeutic applications. Am Heart J 1979; 98:119-31.
6. Barrett AM, Carter J. Comparative chronotropic activity of β-adrenoceptive antagonists. Br J Pharmacol 1970; 40:373-81.

7. Cocco G, Burkart F, Chu D, Follath F. Intrinsic sympathomimetic activity of β-adrenoceptor blocking agents. Eur J Clin Pharmacol 1978; 13:1-4.
8. Man in't Veld AJ, Schalekamp MADH. Pindolol acts as a beta-adrenoceptor agonist in orthostatic hypotension: therapeutic implications. Br Med J 1981; 282:929-31.
9. Koch-Weser J. Metoprolol. N Engl J Med 1979; 301:698-703.
10. Frishman WH. Atenolol and timolol, two new systemic β-adrenoceptor antagonists. N Engl J Med 1982; 306:1456-62.
11. Carruthers SG, Twum-Barima Y. Measurements of partial agonist activity of pindolol. Clin Pharmacol Ther 1981; 30:581-6.
12. Carruthers SG. Cardiac dose-response relationships of oral and intravenous pindolol. Br J Clin Pharmacol 1982; 13: Suppl 2:193s-8s.
13. Kostis JB, Frishman W, Hosler MH, Thorsen NL, Gonasun L, Weinstein J. Treatment of angina pectoris with pindolol: the significance of intrinsic sympathomimetic activity of beta blockers. Am Heart J 1982; 104:496-504.
14. McNeil JJ, Louis WJ. A double-blind crossover comparison of pindolol, metoprolol, atenolol and labetalol in mild to moderate hypertension. Br J Clin Pharmacol 1979; 8: Suppl 2:163s-6s.
15. Gonasun LM. Antihypertensive effects of pindolol. Am Heart J 1982; 104:374-87.
16. Frishman WH, Kostis J. The significance of intrinsic sympathomimetic activity in beta-adrenoceptor blocking drugs. Cardiovasc Rev Rep 1982; 3:503-12.
17. Aellig WH. Pindolol — a β-adrenoceptor blocking drug with partial agonist activity: clinical pharmacological considerations. Br J Clin Pharmacol 1982; 13: Suppl 2:187s-92s.
18. Taylor SH, Silke B, Lee PS. Intravenous beta-blockade in coronary heart disease: is cardioselectivity or intrinsic sympathomimetic activity hemodynamically useful? N Engl J Med 1982; 306:631-5.
19. Hahn B, Strauer BE. The influence of β-adrenoceptor blockade on left ventricular function. Br J Clin Pharmacol 1982; 13: Suppl 2:305s-7s.
20. Heikkilä J, Nieminen MS. Cardiac safety of acute beta blockade: intrinsic sympathomimetic activity is superior to beta-1 selectivity. Am Heart J 1982; 104:464-72.
21. Giudicelli JF, Lhoste F. β-Adrenoceptor blockade and atrioventricular conduction in dogs: role of intrinsic sympathomimetic activity. Br J Clin Pharmacol 1982; 13: Suppl 2:167s-74s.
22. Atterhög JH, Dunér H, Pernow B. Experience with pindolol, a betareceptor blocker, in the treatment of hypertension. Am J Med 1976; 60:872-6.
23. Svensson A, Gubrandsson T, Sivertsson R, Hansson L. Haemodynamic effects of metoprolol and pindolol: a comparison in hypertensive patients. Br J Clin Pharmacol 1982; 13: Suppl 2:259s-67s.
24. Svendsen TL, Hartling OJ, Trap-Jensen J, McNair A, Bliddal J. Adrenergic beta receptor blockade: hemodynamic importance of intrinsic sympathomimetic activity at rest. Clin Pharmacol Ther 1981; 29:711-8.
25. Thulesius O, Gjöres JE, Berlin E. Vasodilating properties of β-adrenoceptor blockers with intrinsic sympathomimetic activity. Br J Clin Pharmacol 1982; 13: Suppl 2:229s-30s.
26. Hamilton BP, Hamilton J, Kirkendall WM. Pulmonary function in hypertensive patients treated with pindolol: a report of two studies. Am Heart J 1982; 104:432-7.

27. Cannon RE, Slavin RG, Gonasun LM. The effect on asthma of a new beta-blocker, pindolol. Am Heart J 1982; 104:438-45.

28. Frishman W, Davis R, Strom J, et al. Clinical pharmacology of the new beta-adrenergic blocking drugs. 5. Pindolol (LB-46) therapy for supraventricular arrhythmia: a viable alternative to propranolol in patients with bronchospasm. Am Heart J 1979; 98:393-8.

29. Smith RS, Warren DJ. Effect of β-blocking drugs on peripheral blood flow in intermittent claudication. J Cardiovasc Pharmacol 1982; 4:2-4.

30. Rangno RE, Langlois S. Comparison of withdrawal phenomena after propranolol, metoprolol, and pindolol. Am Heart J 1982; 104:473-8.

31. Molinoff PB, Aarons RD, Nies AS, Gerber JG, Wolfe BB, Goens MB. Effects of pindolol and propranolol on β-adrenergic receptors in human lymphocytes. Br J Clin Pharmacol 1982; 13: Suppl 2:365s.

32. Thadani U, Davidson C, Singleton W, Taylor SH. Comparison of the immediate effects of five β-adrenoreceptor blocking drugs with different ancillary properties in angina pectoris. N Engl J Med 1979; 300:750-5.

33. Aronow WS, Uyeyama RR. Treatment of arrhythmias with pindolol. Clin Pharmacol Ther 1972; 13:15-22.

34. Podrid PJ, Lown B. Pindolol for ventricular arrhythmia. Am Heart J 1982; 104:491-6.

35. Prichard BNC. β-Adrenergic receptor blockade in hypertension, past, present and future. Br J Clin Pharmacol 1978; 5:379-99.

36. Frishman WH. Nadolol: a new β-adrenoceptor antagonist. N Engl J Med 1981; 305:678-82.

37. Glassock RJ, Weitzman RE, Bennett CM, et al. Pindolol: effects on blood pressure and plasma renin activity. Am Heart J 1982; 104:421-5.

38. Fanchamps A. Therapeutic trials of pindolol in hypertension: comparison and combination with other drugs. Am Heart J 1982; 104:388-406.

39. Epstein M, Oster JR. Beta-blockers and the kidney. Mineral Electrolyte Metab 1982; 8:237-54.

40. Meier J. Pharmacokinetic comparison of pindolol with other beta-adrenoceptor-blocking agents. Am Heart J 1982; 104:364-73.

41. Frithz G. Once-a-day treatment of hypertension with pindolol. Am Heart J 1982; 104:413-6.

42. Raftery EB, Mann S, BalaSubramanian V, Craig MWM. Once-daily pindolol in hypertension: an ambulatory assessment. Am Heart J 1982; 104:417-20.

43. Schelling JL, Scazziga B, Dufour RF, Milinkovic N, Weber AA. Effect of pindolol, a beta receptor antagonist, in hyperthyroidism. Clin Pharmacol Ther 1973; 14:158-64.

44. Schwarz HJ. Pharmacokinetics of pindolol in humans and several animal species. Am Heart J 1982; 104:357-64.

45. Ohnhaus EE, Heidemann H, Meier J, Maurer G. Metabolism of pindolol in patients with renal failure. Eur J Clin Pharmacol 1982; 22:423-8.

46. Bangah M, Jackman G, Bobik A. Determination of pindolol in human plasma by high-performance liquid chromatography. J Chromatog 1980; 183:255-9.

47. Frishman W, Kostis J, Strom J, et al. Clinical pharmacology of the new beta-adrenergic blocking drugs. 6. A comparison of pindolol and propranolol in treatment

of patients with angina pectoris: the role of intrinsic sympathomimetic activity. Am Heart J 1979; 98:526-35.

48. Gonasun LM, Langrall H. Adverse reactions to pindolol administration. Am Heart J 1982; 104:482-6.

49. Carr A, Mulligan OF, Sherrill LN. Pindolol versus methyldopa for hypertension: comparison of adverse reactions. Am Heart J 1982; 104:479-81.

50. Krupp P, Fanchamps A. Pindolol: experience gained in 10 years of safety monitoring. Am Heart J 1982; 104:486-90.

51. Frishman W, Jacob H, Eisenberg E, Ribner H. Clinical pharmacology of the new beta-adrenergic blocking drugs. 8. Self-poisoning with beta-adrenoceptor blocking agents: recognition and management. Am Heart J 1979; 98:798-811.

| Correspondence

Pindolol and Hyperthyroidism*

To the Editor:
The article by Dr. Frishman (April 21 issue) mentioned that, like all other beta blockers, pindolol, a beta-adrenoceptor antagonist with partial agonist activity, could mask some clinical signs of hyperthyroidism. [1] Propranolol, a beta-blocker without intrinsic sympathetic activity, has been shown to be effective in reducing the heart rate in hyperthyroidism. However, few data are available concerning the effects of pindolol in the treatment of thyrotoxicosis.

Recently we used 24-hour Holter electrocardiography to assess variations in sinus rhythm in patients with hyperthyroidism treated by pindolol. Six patients with Graves' disease who were in stable sinus rhythm, without any cardiac insufficiency, were studied. After a drug-free control period, all patients received pindolol alone (5 mg three times a day) during three days. On the third day, a second Holter recording was performed. The results were based on the magnitude of the variations in mean sinus rate (expressed as percentages) during 10 consecutive daytime hours (9 a.m. to 7 p.m.) and 6 consecutive nighttime hours (12 a.m. to 6 a.m.). Student's t-test was used for statistical analysis. Pindolol did not change the daytime heart rate ($+4.9$ per cent, P not significant) but increased the nighttime heart rate significantly ($+23.4$ per cent, $P<0.001$); furthermore, the variations in the nighttime sinus rate were significantly higher in hyperthyroid subjects than in 21 euthyroid controls monitored after administration of the same dose of pindolol under the same conditions ($+23.4\pm4.9$ per cent vs. $+11.6\pm2.6$ per cent, $P<0.05$).

Therefore, it is suggested that unlike propranolol, pindolol does not mask the tachycardia observed in hyperthyroidism. The major enhancement of the heart rate after administration of pindolol in hyperthyroidism may be due to variations

*Originally published on September 29, 1983 (309:795).

in the number or affinity of beta-adrenergic receptors in this condition, as previously discussed by Dr. Skelton in a recent editorial in the *Journal*.[2]

E. Abadie, M.D.
Hôpital Saint Louis
J. F. Leclercq, M.D.
Hôpital Lariboisière
Ph. Passa, M.D.
Hôpital Saint Louis
75010 Paris, France

1. Frishman WH. Pindolol: a new β-adrenoceptor antagonist with partial agonist activity. N Engl J Med 1983; 308:940-4.
2. Skelton CL. The heart and hyperthyroidism. N Engl J Med 1982; 307:1206-8.

The above letter was referred to the author of the article in question, who offers the following reply:

To the Editor:
The observations of Drs. Abadie et al. are welcome.

In both euthyroid and hyperthyroid patients, one would expect pindolol, a beta-adrenergic blocker with moderate partial agonist activity, to increase or maintain heart rate during sleep. In a state of low "sympathetic tone," such as sleep, the partial agonist activity of the drug could predominate over its beta-blocking effects. However, there should be no effect or a minimal effect of pindolol on heart rate during normal daily activities, and a blunting in heart rate during exercise, when the beta-blocking effects of the drug should predominate. The study of Abadie et al. does not support the contention that tachycardia in hyperthyroidism is never masked by pindolol, and is inconsistent with the observations of other investigators who have successfully used beta-blockers with partial agonism to treat hyperthyroid patients.[1,2] However, on the basis of our own observations, I would agree with Dr. Abadie and his group that pindolol is probably less effective for maximally controlling tachycardia than beta-blockers without partial agonist activity.

William H. Frishman, M.D.
Albert Einstein College of Medicine
Bronx, NY 10461

1. Nelson JK, McDevitt DG. Comparative trial of propranolol and practolol in hyperthyroidism. Br J Clin Pharmacol 1975; 2:411-6.
2. Schelling JL, Scazziga B, Dufour RJ, Milinkovic N, Weber AA. Effect of pindolol, a beta receptor antagonist, in hyperthyroidism. Clin Pharmacol Ther 1973; 14:158-64.

Psychotropic Drug Use in the Elderly

(In Two Parts)

Troy L. Thompson II, M.D.,

Michael G. Moran, M.D.,

and Alan S. Nies, M.D.

E LDERLY persons (by definition, those 65 years of age and older) now make up about 11 per cent of the U.S. population, but about 30 per cent of all prescriptions are written for this group, primarily by internists and family physicians.[1,2] Elderly patients have a higher incidence of psychiatric disorders than younger persons and usually go first to their internist or family physician with their symptoms rather than to a psychiatrist. A disproportionately large percentage of psychotropic medications are prescribed for the elderly,[3-5] and many older people believe that their daily performance depends on the use of such drugs.[6] In addition, they commonly purchase over-the-counter medications: almost 70 per cent of elderly patients regularly use such medications, as compared with about 10 per cent of the general adult population.[7,8] About 55 per cent of the over-the-counter drugs used by the elderly are analgesics. Over-the-counter preparations probably account for at least 40 per cent of all drugs used by the elderly.[9]

Because of their high incidence of medical and psychiatric disorders of all kinds, the elderly are relatively frequent visitors to the offices of internists and family physicians.[10] Their symptoms are often complex and confusing, and physicians commonly use drugs to treat them.[11-14] The pharmacokinetics of some drugs are altered in older patients, and the normal variation in drug effects from one person to another is often accentuated in the elderly by the decreased functioning of pharmacokinetically important organ systems, as well as by changes in target-organ sensitivity to the drug.[15-17] In fact, the elderly constitute the most diverse segment of the population psychosocially, biologically, and pharmacokinetically.[18] Therefore, diagnosis is often very challenging, and treatment must frequently be tailored to the individual for maximal efficacy.

From the Divisions of Liaison Psychiatry, Internal Medicine, and Clinical Pharmacology and Toxicology and the Departments of Psychiatry, Medicine, and Pharmacology, University of Colorado School of Medicine.

Originally published in two parts on January 20, 1983 (308:134-138) and January 27, 1983 (308:194-199).

The elderly part of the population is expected to expand for at least the next several decades and should account for about 12.5 per cent of the total by the year 2000. Patients in this age group have twice the incidence of adverse side effects and drug interactions due to psychotropic medications that younger patients have.[1] Thus, it is important for physicians who treat them to understand how these medications should be used in the elderly.[19-21]

Changes in Psychotropic Drug Pharmacokinetics in the Elderly

The physiologic changes associated with aging and their effects on the absorption, distribution, and elimination of psychotropic drugs are summarized in Table 1.[22-28] Although some vitamins, minerals, and carbohydrates may be more poorly absorbed and the absorption of actively transported drugs may decrease with aging,[29,30] there is essentially no change in the absorption of most psychotropic drugs, since they are passively absorbed.[31-33]

TABLE 1.   Pharmacokinetic Effects of Common Physiologic Changes in Absorption, Distribution, and Elimination of Psychotropic Drugs in the Elderly.

Physiologic Change	Pharmacokinetic Effect
Absorption	
Usually little changed	Usually negligible
Distribution	
Decreased lean body mass and total body water	Increased plasma concentration of water-soluble drugs
Incresed total body fat	Decreaed plasma concentration and slower elimination of fat-soluble drugs
Decresed serum albumin	Higher percentage of unbound, metabolically active drugs
Elimination	
Decreased hepatic enzyme activity and blood flow	Decreased effectiveness of metabolism of foreign substances
Decrease in renal function of 40-50 per cent associated with "normal" creatinine levels	Decreased renal excretion; prolonged half-lives of drugs that are primarily excreted unchanged

The distribution of psychotropic drugs often changes markedly with aging, since the lean body mass and total body water decrease, whereas the percentage of total body fat increases.[30,34,35] Therefore, the serum concentration of water-soluble drugs is relatively higher, and the serum concentration of fat-soluble drugs is lower for any given dose. Serum albumin tends to decrease with age,[36-38] so that a higher percentage of the total drug in the circulation is unbound and pharmacologically active. Some drugs, such as the tricyclic antidepressants, are bound to serum α_1-acid glycoprotein, whose level probably changes little with aging.

The elimination half-life of psychotropic medications often increases with age because of an increased volume of distribution or a reduced clearance associated with diminished functioning of the organs involved in the elimination processes.[39] Cardiac output and renal and splanchnic blood flow may decrease by 30 to 40 per cent with aging.[25] The metabolism of psychotropic drugs is carried out primarily by the hepatic microsomal enzymes, although the gastrointestinal tract, lungs, and kidneys may participate to a lesser degree. Tobacco smoking may cause less induction of hepatic microsomal enzymes in the elderly than in younger patients.[40] Drug metabolism may also be affected by alcohol use, and the elderly as a group tend to use relatively more alcohol than younger persons.[41] Long-term alcohol use can induce hepatic microsomal-enzyme activity and increase the rate of drug metabolism. However, this enzyme system is inhibited while alcohol is still in the blood.[42]

Screening Procedures before Use of Psychotropic Drugs in the Elderly

The basic screening procedures that are recommended before a psychotropic medication is prescribed for an elderly patient are outlined in Table 2.[13,14,43-45] Since

TABLE 2. Routine Screening Procedures Recommended for Elderly Patients in Whom Use of Psychotropic Drugs Is Being Considered.

History

Is a medical illness causing the "psychiatric" symptoms?

Is a drug the patient is currently taking causing the psychiatric symptoms?

Has the patient had these or other psychiatric symptoms in the past? If so, what was the diagnosis and what medication, if any, was therapeutically effective? What side effects, if any, developed?

Physical Examination

Is there evidence of neurologic, renal, hepatic, or other medical disease that would further increase the elderly patient's risk for side effects?

Mental Status

Is there a psychiatric illness of recent onset?

Is there evidence of dementia or delirium?

Laboratory Studies

Is there evidence of decreased hepatic synthesizing function (i.e., decreased serum albumin) or decreased renal function (i.e., decreased creatinine clearance)?

Drug Interactions

What adverse drug interactions might develop if the psychotropic drug was added to medications the patient is currently taking?

many medical illnesses and medications can produce psychiatric symptoms, such possible causes should be considered before the patient is diagnosed as having a primary psychiatric disorder. In some cases, careful management of an underlying medical disorder, discontinuation of a medication, or a change to another medication of the same class that has fewer "psychiatric" side effects may alleviate the symptoms. Since the use of multiple drugs is common in the elderly,[4,46,47] a careful history of drug use, including prescription, over-the-counter, and other drugs, may enable the physician to recommend a decrease in the number and types of medications that are being taken. Such a decrease may eliminate symptoms that are secondary to previously unrecognized adverse drug interactions.

It should be noted that in the elderly a serum creatinine level that would usually be considered normal does not rule out the presence of impaired renal function. Since older persons have a decreased muscle mass, they have a decreased rate of creatinine production. Therefore, a reduced rate of creatinine clearance often coexists with serum creatinine concentrations in the normal range, as defined for young healthy adults.[27,48-50]

Guidelines and Precautions for the Use of Psychotropic Drugs in the Elderly

In general, psychotropic medications should be prescribed at doses 30 to 50 per cent as large as those for younger patients.[51,52] Since the physiologic and pathologic variability in the elderly is so great, a basic rule is to start with a low dose whenever possible and increase the dosage much more gradually than is recommended for younger patients. The therapeutic end point must be defined before a drug is started. Partial improvement, rather than a total elimination of symptoms, is often a realistic end point in the elderly. The dosage should be titrated gradually until the therapeutic goal is reached or until adverse side effects develop and persist to a degree that precludes further increases. If such side effects do persist, the drug should be discontinued, and the same procedure should be repeated with the drug from the same class that has the lowest frequency of the side effects that have developed. In many cases, after therapeutic improvement has been achieved and maintained for one to two months, the drug may be gradually discontinued over several months. If symptoms reappear during this process, the patient may need to remain on a maintenance dose, which may be one third to one half the originally effective therapeutic dose. Periodic attempts at tapering these doses should continue. A final general guideline is that patients should not be continued on a psychotropic drug for which clear-cut therapeutic benefit has not been evident. If in doubt, discontinue the medication.

Specific guidelines and precautions for the use of each of the major classes of psychotropic drugs are discussed below.

Antianxiety Agents

Benzodiazepines are by far the most frequently prescribed anxiolytic agents

(Table 3).[53-55] The Food and Drug Administration has recommended that they be used only for "short-term relief of anxiety" and not to facilitate long-term coping with the stresses of life.[56] Psychotherapy or counseling is the treatment of choice for the latter purpose.

TABLE 3. Selected Benzodiazepines: Pharmacologic Factors of Special Relevance for the Elderly.

Drug	FDA-Approved Use	Half-Life	Usual Initial Dose for the Elderly
Flurazepam	Hypnotic	50–100 hours (Major metabolite)	15 mg at bedtime
Temazepam	Hypnotic	5–15 hours	15 mg at bedtime
Oxazepam	Anxiolytic	5–20 hours	10 mg three times a day
Diazepam	Anxiolytic	20–100 hours (Major metabolite)	2 mg per day or twice a day
Lorazepam	Anxiolytic	10–20 hours	0.5–2 mg per day

Age does not produce any consistent alterations in absorption of benzodiazepines. Once absorbed, the benzodiazepines can produce greater effects on the central nervous system in the elderly than in younger patients.[15-17,31,57] These are due partly to increased target-organ sensitivity to benzodiazepines and partly to impairment of drug disposition in the elderly. The elderly are also more sensitive to barbiturates, which are now rarely used to treat anxiety. Barbiturates are especially prone to produce paradoxical excitement, suppress rapid-eye-movement (REM) sleep, and cause rebound nightmares and insomnia in the elderly.[58] Barbiturates should be avoided in older patients for these reasons and also because of their habituating qualities, their low therapeutic ratio, and the risks associated with overdose.[59]

The effects of aging on the distribution and elimination kinetics of the benzodiazepines depend on the specific compound.[60] Diazepam has a longer half-life in the elderly; the half-life may increase from 20 hours in 20-year-olds to 90 hours in 80-year-olds.[15] The delay in elimination is due to an increased apparent volume of distribution, although the clearance of diazepam from the blood remains unchanged. Chlordiazepoxide also has a prolonged elimination half-life in the elderly; it can increase from 7 hours at 20 years to 40 hours at 80 years.[61] The mechanism for this prolongation is both a reduced hepatic clearance of chlordiazepoxide and an increased distribution volume. In contrast, there are no major changes with aging in the pharmacokinetics of lorazepam and oxazepam.[62-64] This may be due to the lower lipid solubility of these drugs and the fact that they are not metabolized by the hepatic mixed-function oxidase system.

All benzodiazepines, given in repeated doses, will accumulate to some degree and may produce excessive sedation, diminished sexual desire, and a reduction in the general level of energy.[54,65] Such side effects may be overlooked because the elderly person may not volunteer, and the physician may not elicit, a history of sexual changes, or the patient and physician may falsely attribute such changes to the normal aging process. The use of a benzodiazepine in a depressed patient or in a patient with a mild or subclinical dementia may cause a worsening of the depression or dementia and occasionally a florid delirium. Therefore, before a benzodiazepine is prescribed it should routinely be determined whether the elderly patient is depressed, has even a subclinical dementia, or is taking some other medication that is a central-nervous-system depressant.[66]

The extent and severity of drug side effects can be minimized by proper attention to a drug's half-life, dosage, and frequency of administration.[55] The benzodiazepines with longer half-lives are flurazepam, diazepam, chlordiazepoxide, clorazepate, prazepam, and halazepam. They should be prescribed for the elderly in smaller doses and at more widely spaced intervals than is recommended for younger patients.[17] The benzodiazepines with shorter half-lives, such as oxazepam, lorazepam, and alprazolam, also require decreased doses. However, because the pharmacokinetics of these drugs with shorter half-lives are not greatly changed in the elderly, the dosage schedule can be more similar to that in younger patients.[67]

Drug interactions with benzodiazepines may be a factor in the excessive response of some elderly patients to these drugs. Cimetidine and disulfiram have been found to impair the clearance of chlordiazepoxide and diazepam from plasma.[68-70] However, the disposition of oxazepam is not affected in this way by cimetidine or disulfiram.

Sedative–Hypnotic Agents

The elderly often report changes in their sleep patterns from earlier years, and physicians frequently attempt to remedy such changes by pharmacologic means. That this is true is attested to by the fact that the elderly receive almost 40 per cent of all sedative–hypnotic prescriptions,[71] although they constitute only about 11 per cent of the population. Reports of a sleep disturbance should lead the physician to make a careful differential diagnosis, and treatment with medications should be considered only if the disturbance is serious and disruptive to the patient. Even then, sleep medications should generally be prescribed only for short-term insomnia, such as may occur during an acute grief reaction, and their use should be reevaluated at least once a month.

Aging by itself may be associated with several changes in the sleep cycle, including a diminished total sleep time in some patients or more frequent disturbances of sleep continuity. Extreme difficulty falling asleep or early morning awakening in elderly patients who are not napping excessively at other times during the day may be symptoms of depression and should usually be treated with psychotherapy and possibly an antidepressant, not with a sedative–hypnotic. Sedative–hypnotics may be especially dangerous if the sleep disturbance is due to some medical conditions. For example, the use of a sedative in a patient whose sleep disturbance is secondary to chronic obstructive lung disease may have serious consequences, and if the sleep disturbance is secondary to sleep-apnea syndrome, a sedative–hypnotic may be lethal.[72]

The benzodiazepines are the medications most frequently prescribed for sleep disturbances. Flurazepam accounted for over 13 million of the approximately 25 million prescriptions written for hypnotics in this country in a recent year.[71] Flurazepam and its active metabolites have half-lives of up to one week or longer in the elderly, so they may produce excessive daytime sedation or other side effects for a number of days after discontinuation of the medication. Therefore, as with all benzodiazepines, the dosage of flurazepam should be decreased in the elderly.[54,73,74] All the benzodiazepines shown in Table 3 may decrease the amount of Stage 3 and 4 sleep, and flurazepam may also decrease REM time. Central-nervous-system depression and other clinically important side effects were found to occur in 39 per cent of elderly patients who were receiving 30 mg or more of flurazepam per day, which is twice the recommended geriatric dose.[17] Such side effects of excessive dosages of benzodiazepines may be especially dangerous if the elderly person is operating machinery, such as an automobile, or using some other central-nervous-system depressant, such as alcohol. The resultant cerebellar and frontal-lobe dysfunctions may predispose to accidents, including falls, perceptual disturbances, depression, dementia, or delirium.

A benzodiazepine with a shorter half-life, such as temazepam, may have some advantages as a hypnotic for the elderly. Compounds with shorter half-lives will not accumulate to the same degree as compounds with longer half-lives, assuming that both are given in equivalent dosages and at equal intervals. As with flurazepam, the dosage of temazepam recommended for the elderly is 15 mg. Since it sometimes takes one to two hours to reach peak serum levels, temazepam may have to be administered several hours before bedtime.

For the reasons discussed above, there is now little place for the use of barbiturates in treating sleep disturbances, especially in the elderly. Antihistamines are the active ingredients in most over-the-counter sleep preparations, and although often effective, they are associated with a higher risk of delirium than are the benzodiazepines in the elderly. Chloral hydrate may be a useful hypnotic for the older patient. It seldom produces delirium, has little habituation potential, and exerts little adverse effect on normal sleep cycles. However, the benzodiazepines are usually a wiser choice because a principal metabolite of chloral hydrate is a relatively potent displacer of such acidic drugs as warfarin and diphenylhydantoin from plasma proteins. Chloral hydrate may thus induce a sudden increase in the free (unbound) concentrations of such displaced drugs, transiently increase the effects of those drugs, reduce their total plasma concentration, and shorten their elimination half-lives.[75]

Antidepressant Agents

It is important to detect depression in the elderly, since it is often responsive to treatment and since suicide is common in this age group, especially among depressed white widowers.[3,76] Other risk factors for suicide that are found frequently in the elderly include living alone, chronic medical illnesses (which may cause dementia or predispose to delirium), recent loss or bereavement, alcohol or sedative abuse, a sense of hopelessness about problems, and a covert wish by others that the elderly person would die.

Clinically important depression is present at any given time in at least 10 per cent of the elderly. It is important to determine whether depression in the elderly is the primary disorder or is secondary to some other psychiatric or medical disorder or to medication, since such disorders and the use of multiple medications are so common in the elderly.[3] Brain tumors, other cancers (especially pancreatic), hypothyroidism or hyperthyroidism, hepatitis, and viral pneumonia may cause or worsen a depression. In addition, drug-induced depression should always be suspected in elderly patients who are receiving medications for a variety of illnesses.[77]

Depressive symptoms are frequently passed over as a normal slowing down due to aging or are misdiagnosed as dementia. The latter error is so common that the term "pseudodementia" is sometimes used to describe cognitive impairments due to depression in the elderly.[66,78] Other psychiatric disorders that may present as depression in the elderly include paranoia, an exacerbation of preexisting schizophrenia, and grief reactions. The bradykinetic syndrome associated with the use of neuroleptics is often mistaken for the motor retardation of depression in the elderly.

Table 4 gives a list of antidepressants from which the initial drug for treating depression in the elderly is usually chosen.[79-81] These compounds tend to be more effective in patients who have "vegetative" or biologic symptoms of depression. Such symptoms may include multiple somatic complaints, decreased appetite and weight loss, sleep disturbances, decreased sexual drive and energy level, and psychomotor agitation or retardation. Steady-state serum levels of several of these drugs (e.g., amitriptyline, desipramine, and imipramine) tend to be high in the elderly because of reduced clearance.[52] Such drugs should be begun at a lower dose in the elderly than in younger adults, and the dosage increased more slowly, since many bothersome side effects and some potentially dangerous ones are common.[82]

Several laboratory tests, including the dexamethasone suppression test and measurement of the urinary metabolites of norepinephrine — a central-nervous-system neurotransmitter whose level may be altered in some depressions — have recently received attention.[83,84] The latter test may sometimes allow greater specificity in selecting a tricyclic antidepressant.[84] However, these tests are not routinely recommended for elderly patients because the possible effects of aging on their specificity and predictive value have not yet been adequately determined.

Since some antidepressants can produce a variety of cardiac effects, electrocardiography is recommended before treatment and at regular intervals thereafter in patients with cardiac disease. The anticholinergic properties of the tricyclic antidepressants may cause an increase in heart rate. In addition, they may increase the P-R interval, QRS duration, and QTc time and flatten the T wave.[85-87] The changes in P-R interval and T wave are probably benign and may gradually disappear even with continued therapy.

TABLE 4. Selected Antidepressants: Pharmacologic Factors of Special Relevance for the Elderly.

Agent	Category	Relative Anticholinergic Effects	Relative Sedative Effects	Usual Initial Daily Dose for the Elderly
Amitriptyline	Tricyclic tertiary amine	6+	5+	10 mg three times a day and possibly 20 mg at bedtime
Doxepin	Tricyclic tertiary amine	3+	6+	25–50 mg
Imipramine	Tricyclic tertiary amine	4+	3+	30–40 mg
Nortriptyline	Tricyclic secondary amine	3+	2+	25–50 mg
Desipramine	Tricyclic secondary amine	1+	2+	25–50 mg
Maprotiline	Tetracyclic	3+	3+	25 mg per day or twice a day
Amoxapine	Dibenzoxazepine	3+	3+	25 mg three times a day
Trazodone	Triazolopyridine	1+	3+	50–100 mg

It has been suggested that tricyclic antidepressants may increase the risk of arrhythmias and sudden death,[88] but this seems unlikely except in the case of overdoses.[85,89] The Boston Collaborative Drug Surveillance Program found no evidence that tricyclic antidepressants caused arrhythmias or sudden death.[90] Recent reports indicate that imipramine may even be antiarrhythmic in depressed patients,[86,88] and studies on Purkinje's fibers in vitro indicate a membrane-stabilizing effect similar to that of some other antiarrhythmic drugs.[91] Although higher degrees of heart block may develop in an occasional patient with preexisting bundle-branch block who is treated with antidepressants,[92] such medications are usually quite safe even in elderly patients with heart disease, if used at recommended dosages.

Orthostatic hypotension is a common side effect of such antidepressants in elderly patients, particularly if there is any evidence of the condition before therapy.[85,92-95] Traumatic falls, myocardial infarction, and cerebrovascular events result more frequently from such hypotension in the elderly. Nortriptyline and desipramine tend to cause fewer hypotensive episodes than other tricyclics.[93]

The anticholinergic effects of tricyclic antidepressants are responsible in the elderly for changes in mentation (including delirium), impaired visual accommodation, delayed gastric emptying, urinary retention, and decreased sweating and hyperthermic reactions.[96,97] The latter may pose a special problem for patients with dementia or stroke, who may be less attentive to thirst. These medications may also cause sexual dysfunctions, which may frequently be overlooked or discounted in elderly persons.[98,99]

The antidepressants differ in their side-effect profile (Table 4). Amitriptyline is the most anticholinergic drug in this class, and desipramine the least. Amitriptyline and doxepin are the most sedating of these drugs — a property that may decrease the general energy level and libido. Desipramine and doxepin are reported to have a low incidence of cardiovascular effects. However, some of the studies with doxepin may have been conducted in patients with plasma levels inadequate for antidepressant effects.[94] Maprotiline is a tetracyclic antidepressant that has a low incidence of cardiovascular side effects but shares anticholinergic and sedative effects with the tricyclic drugs.[80,87] Amoxapine may have a more rapid onset of action than some other tricyclic antidepressants.[81] However, it is more anticholinergic and sedating than desipramine. In addition, since its 7-hydroxy metabolite has dopamine-receptor blocking activity similar to that of antipsychotic drugs, it may cause extrapyramidal symptoms, amenorrhea, or galactorrhea. It is not yet known whether it also causes tardive dyskinesia. Trazodone, a new antidepressant, has virtually no anticholinergic side effects but may cause cardiac toxicity in patients with preexisting cardiac disease.

Tricyclic antidepressants may inhibit the metabolism of neuroleptic agents, just as the neuroleptics may inhibit the metabolism of tricyclics.[100] Therefore, special care should be taken when both types of drugs are used concomitantly, especially in the initial treatment of an agitated depression in the elderly. Tricyclic antidepressants and chlorpromazine can also antagonize the action of guanethidine.[101]

At least two of the antidepressants from Table 4 should generally be tried before other classes of antidepressants are considered. The tertiary-amine tricyclic antidepressants amitriptyline and imipramine may be effective in the elderly, but because of their anticholinergic and sedative properties, it may be preferable to use their dealkylated metabolites, the secondary amines (i.e., nortriptyline and desipramine, respectively). If the patient has responded favorably to an antidepressant in the past, that agent should be the first drug used. Such treatment should last at least three to four weeks in the elderly at a dosage adequate to produce either some therapeutic effects or persistent side effects. However, if such trials do not produce a good therapeutic response or if bothersome side effects persist, a monoamine oxidase inhibitor should be considered. Monoamine oxidase inhibitors are probably under-prescribed in the United States. They may be especially effective for patients with "atypical" depressions — that is, patients with depressed mood who do not have the vegetative symptoms of a major depression. However, because of the dietary and drug restrictions required during their use and the increased risk associated with hypertensive episodes in the elderly, they must be used judiciously.[102]

Methylphenidate has been found to be effective as an antidepressant in some elderly patients.[103] However, it is usually recommended as the drug of choice only for patients who are unable to tolerate a tricyclic or tetracyclic antidepressant or monoamine oxidase inhibitor, who refuse electroconvulsive therapy, or who have a medical illness that contraindicates the use of these approaches. A low dosage, such as 10 mg twice a day, may then be considered. Methylphenidate has the advantage of a rapid therapeutic response when compared with other antidepressant therapies. However, it may produce adverse effects that are poorly tolerated by the elderly, including anorexia, insomnia, palpitations, and rebound depression if the dosage is decreased or stopped. The combination of methylphenidate and an antidepressant may produce a hypertensive crisis. In addition, methylphenidate may impair the metabolism of other drugs through inhibition of the hepatic microsomal enzymes.[104]

As an alternative to the treatment of depression in the elderly with drugs, electroconvulsive therapy is often the most effective and safest form of treatment.[66] When it is applied unilaterally to the nondominant hemisphere with the assistance of an anesthesiologist skilled in the procedure, electroconvulsive therapy produces relatively few side effects.

Antipsychotic Agents

Antipsychotic medications are indicated to treat chronic schizophrenia and psychotic paranoid states (i.e., the paraphrenias) in the elderly. Neuroleptic drugs are also useful in the treatment of manic-depressive disorders and, in combination with an antidepressant, in the treatment of agitated depression. In low doses they are useful for the management of the agitation and confusion of delirium and dementia. The elderly may be more susceptible to the effects of a given dose of chlorpromazine, since oral therapy with that drug results in higher plasma levels in the elderly.[105]

TABLE 5. Selected Antipsychotics: Pharmacologic Factors of Special Relevance for the Elderly.

Agent	Relative Potency *	Predominant Side Effects	Usual Initial Daily Dose for the Elderly
Chlorpromazine	100	Sedating, anti-cholinergic	10–25 mg twice or three times a day
Thioridazine	95–100	Sedating, anti-cholinergic	10–25 mg twice or three times a day
Thiothixene	5	Extrapyramidal	2–3 mg
Haloperidol	2	Extrapyramidal	0.5–2 mg
Fluphenazine	2	Extrapyramidal	0.5–2 mg

*Chlorpromizine was arbitrarily assigned a potency of 100, for the sake of comparison with other agents.

These agents are equal in therapeutic efficacy if prescribed in dosages of equivalent potency (Table 5).[106] However, the side-effect profile varies with potency. The relatively more potent agents, especially haloperidol and fluphenazine, cause the highest incidence of side effects in the extrapyramidal system, including pseudo-Parkinsonism, akathisias, and dystonias.[106] Because of age-related changes in the central nervous system, the elderly are more prone to have extrapyramidal symptoms of the pseudo-Parkinsonian type,[107] but they are less likely to have dystonias than younger patients. The immediate management of such effects should involve tapering the dosage or discontinuing the drug if possible and using an anticholinergic medication. However, long-term use of anticholinergic medications in this manner is not recommended, since it may increase the risk for tardive dyskinesia[108] and cause other anticholinergic side effects, including delirium.

Tardive dyskinesia may be medically and socially debilitating. Changes in the central nervous system associated with aging increase the risk of tardive dyskinesia, even when neuroleptic doses are small and treatment periods are brief. Patients with early development of other types of extrapyramidal symptoms, such as akathisias or pseudo-Parkinsonism, may also be more likely to acquire tardive dyskinesia.[108] Therefore, it may be wise to use a neuroleptic with a lower potency, such as chlorpromazine or thioridazine, in patients with extrapyramidal side effects. Thioridazine has the lowest incidence of extrapyramidal symptoms and may cause the least dopaminergic blockade in the striatum. If so, it may decrease the risk of tardive dyskinesia or slow its rate of progression in some patients.[109]

The increased incidence of tardive dyskinesia in the elderly underscores the importance of prescribing antipsychotic medications in the smallest effective dose. Other precautionary measures that may reduce the risk of tardive dyskinesia include periodic attempts to taper the dosage, drug holidays for as long as possible, and discontinuation of the drug when possible. These drugs should be discontinued if there is no clear-cut evidence of continuing therapeutic effects. It should also be remembered that there is a 1 to 2 per cent incidence of dyskinesias due to other causes in the elderly.

The least potent antipsychotics (chlorpromazine and thioridazine) tend to be the most sedating and to have the most anticholinergic effects. Therefore, the use of such drugs in combination with an antidepressant that also has high anticholinergic activity may cause toxic anticholinergic reactions, including delirium.[110] Autonomic side effects are also relatively frequent with the less potent neuroleptics, and the resultant hypotensive episodes may predispose to falls, myocardial infarction, or cerebrovascular accidents.

In the elderly patient even the incidence of rare side effects of antipsychotic medications is increased. Skin photosensitivity, most common with chlorpromazine, may develop in about 3 per cent of elderly patients[111] and may signal pigmentary retinopathy. In such cases the neuroleptic should be changed. Dosages of thioridazine as high as 800 mg per day are rarely needed in the older patient, but that dosage should not be exceeded in any patient because of the risk of diminution of visual acuity, brownish coloration of vision, and impairment of night vision due to pigmentary retinopathy.

Agranulocytosis is the most important hematologic side effect of these medications. The overall frequency of this complication is rare (0.1 per cent); the incidence is highest in elderly white women.[112] This syndrome usually develops within the first few months of treatment and usually responds to discontinuing or switching the drug. Therefore, elderly patients taking neuroleptics for long periods should be educated to be alert for persistent pharyngitis, fever, poor wound healing, and other symptoms of leukopenia. Abnormal results of liver-function tests secondary to these agents and chlorpromazine-induced jaundice (seldom seen in recent years) are usually self-limited and respond to discontinuing the drug. Liver disease does not seem to predispose to these side effects.[113]

Lithium Carbonate

Lithium is therapeutic and to some degree prophylactic for manic episodes associated with manic-depressive illness, which often continue into the elderly years. Its mechanism of action may involve modulation of transmembrane movement of calcium.[114] It is often used in combination with an antipsychotic medication in the short-term management of manic conditions, but it may decrease the plasma levels of chlorpromazine.[115] Other conditions that can mimic mania, such as schizophrenia, paranoia, delirium, and drug toxicity, occur much more frequently in the elderly than actual manic-depressive illness and should be carefully ruled out before lithium is begun. Lithium may also be combined with an antidepressant or, rarely, with a monoamine oxidase inhibitor in a manic-depressive elderly patient who is acutely depressed.

Since lithium is excreted through the kidney, renal function (serum creatinine, blood-urea nitrogen, and creatinine clearance) should be assessed before lithium is prescribed. Lithium clearance tends to decrease with aging and is correlated with creatinine clearance.[51,116,117] The half-life of lithium in younger patients is usually 18 to 30 hours, whereas in the elderly it may increase to 36 hours.[118] Therefore, a decrease in dosage of 50 per cent or more may be necessary for older patients.[51] Lithium may produce nephrotoxicity, including focal atrophy and interstitial fibrosis, cause decreased creatinine clearance, and lead to nephrogenic diabetes insipidus.[119,120] If such damage occurs, it is usually gradual and rarely causes severe azotemia.

Because of changes in the central nervous system associated with aging, the elderly are much more susceptible than younger patients to neurologic toxicity secondary to lithium. Determinations of serum lithium levels should generally be made monthly and more frequently if toxic symptoms appear. The most common symptoms of lithium toxicity in the elderly include tremors, indigestion, nausea, abdominal pain, and frequent stools.[121] Toxicity may progress to slurred speech, symptoms of the cerebellar or cranial nerves, confusion, delirium, and coma.[117]

Volume depletion secondary to dietary sodium restriction, sweat loss, decreased intake of water, or diuretic treatment that leads to sodium depletion will cause retention of lithium and increase the serum lithium concentration and the likelihood of toxicity.[120,122-125] Lithium and sodium are reabsorbed in a similar manner in the proximal renal tubules. Therefore, physicians should regularly monitor the lithium level of patients who are being treated with diuretics that may cause sodium depletion (e.g., furosemide, ethacrynic acid, and the thiazides).[116,123] Toxicity may also be provoked by methyldopa or indomethacin, which reduce renal clearance of lithium.[124]

Tests of thyroid function should be performed before treatment with lithium and should probably be repeated every six months to one year in elderly patients who are taking lithium. Because of decreasing thyroid function with age, the elderly are more prone than younger patients to the induction of a goiter and clinical hypothyroidism in response to lithium, and the symptoms and signs of hypothyroidism may be more difficult to recognize than in younger patients.

Electrocardiography should be performed before lithium treatment is begun and periodically thereafter. If serum levels are kept within the therapeutic range, serious cardiac toxicity from lithium is rare. However, T-wave flattening and inversion on the electrocardiogram in response to lithium are not uncommon.

Lithium may also interfere with the euphoria produced by the use of opiate drugs.[125] This interference may both decrease the "high" of opiate usage and, in the therapeutic setting, diminish the desired analgesic response to an administered narcotic.

| Conclusions

As a group, the elderly have the highest incidence of medical and psychiatric disorders and therefore require more medications than younger patients. Because of the physiologic age-related changes in the distribution and elimination of drugs and in sensitivity to medications, adverse side effects develop frequently in the elderly. Therefore, dosages and dosage intervals must be adjusted carefully. In addition, since the elderly often take multiple medications, they frequently have adverse drug interactions. Psychotropic drugs are often involved in such interactions and cause twice the incidence of side effects in elderly patients as in younger patients.

Careful screening should identify the elderly patients who are at the highest risk for such effects. In recent years our knowledge has greatly advanced regarding the guidelines to be followed and the special precautions to be taken in the use of psychotropic medications in the elderly. Physicians should be aware that decreased dosages and increased monitoring for side effects are usually indicated when these medications are prescribed for elderly patients.

All classes of psychotropic medications should be used with well-defined therapeutic goals and in the smallest effective doses, and their use should be reassessed on a regular basis. Attempts should be made to taper these medications periodically, and they should be continued only if therapeutic benefit is clearly evident. In elderly patients the side effects of psychotropic medications often compound the primary disorder for which the medication is being prescribed or are as debilitating as that disorder.

We are indebted to Drs. Robert Freedman and Robert W. Piepho of the University of Colorado and to Dr. Robert E. Vestal of the University of Washington for their helpful comments on this paper.

References

1. Vestal RE. Drug use in the elderly: a review of problems and special considerations. Drugs 1978; 16:358-82.
2. Kovar MG. Health of the elderly and use of health services. Public Health Rep 1977; 92:9-19.
3. Butler RN. Why survive? Being old in America. New York: Harper & Row, 1975:198-200.
4. Lamy PP. Prescribing for the elderly. Littleton, Mass.: PSG Publishing, 1980.
5. Williamson J, Chopin JM. Adverse reactions to prescribed drugs in the elderly: a multicentre investigation. Age Ageing. 1980; 9:73-80.
6. Kalchthaler T, Coccaro E, Lichtiger S. Incidence of polypharmacy in a long-term care facility. J Am Geriatr Soc 1977; 25:308-13.
7. Guttmann D. Patterns of legal drug use by older Americans. Addict Dis 1977; 3:337-56.
8. Parry HJ, Balter MB, Mellinger GD, Cisin IH, Manheimer DI. National patterns of psychotherapeutic drug use. Arch Gen Psychiatry 1973; 28:769-83.
9. Chien CP, Townsend EJ, Ross-Townsend A. Substance use and abuse among the community elderly: the medical aspect. Addict Dis 1978; 3:357-72.
10. Feigenbaum EM. Ambulatory treatment of the elderly. In: Busse EW, Pfeiffer E, eds. Mental illness in later life. Washington, D.C.: American Psychiatric Association, 1973:153-66.
11. Ford CV, Sbordone RJ. Attitudes of psychiatrists toward elderly patients. Am J Psychiatry 1980; 137:571-5.
12. Salzman C, Shader RI. Clinical evaluation of depression in the elderly. In: Raskin A, Jarvik LF, eds. Psychiatric symptoms and cognitive loss in the elderly: evaluation and assessment techniques. Washington, D.C.: Hemisphere Publishing, 1979:39-72.
13. Brocklehurst JC, Carty MH, Leeming JT, Robinson JM. Medical screening of old people accepted for residential care. Lancet 1978; 2:141-2.
14. Williams TF, Hill JG, Fairbank ME, Knox KG. Appropriate placement of the chronically ill and aged: a successful approach by evaluation. JAMA 1973; 226:1332-5.
15. Klotz U, Avant GR, Hoyumpa A, Schenker S, Wilkinson GR. The effects of age and liver disease on the disposition and elimination of diazepam in adult man. J Clin Invest 1975; 55:347-59.
16. Castleden CM, George CF, Marcer D, Hallet C. Increased sensitivity to nitrazepam in old age. Br Med J 1977; 1:10-2.
17. Greenblatt DJ, Allen MD, Shader RI. Toxicity of high-dose flurazepam in the elderly. Clin Pharmacol Ther 1977; 21:355-61.
18. Butler RN. Psychiatry and the elderly: an overview. Am J Psychiatry 1975; 132:893-900.
19. Hicks R, Dysken MW, Davis JM, Lesser J, Ripeckyj A, Lazarus L. The pharmaco-kinetics of psychotropic medication in the elderly: a review. J Clin Psychiatry 1981; 42:374-85.

20. Ouslander JG. Drug therapy in the elderly. Ann Intern Med 1981; 95:711-22.

21. Salzman C. A primer on geriatric psychopharmacology. Am J Psychiatry 1982; 139:67-74.

22. Triggs EJ, Nation RL. Pharmacokinetics in the aged: a review. J Pharmacokinet Biopharm 1975; 3:387-418.

23. Lipton MA, Jobson KO. Psychopharmacology. In: Usdin G, Lewis JM, eds. Psychiatry in general medical practice. New York: McGraw-Hill, 1979:613-6.

24. O'Malley K, Laher M, Cusack B, Kelly JG. Clinical pharmacology and the elderly patient. In: Denham MJ, ed. The treatment of medical problems in the elderly. Baltimore: University Park Press, 1980:7-9.

25. Bender AD. The effect of increasing age on the distribution of peripheral blood flow in man. J Am Geriatr Soc 1965; 13:192-8.

26. Vestal RE, Wood AJJ, Branch RA, Shand DG, Wilkinson GR. Effects of age and cigarette smoking on propranolol disposition. Clin Pharmacol Ther 1979; 26:8-15.

27. Rowe JW, Andres R, Tobin JD, Norris AH, Shock NW. The effect of age on creatinine clearance in men: a cross-sectional and longitudinal study. J Gerontol 1976; 31:155-63.

28. Greenblatt DJ, Sellers EM, Shader RI. Drug disposition in old age. N Engl J Med 1982; 306:1081-8.

29. Cusack B, Kelly J, O'Malley K, Noel J, Lavan J, Horgan J. Digoxin in the elderly: pharmacokinetic consequences of old age. Clin Pharmacol Ther 1979; 25:772-6.

30. Norris AH, Lundy T, Shock NW. Trends in selected indices of body composition in men between the ages of 30 and 80 years. Ann NY Acad Sci 1963; 110:623-39.

31. Crooks J, O'Malley K, Stevenson IH. Pharmacokinetics in the elderly. Clin Pharmacokinet 1976; 1:280-96.

32. Garattini S, Marucci F, Morselli PL, Mussini E. The significance of measuring blood levels of benzodiazepines. In: Davies DS, Prichard BNC, eds. Biological effects of drugs in relation to their plasma concentrations. Baltimore: University Park Press, 1973:211-25.

33. Shader RI, Greenblatt DJ, Harmatz JS, Franke K, Koch-Weser J. Absorption and disposition of chlordiazepoxide of young and elderly male volunteers. J Clin Pharmacol 1977; 17:709-18.

34. Novak LP. Aging, total body potassium, fat-free mass, and cell mass in males and females between ages 18 and 85 years. J Gerontol 1972; 27:438-43.

35. Forbes GB, Reina AJC. Adult lean body mass declines with age: some longitudinal observations. Metabolism 1970; 19:653-63.

36. Wallace S, Whiting B, Runcie J. Factors affecting drug binding in plasma of elderly patients. Br J Clin Pharmacol 1976; 3:327-30.

37. Hayes MJ, Langman MJS, Short AH. Changes in drug metabolism with increasing age: 1. Warfarin binding and plasma proteins. Br J Clin Pharmacol 1975; 2:69-72.

38. Misra DP, Loudon JM, Staddon GE. Albumin metabolism in elderly patients. J Gerontol 1975; 30:304-6.

39. Shader RI, Greenblatt DJ. Pharmacokinetics and clinical drug effects in the elderly. Psychopharmacol Bull 1979; 15(2):8-14.

40. Vestal RE, Wood AJJ. Influence of age and smoking on drug kinetics in man: studies using model compounds. Clin Pharmacokinet 1980; 5:309-19.

41. Schuckit MA, Morrissey ER, O'Leary MR. Alcohol problems in elderly men and women. Addict Dis 1978; 3:405-16.

42. Nies AS. Drug interactions. Med Clin North Am 1974; 58:965-75.

43. Special Committee on Aging, United States Senate. Nursing home care in the United States: failure in public policy. Washington, D.C.: Government Printing Office, 1974.

44. Atkinson L, Gibson I, Andrews J. An investigation into the ability of elderly patients continuing to take prescribed drugs after discharge from hospital and recommendations concerning improving the situation. Gerontology 1978; 24:225-34.

45. Wandless I, Davie JW. Can drug compliance in the elderly be improved? Br Med J 1977; 1:359-61.

46. Shader RI. Problems of polypharmacy in depression. Dis Nerv Syst 1976; 37(3: Section 2):30-4.

47. Nitham CJ, Parkhurst YE, Sommers EB. Physicians' prescribing habits: effects of Medicare. JAMA 1971; 217:585-7.

48. Rowe JW, Andres R, Tobin JD, Norris AH, Shock NW. Age-adjusted standards for creatinine clearance. Ann Intern Med 1976; 84:567-9.

49. Kampmann J, Siesbaek-Nielsen K, Kristensen M, Mølholm-Hansen J. Rapid evaluation of creatinine clearance. Acta Med Scand 1974; 196:517-20.

50. Cockroft DW, Gault MH. Prediction of creatinine clearance from serum creatinine. Nephron 1976; 16:31-41.

51. Hewick DDS, Newbury PA, Hopwood S, Naylor G, Moody J. Age as a factor affecting lithium therapy. Br J Clin Pharmacol 1977; 4:201-5.

52. Nies A, Robinson DS, Friedman MJ, et al. Relationship between age and tricyclic antidepressant plasma levels. Am J Psychiatry 1977; 134:790-3.

53. Cohen S. A clinical appraisal of diazepam. Psychosomatics 1981; 22:761-9.

54. Kaplan SA, de Silva JAF, Jack ML, et al. Blood level profile in man following chronic oral administration of flurazepam hydrochloride. J Pharm Sci 1973;.62:1932-5.

55. Harvey SC. Hypnotics and sedatives. In: Gilman AG, Goodman LS, Gilman A, eds. The pharmacological basis of therapeutics. 6th ed. New York: Macmillan, 1980:342-75.

56. Datloff EH, ed. Drug news. Drug Ther Clin Ther 1981; 6:13.

57. Reidenberg MM, Levy M, Warner H, et al. Relationship between diazepam dose, plasma level, age, and central nervous system depression. Clin Pharmacol Ther 1978; 23:371-4.

58. Kales A, Kales JD. Sleep disorders: recent findings in the diagnosis and treatment of disturbed sleep. N Engl J Med 1974; 280:487-99.

59. Kenny D. How to avoid pitfalls with commonly used drugs. Drug Ther Clin Ther 1980; 5:96-106.

60. Wilkinson GR. Effects of aging on the disposition of benzodiazepines in human beings: binding and distribution considerations. In: Raskin A, Robinson DS, Levine J, eds. Age and the pharmacology of psychoactive drugs. New York: Elsevier, 1981:3-15.

61. Roberts RK, Wilkinson GR, Branch RA, Schenker S. Effects of age and parenchymal liver disease on the disposition and elimination of chlordiazepoxide (librium). Gastroenterology 1978; 75:479-85.

62. Shull HJ Jr, Wilkinson GR, Johnson R, Schenker S. Normal disposition of oxazepam in acute viral hepatitis and cirrhosis. Ann Intern Med 1976; 84:420-5.

63. Greenblatt DJ, Shader RI, Koch-Weser J. Pharmacokinetics in clinical medicine: oxazepam versus other benzodiazepines. Dis Nerv Syst 1975; 36(5: Section 2):6-13.

64. Kraus JW, Desmond PV, Marshall JP, Johnson RF, Schenker S, Wilkinson GR. Effects of aging and liver disease on disposition of lorazepam. Clin Pharmacol Ther 1978; 24:411-9.

65. Hughes JM. Failure to ejaculate with chlordiazepoxide. Am J Psychiatry 1964; 121:610-1.

66. Finlayson RE, Martin LM. Recognition and management of depression in the elderly. Mayo Clin Proc 1982; 57:115-20.

67. Merlis S, Koepke HH. The use of oxazepam in elderly patients. Dis Nerv Syst 1975; 36(5: Section 2):27-9.

68. Desmond PV, Patwardhan RV, Schenker S, Speeg KV Jr. Cimetidine impairs elimination of chlordiazepoxide (Librium) in man. Ann Intern Med 1980; 93:266-8.

69. MacLeod SM, Sellers EM, Giles HG, et al. Interaction of disulfiram with benzodiazepines. Clin Pharmacol Ther 1978; 24:583-9.

70. Klotz U, Reimann I. Influence of cimetidine on the pharmacokinetics of desmethyldiazepam and oxazepam. Eur J Clin Pharmacol 1980; 18:517-20.

71. Solomon F, White CC, Parron DL, Mendelson WB. Sleeping pills, insomnia and medical practice. N Engl J Med 1979; 300:803-8.

72. Dement W, Guilleminautt C. Sleep apnea syndromes. New York: Alan R Liss, 1978:1-93.

73. Greenblatt DJ, Shader RI. Pharmacokinetic understanding of antianxiety drug therapy. South Med J 1978; 71: Suppl 2:2-9.

74. Clinical depression of the central nervous system due to diazepam and chlordiazepoxide in relation to cigarette smoking and age: a report from the Boston Collaborative Drug Surveillance Program, Boston University Medical Center. N Engl J Med 1973; 288:277-80.

75. Greenblatt DJ, Miller RR. Rational use of psychotropic drugs. I. Hypnotics. Am J Hosp Pharm 1974; 31:990-5.

76. Frederick CJ. Current trends in suicidal behavior in the United States. Am J Psychotherapy 1978; 32:172-200.

77. Johnson DAW. Drug-induced psychiatric disorders. Drugs 1981; 22:57-69.

78. Wells CE. Chronic brain disease: an overview. Am J Psychiatry 1978; 135:1-12.

79. Gershon S, Newton R. Lack of anticholinergic side effects with a new antidepressant — trazodone. J Clin Psychiatry 1980; 41:100-4.

80. Pinder RM, Brogden RN, Speight TM, Avery GS. Maprotiline: a review of its pharmacological properties and therapeutic efficacy in mental depressive states. Drugs 1977; 13:321-52.

81. Hekimian LT, Friedhoff AJ, Deever E. A comparison of the onset of action and therapeutic efficacy of amoxapine and amitriptyline. J Clin Psychiatry 1978; 39:633-7.

82. Hollister LE. Treatment of depression with drugs. Ann Intern Med 1978; 89:78-84.

83. Kalin NH, Risch SC, Janowsky DS, Murphy DL. Use of the dexamethasone suppression test in clinical psychiatry. J Clin Psychopharmacol 1981; 1:64-9.

84. Maas JW. Biogenic amines and depression: biochemical and pharmacological separation of two types of depression. Arch Gen Psychiatry 1975; 32:1357-61.

85. Kantor SJ, Glassman AH, Bigger JT Jr, Perel JM, Giardina EV. The cardiac effects of therapeutic plasma concentrations of imipramine. Am J Psychiatry 1978; 135:534-8.

86. Giardina E-GV, Bigger JT Jr, Glassman AH, Perel JM, Kantor SJ. The electrocardiographic and and antiarrhythmic effects of imipramine hydrochloride at therapeutic plasma concentrations. Circulation 1979; 60:1045-52.

87. Burckhardt D, Raeder E, Müller V, Imhof P, Neubauer H. Cardiovascular effects of tricyclic and tetracyclic antidepressants. JAMA 1978; 239:213-6.

88. Moir DC, Crooks J, Cornwell WB, et al. Cardiotoxicity of amitriptyline. Lancet 1972; 2:561-4.

89. Veith RC, Raskind MA, Caldwell JH, Barnes RF, Gumbrecht G, Ritchie JL. Cardiovascular effects of tricyclic antidepressants in depressed patients with chronic heart disease. N Engl J Med 1982; 306:954-9.

90. Adverse reactions to the tricyclic-antidepressant drugs: report from Boston Collaborative Drug Surveillance Program. Lancet 1972; 1:529-31.

91. Rawling DA, Fozzard HA. Effects of imipramine on cellular electrophysiological properties of cardiac Purkinje fibers. J Pharmacol Exp Ther 1979; 209:371-5.

92. Bigger JT Jr, Kantor SJ, Glassman AH, Perel JM. Cardiovascular effects of tricyclic antidepressant drugs. In: Lipton MA, Dimascio A, Killiam KF, eds. Psychopharmacology: a generation of progress. New York: Raven Press, 1978:1033-46.

93. Roose SP, Glassman AH, Siris SG, Walsh BT, Bruno RL, Wright LB. Comparison of imipramine- and nortriptyline-induced orthostatic hypotension: a meaningful difference. J Clin Psychopharmacol 1981; 1:316-21.

94. Vohra J, Burrows GD, Sloman G. Assessment of cardiovascular side effects of therapeutic doses of tricyclic anti-depressant drugs. Aust NZ J Med 1975; 5:7-11.

95. Hayes JR, Born GF, Rosenbaum AH. Incidence of orthostatic hypotension in patients with primary affective disorders treated with tricyclic antidepressants. Mayo Clin Proc 1977; 52:509-12.

96. Morgan JP, Rivera-Calimlim L, Messiha F, Sundaresan PR, Trabert N. Imipramine-mediated interference with levodopa absorption from the gastrointestinal tract in man. Neurology (Minneap) 1975; 25:1029-34.

97. Consolo S, Morselli PL, Zaccala M, Garattini S. Delayed absorption of phenylbutazone caused by desmethylimipramine in humans. Eur J Pharmacol 1970; 10:239-42.

98. Nininger JE. Inhibition of ejaculation by amitriptyline. Am J Psychiatry 1978; 135:750-1.

99. Greenberg HR. Erectile impotence during the course of Tofrānil therapy. Am J Psychiatry 1965; 121:1021.

100. El-Yousef MK, Manier DH. Tricyclic antidepressants and phenothiazines. JAMA 1974; 229:1419.

101. Woosley RL, Nies AS. Guanethidine. N Engl J Med 1976; 295:1053-7.

102. Baldessarini RJ. Chemotherapy in psychiatry. Cambridge, Mass.: Harvard University Press, 1977:103-12.

103. Katon W, Raskind M. Treatment of depression in the medically ill elderly with methylphenidate. Am J Psychiatry 1980; 137:963-5.

104. Davis JM, Sekerke J, Janowsky DS. Drug interactions involving the drugs of abuse. Drug Interact Clin Pharmacol 1974; 8:12-41.

105. Rivera-Calimlim L, Nasrallah H, Gift T, Kerzner B, Griesbach PH, Wyatt RJ. Plasma levels of chlorpromazine: effect of age, chronicity of disease, and duration of treatment. Clin Pharmacol Ther 1977; 21:115-6. abstract.

106. Thompson TL II. Psychosocial and psychiatric problems in the aged. In: Schrier RW, ed. Clinical internal medicine in the aged. Philadelphia: WB Saunders, 1982:29-40.

107. Hamilton LD. Aged brain and the phenothiazines. Geriatrics 1966; 21(5):131-8.

108. Task Force on Late Neurological Effects of Antipsychotic Drugs. Tardive dyskinesia: summary of a task force report of the American Psychiatric Association. Am J Psychiatry 1980; 137:1163-72.

109. Klawans HL, Goetz CG, Perlik S. Tardive dyskinesia: review and update. Am J Psychiatry 1980; 137:900-8.

110. Hall RCW, Feinsilver DL, Holt RE. Anticholinergic psychosis: differential diagnosis and management. Psychosomatics 1981; 22:581-7.

111. Salzman C, van der Kolk B, Shader RI. Psychopharmacology and the geriatric patient. In: Shader RI, ed. Manual of psychiatric therapeutics: practical psychopharmacology and psychiatry. Boston: Little, Brown, 1975:171-84.

112. Shader RI, Jackson AH. Approaches to schizophrenia. In: Shader RI, ed. Manual of psychiatric therapeutics: practical psychopharmacology and psychiatry. Boston: Little, Brown, 1975:63-100.

113. Maxwell JD, Carrella M, Parkes JD, Williams R, Mould GP, Curry SH. Plasma disappearance and cerebral effects of chlorpromazine in cirrhosis. Clin Sci 1972; 43:143-51.

114. Carman JS, Wyatt RJ. Calcium: bivalent cation in the bivalent psychoses. Biol Psychiatry 1979; 14:295-336.

115. Kerzner B, Rivera-Calimlim L. Lithium and chlorpromazine (CPZ) interaction. Clin Pharmacol Ther 1976; 19:109. abstract.

116. Jefferson JW, Greist JH. Lithium and the kidney. In: Davis JM, Greenblatt DJ, eds. Psychopharmacology update: new and neglected areas. New York: Grune and Stratton, 1979:81-104.

117. Davis JM, Fann WE, El-Yousef MK, Janowsky DS. Clinical problems in treating the aged with psychotropic drugs. In: Eisdorfer C, Fann WE, eds. Psychopharmacology and aging. New York: Plenum Press, 1973:111-25.

118. Schou M. Lithium in psychiatric therapy and prophylaxis. J Psychiatr Res 1968; 6:67-95.

119. Hestbech J, Hansen HE, Amdisen A, Olsen S. Chronic renal lesions following long-term treatment with lithium. Kidney Int 1977; 12:205-13.

120. Burrow GD, Davies B, Kincaid-Smith P. Unique tubular lesion after lithium. Lancet 1978; 1:1310.

121. van der Velde CD. Toxicity of lithium carbonate in elderly patients. Am J Psychiatry 1971; 127:1075-7.

122. Israili ZH. Age-related change in the pharmacokinetics of some psychotropic drugs and its clinical implications. In: Nandy K, ed. Geriatric psychopharmacology. New York: Elsevier/North-Holland, 1979:31-62.

123. Himmelhoch J, Poust RI, Mallinger AG, Hanin I, Neil JF. Adjustment of lithium dose during lithium-chlorthiazide therapy. Clin Pharmacol Ther 1977; 22:225-7.

124. Ayd F. Broadening the clinical uses of lithium: coadministering lithium and thiazide diuretics. Int Drug Ther Newslett 1977; 12:25-7.

125. Jefferson JW, Greist JN. Primer of lithium therapy. Baltimore: Williams & Wilkins, 1977:46-8.

Correspondence

Caution in the Use of Drugs in the Elderly*

To the Editor:

In their article on psychotropic drug use in the elderly, Thompson et al. (Jan. 27 issue)† emphasize the reduced clearance of antidepressant drugs in the elderly and recommend low initial doses. However, they do not address the problem of underdosage.

Antidepressant pharmacokinetics show great interindividual variation, and it is not uncommon to see elderly patients who have inadequate serum levels of tricyclic antidepressants while they are taking conventional adult dosages, let alone the reduced dosages recommended for the elderly. For example, a 68-year-old woman treated recently for retarded depression had no response to 250 mg of desipramine per day but had a complete response to 400 mg per day. The desipramine blood level was 83 ng per milliliter with the former dose and 225 ng per milliliter with the latter dose. If dosages are increased in small, infrequent increments, it may take some patients many weeks to reach an adequate level of medication, during which time they may have serious morbidity. In the outpatient setting, adequate levels may never be reached, because the patient may give up or the doctor, observing the lack of response, may switch drugs.

The optimal care of seriously depressed elderly patients is best accomplished with frequent clinical reassessment and judicious consideration of blood levels of antidepressants. Moreover, respect for their pharmacokinetic variability should be added to the list of our senior citizens' rights.

Barry S. Fogel, M.D.
Rhode Island Hospital
Providence, RI 02902

To the Editor:

In their review of psychotropic drug use in the elderly, Thompson et al. (Jan. 20 issue),[1] discussed the increased sensitivity of geriatric patients to benzodiazepines.

We recently completed a study of diazepam's effects on memory and psychomotor performance in 12 normal geriatric volunteers (7 men and 5 women; mean age, 70.4 years; range, 60 to 77) who were free of serious medical or psychiatric illness as determined by physical examination, psychiatric interview, and routine laboratory tests. Neuropsychologic screening was also done to exclude the presence of cognitive impairment.

In separate sessions, these subjects received doses of 2.5 mg of diazepam, 5.0 mg of diazepam, and placebo under double-blind conditions. In a fourth

*Originally published on June 30, 1983 (308:1600-1601).

†Thompson TL II, Moran MG, Nies AS. Psychotropic drug use in the elderly (second of two parts). N Engl J Med 1983; 308:194-9.

session, they received 10 mg of diazepam. At base line and at one and three hours after the drug, immediate and delayed recall were assessed on the Buschke selective-reminding task[2] (a multiple-trial verbal free-recall task) and on a single-trial visual-memory task. Digit span/supraspan, discriminant reaction time, and critical flicker fusion tasks were given as well.

Diazepam impaired memory in both immediate and delayed testing on the Buschke task and in delayed testing on the visual-memory task. Diazepam also slowed discriminant reaction time. The mean percentage changes in performance on these measures are shown in Table 1. The most striking finding was that performance in these tasks was markedly impaired at each dose level, including the lowest (2.5 mg). Most studies of the effects of diazepam on the performance of younger subjects have used doses of 5 to 20 mg or more.[3,4]

TABLE 1. Percentage Changes from Base-Line Performance after Diazepam.*

Task	Placebo		Diazepam					
			2.5 mg		5 mg		10 mg	
			hours after treatment					
	1	3	1	3	1	3	1	3
Buschke task, immediate recall	−4	−10	−15	−11	−17	−7	−29	−14
Buschke task, delayed recall	−5	−11	−20	−17	−23	−10	−35	−21
Visual memory, delayed recall	−4	−16	−29	−13	−32	−24	−44	−31
Discriminant reaction time †	−1	−3	+6	+3	+5	0	+13	+5

*Mean percentage changes from pretreatment base-line performance are shown for each dose and time of assessment. For all measures shown, changes in comparison to placebo were statistically significant for the 2.5-mg, 5-mg, and 10-mg doses analyzed individually and for all doses analyzed together ($P<0.05$ or less).

†Positive values indicate slowing performance.

As Thompson et al. emphasize, elderly patients with depression or mild or subclinical dementia may be at even greater risk of adverse effects. Since low doses of diazepam may impair memory and psychomotor skills, such as those required in driving or operating machinery, elderly persons should avoid even the lowest doses of these agents before engaging in such activities.

NUNZIO POMARA, M.D., BARBARA STANLEY, PH.D.,
ROBERT BLOCK, PH.D., JEANINE GUIDO, M.A.,
DEBORAH RUSS, B.S., AND MICHAEL STANLEY, PH.D.
Wayne State University School of Medicine
Detroit, MI 48207

1. Thompson TL II, Moran MG, Nies AS. Psychotropic drug use in the elderly (first of two parts). N Engl J Med 1983; 308:134-8.

2. Buschke H. Selective reminding for analysis of memory and learning. J Verb Learn Verb Behav 1973; 12:543-50.

3. Salzman C, Shader RI, Harmatz J, Robertson L. Psychopharmacologic investigations in elderly volunteers: effect of diazepam in males. J Am Geriatr Soc 1975; 23:451-7.

4. O'Hanlon JF, Haak TW, Blaauw GJ, Riemersma JBJ. Diazepam impairs lateral position control in highway driving. Science 1982; 217:79-81.

The above letters were referred to the authors of the article in question, who offer the following reply:

To the Editor:

We agree with Dr. Fogel's suggestion that the variable effects of drugs in the elderly should be carefully considered. We hoped to emphasize that point by placing it in the second paragraph of our article, stating, "[T]he normal variation in drug effects from one person to another is often accentuated in the elderly. . . . In fact, the elderly constitute the most diverse segment of the population . . . pharmacokinetically. Therefore . . . treatment must frequently be tailored to the individual for maximal efficacy."

We address the problem of underdosage in the general guidelines section of our paper, stating, "The dosage should be titrated gradually until the therapeutic goal is reached or until adverse side effects develop and persist to a degree that precludes further increases." However, we find "overdosage" of all types of psychotropic drugs a much more frequent problem for the elderly. The risks of multiple serious side effects due to unnecessarily large dosages of the tricyclic antidepressants in the elderly led us to devote twice the space to them as to any other class of psychotropic drug. In addition, side effects that develop must be carefully distinguished from somatic complaints associated with the underlying depressive illness.

Therefore, the cases Dr. Fogel presents are exceptions to the usual problem with elderly patients. Nevertheless, this subset of the "pharmacologically resistant" elderly should be recognized in order to ensure maximally effective treatment.

The results of the study by Dr. Pomara and colleagues clearly emphasize the increased sensitivity of normal elderly persons to benzodiazepines. More such clinical trials in the elderly are needed for all psychotropic drugs. It should be obvious that the conscientious physician who carefully follows package-insert instructions and uses quite small dosages of benzodiazepine may nevertheless be causing iatrogenous objective cognitive and psychomotor impairments in elderly patients. Their results undoubtedly would have been even more striking if the drug had been given to elderly patients who were medically or psychiatrically ill. In addition, it would be instructive to restudy such a group after a week or two of the typical multiple daily dosages of one of the benzodiazepines with a long half-life, when the drug had had time to accumulate in the patient's system.

TROY L. THOMPSON II, M.D.
MICHAEL G. MORAN, M.D.
ALAN S. NIES, M.D.
University of Colorado School of Medicine
Denver, CO 80262

Psychotropic Drug Use in the Elderly*

To the Editor:

While reading the article on psychotropic drug use in the elderly, Part 2, by Thompson et al. (Jan. 27, 1983, issue)[1] I found an error in Table 5 (page 196), which was not corrected in subsequent issues of the *Journal*.

In the second column, under "relative potency," chlorpromazine was arbitrarily assigned a potency of 100, as mentioned in the footnote, and the relative potency of the other compounds compared with chlorpromazine were: thioridazine, 95 to 100; thiothixene, 5; halperidol, 2; and fluphenazine, 2. One concludes from this comparison that chlorpromazine is the most potent antipsychotic and that haloperidol and fluphenazine are the least potent.

In fact, this is not correct. Haloperidol and fluphenazine are the most potent antipsychotic agents; they are about 50 times more potent than chlorpromazine in their antipsychotic action, on a milligram-for-milligram basis.[2-4] This is clearly shown in the article itself in line 13, second column, page 196, and in line 9, first column, page 197, and in the fourth column of the same table, where it is shown that equipotent doses of haloperidol are much smaller than those of chlorpromazine: 0.5 to 2 mg per day versus 10 to 25 mg two or three times a day, respectively.

So, I think that the numbers in the second column of Table 5, under "relative potency," should be corrected as follows:

Agent	Relative Potency
Chlorpromazine	2
Thioridazine	2–2.1
Thiothixene	40
Haloperidol	100
Fluphenazine	100

And the word "chlorpromazine" in the footnote should be changed to "haloperidol."

SUHAIL H. ZAVARO, M.D.
Miriam Hospital
Providence, RI 02906

*Originally published on March 7, 1985 (312:652)

1. Thompson TL II, Moran MG, Nies AS. Psychotropic drug use in the elderly. Part 2. N Engl J Med 1983; 308:194-9.
2. Gilman AG, Goodman LS, Gilman A, eds. The pharmacological basis of therapeutics. 6th ed. New York: Macmillan, 1980:408-10.
3. Kane RL, Ouslander JG, Abrass IB. Essentials of clinical geriatrics. New York: McGraw-Hill, 1984:279.
4. Salzman C. Clinical geriatric psychopharmacology. New York: McGraw-Hill, 1984:62.

The above letter was referred to the authors of the article in question, who offer the following reply:

To the Editor:

We thank Dr. Zavaro for his very careful reading of our paper and for calling to our attention possible confusion due to our use of the word "potency" in Table 5.

As he stated, the article does discuss in several places what was meant by the second column in Table 5, and the "usual initial daily dose" column supports those explanations. However, we understand how the heading "relative potency" might be misleading. A clearer heading might have been "milligrams equivalency," as used by other authors in making this point.*

Since most physicians tend to think in terms of the dosages that they prescribe instead of inverting them to calculate potency, we recommend changing our heading (as below) and leaving the numbers as they were in the table rather than leaving our heading and inverting the numbers, as Dr. Zavaro did.

Agent	Equivalency (in milligrams)
Chlorpromazine	100
Thioridazine	95–100
Thiothixene	5
Haloperidol	2
Fluphenazine	2

TROY L. THOMPSON II, M.D.
MICHAEL G. MORAN, M.D.
ALAN S. NIES, M.D.
University of Colorado School of Medicine
Denver, CO 80262

*Bernstein JG. Handbook of drug therapy in psychiatry. Littleton, Mass.: John Wright/PSG, 1983:54.

Rate-Controlled Drug Delivery

Peter Goldman, M.D.

T HE goal of pharmaceutical research is to find drugs with desirable therapeutic properties and low risks of undesirable side effects. Drugs with such high
therapeutic ratios are usually sought as new chemical entities — molecules designed to produce the desirable effects without the undesirable ones. However,
another method of achieving the goal of pharmaceutical research is through the
development of drug-delivery systems that achieve pharmacologic selectivity not
solely on the basis of chemical structure but also on the basis of pharmacokinetic
principles. Drug products achieving controlled rates of delivery offer one such
approach. A few of these are already available for clinical application, and more
can be expected in the future. The principles underlying such rate-controlled
delivery systems and some of their applications are the subject of this review.

Basic Principles

The relation between the amount of drug taken and the resultant beneficial or
adverse effect is best portrayed by the dose-response curve. Figure 1A shows this
relation for a typical drug. If the drug is digoxin, for example, the benefit may be
an increased cardiac output, whereas an undesirable or adverse side effect may be
an increased number of premature ventricular contractions. A dose high enough to
maximize the beneficial effect yet not high enough to provoke undesirable side
effects provides optimal therapy.

Obviously, the dose need not be rigidly stipulated when benefit and hazard
are widely separated in this dose-response formulation. A problem arises, however, in the case of a drug (such as digoxin) whose dose for optimal benefit may be
close to that producing adverse effects. Careful dosage adjustment is then required
to penetrate what has been termed a narrow therapeutic window. Adjusting the
dose to a desirable serum digoxin concentration is one strategy for penetrating this
window. The serum concentration is useful because at the steady state it reflects
the amount of drug in the body — a measure that is more indicative of the drug's
effect than is its dose.[1] Thus, one may portray the therapeutic problem by
referring to the serum drug concentration (Fig. 1B) rather than to the dose

From the Division of Clinical Pharmacology, Department of Pharmacology, Harvard Medical School,
the Charles A. Dana Research Institute, and the Harvard–Thorndike Laboratory, Department of
Medicine, Beth Israel Hospital, Boston.

Originally published on July 29, 1982 (307:286-290).

(Fig. 1A). In these terms, we seek a dose that will provide the drug concentration yielding the optimal compromise between beneficial and adverse effects. This concentration is represented by the dotted line in Figure 1B.

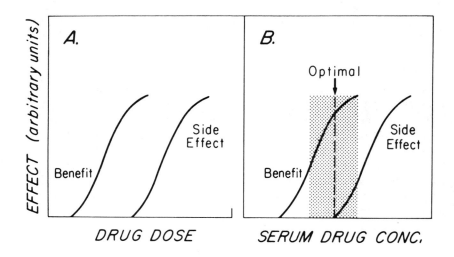

Figure 1. *Relation between Drug Dose (Panel A) or Serum Concentration (Panel B) and Both Benefits and Side Effects.*

Panel B indicates the optimal serum drug concentration by a dotted line and its variation during the dosage interval as a shaded area.

The optimal drug concentration is a theoretical concept, a goal that is not realizable in practice unless the dosage form maintains an invariant drug concentration throughout the dosage interval. Traditional dosage forms such as tablets, capsules, and elixirs do not do this. They inevitably provide a peak in the serum drug concentration after each dose and thus a series of peaks and valleys that correspond to the intervals between doses. Digoxin, for example, with a half-life of approximately 40 hours, will undergo a 30 per cent fluctuation in the amount of drug in the body when administered as a single daily tablet. This variation is inherent for any dosage form that does not release the drug to the systemic circulation at a constant rate.

The shaded area of Figure 1B represents these inevitable fluctuations in the amount of drug in the body, as reflected in the serum drug concentration during the dosage interval. These considerations suggest that a single daily dose of digoxin may provide a range of drug concentrations in cardiac muscle during the dosage interval that may vary between toxic and subtherapeutic values. That these variations may engender intervals of digoxin toxicity is suggested by a study that found transient cardiac arrhythmias in patients within a few hours of their daily dose of digoxin[2] — a time when pharmacokinetic considerations suggest that the concentration of digoxin in the myocardium is highest. Presumably, these manifestations of excess dosage would not occur if transient peaks in the body's digoxin level were avoided.

Clinical studies have shown that the various effects of a drug may be dissociated at different serum concentrations. Thus, the antihistaminic activity of diphenhydramine occurs at lower serum concentrations than its sedative effects.[3] Similarly, when drugs are administered so as to eliminate peaks, their beneficial effects may be separated from the undesirable ones. Postoperative pain, for example, was better controlled by low doses of morphine administered by intravenous infusion than by higher doses given intramuscularly.[4] This result was of particular interest for achieving optimal therapy, because patients receiving morphine by continuous infusion also had better respiratory function. Although diuretics are usually administered once a day, changes in the dosage schedule have been found to alter the pattern of urinary water and electrolyte excretion induced by furosemide[5] and the apparent potency of chlorothiazide.[6] Similarly, deferoxamine is more effective in removing iron from patients with siderosis when administered continuously.[7]

These examples tend to justify the prediction that clinically important differences in drug effects may arise from changes in dosage programs. More examples might be found if the drugs in our pharmacopeia were not already selected to meet standards of safety and efficacy even when administered by traditional dosage forms. Obviously, there is little incentive to undertake studies that might improve the performance of drugs that are already perceived to be satisfactory.

Rate-Controlled Release Systems

Pumps

The most familiar form of a controlled-release drug-delivery system is an intravenous infusion that is monitored by an infusion pump or drop counter. Such systems have become the standard means of administering a number of drugs, including lidocaine, nitroprusside, and dobutamine, to hospitalized patients. The system consists of the following elements: a drug reservoir (the drug solution in a bottle or bag), an energy source (gravity or a pump), a rate-controlling element (the pump or a drop counter), and the delivery portal (the intravenous needle or catheter). These elements external to the patient (including the bedside pole) constitute the drug-delivery platform.

Pumps and reservoirs, which are compact enough to be worn externally[8] or to be implanted under the skin,[9] are the basis for a platform that provides rate-controlled drug delivery for ambulatory patients. Thus far, only experimental studies have been conducted with these devices, but the results suggest that the administration of several well-known drugs by sustained infusion may increase their therapeutic benefits. The programmed infusion of insulin may offer a more reliable means of correcting the metabolic abnormalities of diabetes mellitus,[8, 10] whereas heparin may be more effective in preventing thrombosis[11] when administered by constant infusion. Pumps are also being used experimentally to perfuse selected sites such as the liver[12, 13] or the central nervous system[14] with cancer chemotherapeutic agents. The narrow therapeutic window characteristic of most of these drugs makes them particularly attractive for administration by rate-controlled methods either to the vasculature of specific organs or to the systemic circulation.

Transdermal Devices

Devices that provide rate-controlled administration of drugs by the transdermal route are a novel application of the principles discussed. One of these devices enables scopolamine to be adapted to the control of motion sickness. Tight control of the serum scopolamine concentration allows control of nausea with a tolerable frequency of minor adverse effects such as dry mouth and drowsiness and with only a rare instance of major reactions such as failure of accommodation, tachycardia, and hallucinations. The transdermal therapeutic system Transderm-V, which contains 1.5 mg of scopolamine and delivers 0.5 mg at a constant rate over a period of three days, significantly decreased motion sickness as compared with both placebo and a conventional dosage form of diphenhydramine. Although blurred vision and drowsiness were noted by some subjects, dry mouth was the only side effect reported to occur at a significantly greater frequency than in control subjects.[15]

The transdermal device used for scopolamine functions by permitting the drug, which is highly concentrated in a small reservoir, to diffuse through a dense or microporous rate-controlling membrane. The driving force for this system, the concentration gradient of drug across the membrane, is established by the difference between the concentration of drug in the reservoir and that outside the membrane. The rate of drug release is determined by the properties of the membrane and the difference in drug concentration across the membrane. It is assumed in calibrating these devices that the concentration of drug remains negligible between the microporous membrane and the skin. Thus, to ensure that drug delivery remains constant at the specified rate, the skin must be capable of removing the drug at a rate faster than that of its release from the device. For this reason it is important that the transdermal therapeutic system be placed at an appropriate skin site. Placement behind the ear is recommended for the scopolamine device because the skin there can absorb the drug at a rate considerably greater than that of its passage through the rate-controlling membrane. Thus, after a day in this position, the transdermal device provides the functional equivalent of scopolamine infused intravenously at a rate of approximately 5 μg per hour.[16]

Because nitroglycerin affects the tone of blood vessels in both venous and arterial circulations[17] with different dose-response relations,[18] it is theoretically possible to find a serum concentration at which the vascular changes responsible for adverse side effects are dissociated from those responsible for the beneficial decrease in cardiac work. Ordinarily it is difficult to maintain such a concentration, because nitroglycerin is rapidly metabolized by the liver and other tissues and thus has a half-life of only a few minutes.[19,20] On the other hand, nitroglycerin rapidly gains entry to the body when administered by the sublingual route. This combination of rapid absorption and rapid clearance permits the administration of a bolus of drug that is sufficient to abort an anginal attack.[19] Nitroglycerin administered in this way, however, is not suitable for anginal prophylaxis and furthermore is likely to cause hemodynamic changes responsible for side effects. These problems might be avoided if nitroglycerin were released at a constant rate to the systemic circulation.

A dependable form of administration of nitroglycerin by the oral route is not feasible because of a large first-pass effect. The liver can be bypassed, however, and the systemic circulation entered directly by nitroglycerin that is incorporated into a paste and applied to the skin. Although this dosage form provides sustained release, it is neither dependable nor convenient, and thus attention has turned to devices that provide controlled release of nitroglycerin by the transdermal route. These devices use the pharmaceutical principles discussed previously, or some variation of them, and provide nitroglycerin to the body at a constant rate and thus maintain a constant serum concentration.

Transdermal devices contain sufficient nitroglycerin to maintain delivery for 24 hours at a rate determined by the surface area either of the rate-controlling membrane or of the other means used to control drug release. Indeed, the relative "strengths" of the devices of various manufacturers are specified in terms of the surface area of the device. Only one device, the Transderm Nitro, also specifies that nitroglycerin is released at a rate of either 5 or 10 mg per 24 hours. Labeling in this manner is important because it emphasizes the concept of specifying dosage strength as a rate of drug release. The traditional prescription, on the other hand, specifies the amount of drug in the dosage form and leaves the matter of rate to be implied in the directions for taking the dosage form.

The failure to provide labeling of the rate of nitroglycerin delivery in all devices is unfortunate because it prevents the patient from interchanging the devices of various manufacturers. In any case, the appropriate device size is determined by successive application of devices with increasing rates of delivery until one is found that provides optimal control of anginal attacks with acceptable side effects. Efficacy may be ascertained either directly in terms of the number of attacks or indirectly in terms of the requirement for additional sublingual doses of nitroglycerin.

The administration of drugs by the transdermal route may find more applications in the future. A recent preliminary report, for example, indicates that the administration of clonidine by a rate-controlled transdermal device lowers the blood pressure to the same extent as the oral dosage form, but with fewer side effects.[21]

Local Delivery Systems

Systems have been developed to apply principles of rate-controlled release for the delivery of drugs to specific organs. These systems not only restrict the drug to the site where its effects are sought but may also enable the desirable effects to be accentuated within the site itself. This advantage is illustrated in the rate-controlled delivery of pilocarpine for the treatment of glaucoma. Although pilocarpine has the desirable effect of decreasing intraocular pressure, it also causes decreased visual activity as the result of miosis and myopia. That these side effects occur within the first hour after the administration of pilocarpine eye drops suggests that they are due to excessive pilocarpine. When administered at controlled rates, pilocarpine can effect a substantial lowering of intraocular pressure, with only minimal miosis and myopia.[22]

In many respects, the problems of adapting pilocarpine for the control of glaucoma poses challenges that are similar to those already discussed for the use of nitroglycerin in the prophylaxis of angina pectoris. Pilocarpine is rapidly cleared from the eye, not by metabolism but by the tear flow through the lacrimal duct. As a result, frequent administration is necessary to maintain an adequate drug concentration in the tear film. Frequent administration of eye drops is not only inconvenient but also causes wide swings in drug concentration that make it impossible to sustain the desired effects without incurring the undesirable ones.

Sustained drug release is provided by the Ocusert, a device that can be placed under the lower eyelid by the patient to release pilocarpine at a rate of either 20 or 40 μg per hour for one week. By maintaining a uniform concentration of pilocarpine in the tear film, it is possible to have sustained control of intraocular pressure with a lower incidence of side effects. Furthermore, these goals are achieved at a total dose of pilocarpine that is lower than that required when the drug is administered in the form of conventional eye drops. The use of less drug and the avoidance of bolus administration tend to diminish the possibility of systemic drug effects.

It may be desirable to administer other ophthalmic drugs by intraocular delivery systems in the future both to ensure constant local effects and to avoid the possibility of systemic side effects. One candidate for this technology may be the β-adrenergic blocker timolol, which in the form of eye drops provides effective control of intraocular pressure in glaucoma but may also provoke side effects such as asthma in susceptible patients.[23]

Rate-controlled delivery of progesterone from an intrauterine device (Progestasert) offers a method of birth control that limits the systemic effects of the hormone by confining its effects to the uterus. One of these intrauterine devices contains sufficient hormone to last one year, at which time it must be replaced.[24]

Oral Drug Delivery

Although the transdermal route has been used to administer drugs systematically in several of these early applications of rate-controlled delivery, this route of administration is impractical unless a drug is highly potent and the skin is readily permeable to it. Thus, it seems likely that in the future, as in the past, many drugs will still be administered by the oral route.

One way of smoothing out the peaks and valleys in the serum drug concentration that are caused by the usual oral drug preparations has been to formulate drugs into slow-release preparations. This application of the pharmacokinetic principles discussed here will be the topic of a future Drug Therapy article.

| The Future

A rate-controlled device resembling a tablet has been used experimentally to provide a constant rate of drug delivery within the gastrointestinal tract. The energy for drug release in this device is provided by the osmotic pressure that is obtained when water is absorbed through a membrane impermeable to the drug.[25] Drug is then released at a controlled rate through a small, calibrated orifice. When acetazolamide is administered by this device, there is moderation of the peaks and valleys of serum concentrations incurred with the usual tablet formulation.[26] This technology may therefore be useful for improving the therapeutic properties of drugs that rely on the gastrointestinal tract as a means of entry to the systemic circulation. Devices of this kind may also be designed that will permit drugs to be selectively released at specific sites within the gastrointestinal tract.

The greatest potential applications of rate-controlled delivery are to be found in drugs with poor therapeutic ratios. Many drugs with this limitation are used in cancer chemotherapy, and it is therefore surprising that rate-controlled delivery has not received more attention as a means of improving results with these drugs. The possible benefit of this technology is suggested by a report that tumor response was improved, and pulmonary toxicity apparently decreased, when mice with Lewis lung carcinoma received bleomycin by continuous infusion rather than by injections twice daily.[27]

The principles of rate-controlled drug delivery will have relatively little impact on therapeutics until they are incorporated into the tests that are part of the preclinical and early clinical phases of drug development. If potential new drugs were tested by rate-controlled methods, it is possible that a different and probably larger group of drugs would survive the demanding process of drug development. Drugs with lower therapeutic ratios might become more acceptable if they were administered by rate-controlled methods, and potent drugs that could readily be incorporated into small devices of the kind discussed previously would become more desirable. Obviously, novel dosage forms may be obligatory if certain experimental compounds, such as the biologically active peptides, are to be useful clinically.

Rate-controlled delivery may also change our perception of the value of animal studies that are often used for predicting a drug's effects on human subjects. Sometimes such tests are discredited because their results seem to bear little resemblance to human experience. Many drugs causing teratism in animals, for example, seem to have no discernible effect on the human fetus. A recent report calls attention to a possible reason for this poor correlation. It was found that a constant infusion of valproic acid, which yielded drug concentrations in pregnant mice comparable to those in human beings, had fewer serious consequences for the embryo than the same amount of drug administered in daily boluses.[26] Thus, high peaks of serum drug concentrations, inevitable with standard methods of animal dosing, may cause misleading results and thus unwarranted concern about potential toxicity to human beings.

Although the conceptual advantages of rate-controlled delivery have been recognized for years, only recently has the concept become technically feasible. So far, the technology has been restricted merely to improving the therapeutic properties of well-known drugs. If the concept of rate-controlled delivery becomes incorporated into the search for new drugs, it may change the kinds of drugs that become available as well as their use.

References

1. Koch-Weser J. Serum drug concentrations as therapeutic guides. N Engl J Med 1972; 287:227-31.
2. Manninen V, Reissell P, Paukkala E. Transient cardiac arrhythmias after single daily maintenance doses of digoxin. Clin Pharmacol Ther 1976; 20:266-8.
3. Carruthers SG, Shoeman DW, Hignite CE, Azarnoff DL. Correlation between plasma diphenhydramine level and sedative and antihistamine effects. Clin Pharmacol Ther 1978; 23:375-82.
4. Rutter PC, Murphy F, Dudley HAF. Morphine: controlled trial of different methods of administration for postoperative pain relief. Br Med J 1980; 280:12-3.
5. Wilson TW, Falk KJ, Labelle JL, Nguyen KB. Effect of dosage regimen on natriuretic response to furosemide. Clin Pharmacol Ther 1975; 18:165-9.
6. Murphy J, Casey W, Lasagna L. The effect of dosage regimen on the diuretic efficacy of chlorothiazide in human subjects. J Pharmacol Exp Ther 1961; 134:286-90.
7. Propper RD, Cooper B, Rufo RR, et al. Continuous subcutaneous administration of deferoxamine in patients with iron overload. N Engl J Med 1977; 297:418-23.
8. Tamborlane WV, Sherwin RS, Genel M, Felig P. Restoration of normal lipid and aminoacid metabolism in diabetic patients treated with a portable insulin-infusion pump. Lancet 1979; 1:1258-61.
9. Blackshear PJ, Dorman FD, Blackshear PL, Varco RL, Buchwald H. The design and initial testing of an implantable infusion pump. Surg Gynecol Obstet 1972; 134:51-6.
10. Rupp WM, Barbosa JJ, Blackshear PJ, et al. The use of an implantable insulin pump in the treatment of Type II diabetes. N Engl J Med 1982; 307:265-7.
11. Buchwald H, Rohde TD, Schneider PD, Varco RL, Blackshear PJ. Long term, continuous intravenous heparin administration by an implantable infusion pump in ambulatory patients with recurrent venous thrombosis. Surgery 1980; 88:507-16.
12. Buchwald H, Grage TB, Vassilopoulos PP, Rohde TD, Varco RL, Blackshear PJ. Intraarterial infusion chemotherapy for hepatic carcinoma using a totally implantable infusion pump. Cancer 1980; 45:866-9.

13. Ensminger W, Niederhuber J, Dakhil S, Thrall J, Wheeler R. Totally implanted drug delivery system for hepatic arterial chemotherapy. Cancer Treat Rep 1981; 65:393-400.

14. Dakhil S, Ensminger W, Kindt G, et al. Implanted system for intraventricular drug infusion in central nervous system tumors. Cancer Treat Rep 1981; 65:401-11.

15. Price NM, Schmitt LG, McGuire J, Shaw JE, Trogough G. Transdermal scopolamine in the prevention of motion sickness at sea. Clin Pharmacol Ther 1981; 29:414-9.

16. Shaw JE, Chandrasekaran SK. Transdermal therapeutic systems. In: Prescott LF, Nimmo WS, eds. Drug absorption: proceedings of the International Conference on Drug Absorption. Edinburgh, September, 1979. New York: ADIS Press, 1979:186-93.

17. Abrams J. Nitroglycerin and long-acting nitrates. N Engl J Med 1980; 302: 1234-7.

18. Imhof PR, Ott B, Frankhauser P, Chu L-C, Hodler J. Difference in nitroglycerin dose-response in the venous and arterial beds. Eur J Clin Pharmacol 1980; 18:455-60.

19. Armstrong PW, Armstrong JA, Marks GS. Blood levels after sublingual nitroglycerin. Circulation 1979; 59:585-8.

20. McNiff EF, Yacobi A, Young-Chang FM, Golden LH, Goldfarb A, Fung H-L. Nitroglycerin pharmacokinetics after intravenous infusion in normal subjects. J Pharm Sci 1981; 70:1054-8.

21. Mroczek WJ, Ulrych M, Yoder S. Weekly transdermal clonidine administration in hypertensive patients. Clin Pharmacol Ther 1982; 31:252. abstract.

22. Urquhart J. Case Study 2: development of the OCUSERT® pilocarpine ocular therapeutic systems: a case history in ophthalmic product development. In: Robinson JR, ed. Ophthalmic drug delivery systems. Washington, D.C.: American Pharmaceutical Association, 1979:105-8.

23. Additions to timoptic contraindications. FDA Drug Bull 1981; 11:17-8.

24. Martinez-Manautou J. Contraception by intrauterine release of progesterone: clinical results. J Steroid Biochem 1975; 6:889-94.

25. Theeuwes F. Drug delivery systems. Pharmacol Ther 1981; 13:149-91.

26. Theeuwes F, Bayne W, McGuire J. Gastrointestinal therapeutic system for acetazolamide: efficacy and side effects. Arch Ophthalmol 1978; 96:2219-21.

27. Sikic BI, Collins JM, Mimnaugh EG, Gram TE. Improved therapeutic index of bleomycin when administered by continuous infusion in mice. Cancer Treat Rep 1978; 62:2011-17.

28. Nau H, Zierer R, Spielmann H, Neubert D, Gansau C. A new model for embryotoxicity testing: teratogenicity and pharmacokinetics of valproic acid following constant-rate administration in the mouse using human therapeutic drug and metabolite concentrations. Life Sci 1981; 29:2803-13.

Correspondence

Rate-Controlled Drug Delivery*

To the Editor:

Dr. Goldman's excellent review in the July 29 issue of the *Journal* highlights the important technical advances taking place in the field of drug-delivery systems.[1]

---

*Originally published on December 16, 1982 (307:1580).

The possibility of drug implantation has been revitalized by the development of nontoxic biodegradable polymers. Drugs can be combined with polymers, such as polylactic glycolic acid. Solid rods of this material, implanted subcutaneously, will break down at a steady and predictable rate and release the bound drug into the circulation.[2] Animal studies have demonstrated that drug–polymer implants can deliver rate-controlled doses of contraceptives,[3] antimalarials,[4] and narcotic antagonists[5] for periods of 90 days or more. Although this technique has not yet been evaluated in human beings, it appears to be an exciting new approach to the old problem of ensuring compliance with drug therapy.

MICHAEL PHILLIPS, M.R.C.P.
Georgetown University Hospital
Washington, DC 20007

1. Goldman P. Rate-controlled drug delivery. N Engl J Med 1982; 307:286-90.
2. Wise DL, Fellmann TD, Sanderson JE, Wentworth RL. Lactic/glycolic acid polymers. In: Gregoriadis G, ed. Drug carriers in biology and medicine. New York: Academic Press, 1979:237-70.
3. Gresser JD, Wise DL, Beck LR, Howes JF. Larger animal testing of an injectable sustained release fertility control system. Contraception 1978; 17:253-66.
4. Wise DL, Gresser JD, McCormick GJ. Sustained release of a dual antimalarial system. J Pharm Pharmacol 1979; 31:201-4.
5. Schwope AD, Wise DL, Howes JF. Development of polylactic/glycolic acid delivery systems for use in treatment of narcotic addiction. In: Willette RE, ed. Narcotic antagonists: the search for long-acting preparations. Rockville, Md.: National Institute of Drug Abuse, 1976.

The above letter was referred to the author of the article in question, who offers the following reply:

To the Editor:
Since implantable drug-delivery systems require a biodegradable matrix of at least twice the drug's weight to ensure reliable drug release, it must be emphasized that the concepts mentioned by Dr. Phillips are likely to be implemented only for drugs of very high potency.

PETER GOLDMAN, M.D.
Beth Israel Hospital
Boston, MA 02215

Atenolol and Timolol, Two New Systemic β-Adrenoceptor Antagonists

Willaim H. Frishman, M.D.

ATENOLOL (Tenormin) and timolol (Blocadren) are two β-adrenoceptor antagonists recently released for clinical use in the United States (Fig. 1). They are the fourth and fifth systemic β-blockers to be approved by the Food and Drug Administration for the treatment of hypertension. Atenolol was released in 1981; like metoprolol, it is a β_1-selective adrenergic blocker. However, unlike metoprolol, it has a long plasma half-life, which allows single daily doses in the treatment of hypertension.[1-3] Timolol is a nonselective β-adrenergic blocker that has characteristics similar to those of propranolol but lacks membrane-stabilizing activity.[1] It was approved by the FDA in 1978 under the trade name of Timoptic for the topical treatment of elevated intraocular pressure. On the basis of the results of the Norwegian Multicenter Study Group,[4] the FDA has now approved timolol for the reduction of cardiovascular mortality and reinfarction in survivors of acute myocardial infarction. Propranolol will also receive FDA approval for this indication.

β-Adrenergic blockers have been shown to have similar effects in the treatment of cardiovascular disease.[1,5] It is widely assumed that the therapeutic actions of the currently available agents — atenolol, metoprolol, nadolol, propranolol, and timolol — stem from β-adrenoceptor blockade. However, since this has not been conclusively established, the FDA requires that the effectiveness and safety of each new β-receptor antagonist be specifically established for each therapeutic indication.

Atenolol

Clinical Effectiveness

Atenolol has no intrinsic sympathomimetic activity (partial agonist effect) or membrane-stabilizing properties.[1,3] When given orally, it is about as potent as

From the Division of Cardiology, Department of Medicine, Albert Einstein College of Medicine, Bronx, New York.

Supported by a grant (HL 00653-2) from the National Institutes of Health. Dr. Frishman is a Teaching Scholar of the American Heart Association.

Originally published on June 17, 1982 (306:1456-1462).

TIMOLOL

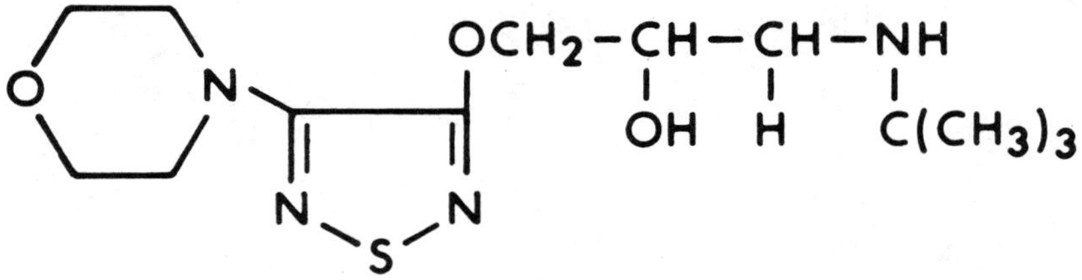

ATENOLOL

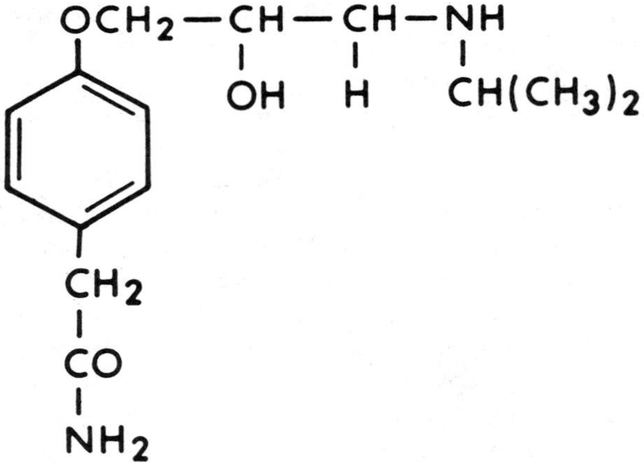

Figure 1. Molecular Structures of Timolol and Atenolol.

metoprolol, nadolol, and propranolol in inhibiting isoproterenol-induced tachy-cardia.[1] Like metoprolol,[6] it appears to be relatively selective for cardiac β_1-receptors.[3] Some deterioration in airway function can occur in patients with asthma who are receiving these drugs, but this is clearly less severe than that occurring with nonselective β-blockers, such as propranolol.[7] Furthermore, β_1-selective agents in low doses may not block β_2-receptors that mediate di-lation of arterioles.[6] This property might provide an advantage in the treatment of hypertension with relatively low doses of metoprolol or atenolol, but this has not been demonstrated.[1] Like that of metoprolol, the relative β_1-selectivity of atenolol diminishes with higher doses, so that peripheral β_2-receptors are blocked. [1,6]

Hypertension

The antihypertensive effectiveness of atenolol in doses taken once a day has been well established in numerous placebo-controlled clinical trials. [3,8-11] Its antihypertensive action appears to be quantitatively similar to those of other β-blockers, [12,13] methyldopa, [14] and thiazide diuretics. [3]

When administered to hypertensive patients (usually with mild to moderate hypertension), atenolol reduces both systolic and diastolic pressure by about 15 per cent. [3,15] The drug is equally effective in the supine and standing positions, and postural hypotension has only rarely been observed. The dose-response curve for atenolol in hypertension is relatively flat, with the maximal effect of the drug usually occurring by the third day of treatment with a dose of 100 mg per day. [3,10] There is some evidence that the response to atenolol may increase slightly after several weeks of treatment. [3] As with other β-blockers, the reduction in blood pressure with atenolol is consistently accompanied by a 20 per cent reduction in heart rate and cardiac output. [3,15] In studies assessing the control of blood pressure with a single dose of atenolol over a 24-hour period, the peak effect (measured at three hours) and the trough effect (measured at 24 hours) has not differed significantly. [16] There are large differences between patients in the response of blood pressure to atenolol, as is true for all β-blockers and other antihypertensive drugs.

Atenolol is more effective when combined with a diuretic, and this may permit reduction of the atenolol dose. [17] The addition of methyldopa, [14] hydralazine, [18] or prazosin [19] to atenolol enhances the reduction in blood pressure. The drug appears to be safe and effective in the treatment of hypertension in patients with renal damage. [3] Atenolol reduces blood pressure in patients with low, normal, or elevated plasma renin activity, and drug tolerance does not develop with prolonged use. [3,18]

Since atenolol can be taken once daily for the treatment of hypertension, patients' compliance may be high. The antihypertensive efficacy of nadolol and that of atenolol, each given once daily, have not been compared. In addition, it remains possible that shorter-acting β-blockers can also be taken once a day in the treatment of hypertension.

Ischemic Heart Disease

Like other β-blockers, atenolol may be expected to protect the heart from some deleterious effects of physiologic and psychological stress. [20] In patients with angina pectoris, atenolol (50 to 200 mg administered once daily) decreases the heart rate, reduces the elevation of the heart rate and blood pressure in response to stress or exercise, prevents or reverses ischemic electrocardiographic changes, and increases exercise tolerance. [21] Atenolol is used in many countries for the long-term treatment of angina, [3] but this indication has not been approved in the United States. [3]

An exciting application of β-adrenoceptor antagonists is their potential use as cardioprotective agents in acute myocardial infarction and as secondary prophylaxis against death and reinfarction. The effects of intravenous atenolol were compared with those of placebo in a double-blind, controlled study of 214 patients with threatened or definite myocardial infarctions.[22] Patients were seen within 12 hours of the onset of symptoms. In this study, atenolol reduced the incidence of completed infarction in patients presenting with threatened infarctions. In patients who presented with definite myocardial infarcts, the drug may have also influenced infarct size, as judged by electrocardiographic changes and creatine kinase measurements. Moreover, the patients treated wth intravenous atenolol had fewer long-term complications (e.g., congestive heart failure or arrhythmia) than those given placebo treatment. The effects of oral atenolol and propranolol on total mortality in survivors of acute myocardial infarction were assessed in a placebo-controlled, randomized, double-blind trial in 388 patients.[23] After one year of treatment, total mortality was the same in patients treated with each β-blocker and with placebo.[23] Atenolol is not available in intravenous form in the United States and is not approved for use as prophylactic treatment for reducing the incidence of reinfarction and death in survivors of acute myocardial infarction.

Arrhythmia

Like other β-adrenergic blockers, atenolol has antiarrhythmic properties that stem from its ability to antagonize the effects of catecholamines on cardiac automaticity and conductivity.[20,24,25] Although the electrophysiologic properties of atenolol are known, there are few recorded clinical data on its antiarrhythmic effects, and the drug is not yet approved for this indication.

Pharmacokinetics

Atenolol is rapidly absorbed from the gastrointestinal tract, and absorption of the drug is not significantly influenced by the presence of food.[3,26,27] Approximately 50 per cent of an oral dose is absorbed, with the remainder excreted unchanged in the feces, and peak blood levels (proportional to the oral dose) are reached between two and four hours after ingestion.[26,28] Unlike propranolol and metoprolol, but like nadolol, atenolol undergoes little or no hepatic metabolism.[3,27] The absorbed portion of the drug is eliminated primarily by renal excretion and to a lesser extent by nonrenal routes.[27] After a single dose, there is a fourfold variation in plasma drug levels among patients.[1]

Like nadolol, atenolol is more hydrophilic than propranolol and metoprolol, which are highly lipid-soluble.[29] In human plasma less than 5 per cent of atenolol is bound to plasma proteins[30]; the drug has a volume of distribution of 0.7 liter per kilogram of body weight.[3,29] Atenolol crosses the placenta and is also excreted in milk in measurable amounts.[31] Because of its low lipid solubility, atenolol penetrates poorly into the central nervous system, and during long-term therapy the concentrations of the drug in the brain are substantially lower than those in the peripheral blood.[24,32] It has been suggested that because of this property atenolol may have fewer side effects on the central nervous system than the lipid-soluble β-blockers do, but this remains to be proved.[2,29] The plasma concentrations of atenolol decline biexponentially, with a terminal half-life of six to nine hours in patients with normal renal function.[2] There is no alteration of the kinetic profile with long-term administration.[26] During once-daily dosage, steady-state plasma concentrations are attained in approximately two days. Elimination of atenolol is markedly reduced in patients with moderate or severe renal dysfunction.[33] Dosage adjustments are therefore necessary in patients with impaired renal function. Unlike propranolol, atenolol can be removed from the body by hemodialysis.[34] Differences in plasma levels among patients with normal renal function are less pronounced with atenolol than with shorter-acting β-adrenoceptor-blocking drugs such as propranolol, which are metabolized in the liver.[29]

Any increase of the atenolol dose within the therapeutic range can be expected to cause a proportional increase in the drug concentration of the body (dose-dependent pharmacokinetics).[3] Gas-chromatographic methods for determining plasma levels of atenolol are available, but as with all β-blockers, such measurements have little to offer as therapeutic guides except for checking compliance or treating patients with renal impairment. Like those of other β-blockers, the effect of atenolol on the heart rate during exercise is linearly related to the logarithm of plasma concentration, but there is only a weak correlation between the plasma level and the antihypertensive effect.[35] Since the blood pressure and the heart rate are easily measured, the atenolol dose can be "titrated" against changes in these vital signs.

Clinical Use

Because of atenolol's relatively long plasma half-life and even longer pharmacodynamic half-life, it is approved in once-daily dosage for the treatment of hypertension. It is available in tablets containing 50 and 100 mg (the cost of atenolol is compared with that of other β-blockers in Table 1). Since there is no consistent correlation between the dose of atenolol and the therapeutic response in different patients, doses must be individualized. For the treatment of hypertension, the recommended initial adult dose of atenolol is 50 mg daily, given alone or added to diuretic therapy. The full effect of this dose will usually be seen within one to two weeks.[3] If an optimal response is not achieved, the dose should be increased to 100 mg, given as one tablet a day. Increasing the dose beyond 100 mg a day is unlikely to produce any further benefit.[3,10] Atenolol may be used concomitantly with other antihypertensive agents, including thiazide-type diuretics,[17] hydralazine,[18] prazosin,[19] and methyldopa.[14]

In patients with renal impairment the dosage should be adjusted (Table 2). No substantial accumulation of atenolol occurs until creatinine clearance falls below 35 ml per minute.[33] As with other β-blockers, treatment should not be

TABLE 1. Comparative Costs of β-Adrenoceptor-Blocking Drugs Used in the Treatment of Hypertension.

Drug	Relative β₁ Selectivity	Available Tablet Forms	Cost ($) per Tablet*	Recommended Daily Dose Range	Cost of an Equivalent β-Blocker Daily Dose †
Atenolol	Yes	50 mg, 100 mg	0.29, 0.43	50–200 mg (one dose)	100 mg: $0.43
Metoprolol	Yes	50 mg, 100 mg	0.13, 0.23	100–400 mg (two divided doses)	200 mg: 0.46
Nadolol	No	40 mg, 80 mg, 120 mg, 160 mg	0.24, 0.32, 0.42, 0.56	40–320 mg (one dose)	120 mg: 0.42
Propranolol	No	10 mg, 20 mg, 40 mg, 80 mg	0.05, 0.07, 0.10, 0.17	40–320 mg (two divided doses)	160 mg: 0.34
Timolol	No	10 mg, 20 mg	0.17, 0.32	20–60 mg (two divided doses)	20 mg: 0.34

*Based on 1982 standard wholesale costs per 100-tablet order.

†Daily costs may differ, depending on the comparative dose strengths used.

stopped abruptly, and patients should be cautioned against interrupting therapy on their own. When discontinuation of atenolol is planned, the patient should be carefully observed. Atenolol appears to be safe when used during pregnancy and lactation, but the clinical experience is still limited. Its effectiveness and safety in children have not been established.

TABLE 2. Adjustment of Dosage and Dose Interval of Oral Atenolol in Patients with Renal Dysfunction, According to Creatinine Clearance.

Creatinine Clearance	Elimination Half-Life	Maximum Dosage
ml/min/1.73 m²	*hr*	
15–35	16–27	50 mg daily
<15	>27	50 mg every other day

Like other β-adrenergic antagonists, atenolol is contraindicated in clinical situations in which blockade of adrenergic stimulation of the heart may be poorly tolerated.[1,36] Contraindications include marked bradycardia, partial or complete atrioventricular block, cardiogenic shock, and congestive heart failure.[3] In hypertensive patients who have congestive heart failure that is controlled by digitalis and diuretics, atenolol should be administered cautiously.

Patients with bronchospastic disease should generally not be treated with β-adrenergic-blocking drugs.[1,6] Because of its relative β_1-selectivity, however, atenolol may be used with caution in patients with bronchospastic disease who do not respond to other antihypertensive treatment or cannot tolerate it. Since β_1-selectivity is not absolute, the lower dose of atenolol should be used in initiating treatment.[3] Should bronchospasm occur, it is also possible to use both atenolol (at the low dose) and a β_2-selective agonist (such as albuterol) in certain patients.[7] If the dose of atenolol must be increased in patients with bronchospastic disease, dividing the daily dose will provide lower peak blood levels.

Changing from other oral β-blockers to oral atenolol must be done with care because of pharmacokinetic differences between the drugs.[1] The manufacturer recommends starting with a 50-mg dose of atenolol, given once daily, when switching a patient from moderate daily doses of metoprolol, nadolol, propranolol, or timolol. If the patient has previously been receiving larger daily doses of one of these drugs (200 mg of metoprolol, 240 mg of nadolol, 320 mg of propranolol, or 60 mg of timolol) then a single daily 100-mg dose of atenolol should be used. When switching patients from methyldopa or prazosin, it is recommended that administration of these drugs be stopped for 24 hours before atenolol therapy is started at 50 mg once daily.

Side Effects

Any serious side effects of atenolol are related to its β-adrenergic-blocking actions and are similar to those of all available β-adrenergic-blocking drugs.[1,36] The occurrence of unwanted depression of left ventricular function and cardiac electrical activity by atenolol and other β-adrenergic blockers used in therapeutic doses is related to the dependence of these functions on adrenergic stimulation in some patients.[1] Similarly, high-dose atenolol will interfere with ventilatory function in patients who are dependent on adrenergic stimulation of β_2-receptors.[7] Other side effects of atenolol are rather uncommon and are generally mild and transient. Generally, the profile of adverse effects is similar to that of propranolol.[37] Nausea, diarrhea, abdominal discomfort, and constipation are seen in about 2 per cent of patients. Rarely, skin rashes, dry eyes, and postural hypotension have been reported. Although a single case of retroperitoneal fibrosis has been described in a patient receiving therapeutic doses of atenolol, a causal relation was not clearly established.[38] There is also no evidence to date to suggest that atenolol can cause a generalized oculomucocutaneous syndrome like that seen with practolol. Indeed, in 19 patients with such a reaction induced by practolol, the lesions healed after a switch to atenolol treatment.[39] Like other β-blockers, atenolol can mask some clinical signs of hypoglycemia or hyperthyroidism, particularly tachycardia. Atenolol, like metoprolol, does not potentiate insulin-induced hypoglycemia; unlike nonselective β-blockers, it does not delay the recovery of blood glucose to normal levels.[1,6,40] The package insert still advises that the drug be used cautiously in patients with diabetes. Treatment for overdosage of atenolol should follow that of other β-adrenergic blocking drugs.[40] The long half-life of atenolol should be considered in the event of an overdosage and suggests that supportive measures may be needed for a long period.[2,41] Clearly, atenolol, like other β-blockers, has an enormous margin of safety in patients not dependent on functioning β-receptors.

| Timolol

Clinical Effectiveness

Timolol maleate is an orally active β-adrenoceptor-blocking drug that lacks both intrinsic sympathomimetic activity and membrane-stabilizing properties.[1] It is the only β-adrenoceptor-blocking drug that has proved to be safe and clinically efficacious in reducing elevated intraocular pressure when used topically, raising the possibility that all β-blockers may not be alike in their clinical effectiveness.[1] Moreover, unlike other β-blockers, timolol is presented as a maleate and only in the levorotatory form.[42] When given orally to human beings, it is about six to eight times more potent than propranolol.[1]

Hypertension

The antihypertensive effectiveness of timolol taken twice daily has been well established in numerous placebo-controlled trials.[43,44] Its antihypertensive action appears to be quantitatively similar to that of other β-blockers, thiazides, and methyldopa.

When administered to patients with hypertension, timolol reduces both systolic and diastolic blood pressure by about 15 per cent.[44] The drug is equally effective in the supine and standing positions; postural hypotension has rarely been described.[44] Administration of timolol initially results in a decrease in cardiac output, little immediate change in blood pressure, and an increase in calculated peripheral vascular resistance.[45] With continued administration of timolol, blood pressure decreases within a few days, cardiac output usually remains reduced, and peripheral resistance falls toward pretreatment levels.[45] Plasma volume may decrease or remain unchanged. In the majority of patients timolol also decreases plasma renin activity; however, blood pressure is reduced in hypertensive patients with low, normal, or elevated pretreatment renin levels.[45,46] Dosage adjustment to achieve an optimal antihypertensive effect may require a few weeks.[44] When therapy with timolol is discontinued, the blood pressure tends to return gradually to pretreatment levels.[44] In most patients drug tolerance does not develop with long-term therapy.[44]

As is true for other β-blockers used to treat hypertension, there are large differences between patients in the response of blood pressure to timolol.[44] The drug is more effective when combined with a diuretic; this may permit reduction of the timolol dose.[47,48] The addition of methyldopa and hydralazine[49] to timolol enhances the reduction in blood pressure. The drug appears to be safe and effective for the treatment of hypertension in patients with renal dysfunction. However, the dose may have to be reduced in most patients undergoing hemodialysis, as is true with any other antihypertensive medication. Despite its relatively short plasma half-life, timolol has been used once daily in the treatment of hypertension,[50] but more clinical data are required to substantiate the efficacy of this regimen.

Ischemic Heart Disease

Timolol protects the heart from the deleterious effects of physiologic and psychological stresses.[20] In patients with angina pectoris, timolol (10 to 30 mg administered twice daily) decreases the heart rate, reduces the elevation of the heart rate and blood pressure in response to stress or exercise, prevents or reverses ischemic electrocardiographic changes, and improves exercise tolerance.[51-53] Timolol is used in many countries for the treatment of anginal pectoris but is not yet approved for this indication in the United States.

It was recently demonstrated that timolol can reduce the long-term risk of cardiovascular mortality and reinfarction in stabilized survivors of acute myocardial infarction.[4] It is the first β-blocker to be approved by the FDA for this indication; approval was based on the results of a Norwegian multicenter double-blind study that compared the effects of timolol with those of placebo in 1884 patients who had survived the acute phase of a myocardial infarction.[4] This new indication for β-adrenergic blockade will be discussed in a future Drug Therapy article.

Arrhythmia

Timolol has antiarrhythmic properties that result from its ability to antagonize the effects of catecholamines on cardiac automaticity and conductivity.[52] There are few recorded clinical data on timolol used as an antiarrhythmic agent, and the drug is not yet approved for this indication.

Pharmacokinetics

Timolol is rapidly and nearly completely absorbed (about 90 per cent) after oral ingestion, and absorption is not influenced by the presence of food.[54] Detectable blood levels of timolol occur within half an hour, and peak plasma levels occur in about one to two hours.[54] The drug's half-life in plasma is approximately three to four hours (similar to those of propranolol and metoprolol)[54] and is essentially unchanged in patients with moderate renal insufficiency. Timolol is largely metabolized by the liver (80 per cent), and the drug and its inactive metabolites are excreted by the kidney.[54] Unlike propranolol, timolol is not extensively bound to plasma proteins (approximately 10 per cent).[42] Plama levels of timolol after oral administration are about half those after intravenous administration, indicating approximately 50 per cent first-pass hepatic metabolism. At a given dose, there is a sevenfold variation between patients in plasma levels of the drug.[1,55] Timolol is less lipid-soluble than propranolol or metoprolol. Thus, it may penetrate less into the brain and cause fewer side effects on the central nervous system,[1,29,56] but this suggestion remains to be proved.

The level of β-sympathetic activity varies widely among persons, and no simple relation exists between the dose of timolol, the plasma level, and the therapeutic activity. Therefore, objective measurements of the heart rate or blood pressure or both should be used as guides in determining the optimal dosage for each patient.

Clinical Use

Timolol maleate is available in tablets containing 10 mg or 20 mg (comparative wholesale costs are shown in Table 1). For the treatment of hypertension, the recommended initial adult dose is 10 mg given twice a day, whether it is used alone or added to diuretic therapy. Depending on the blood pressure and pulse rate, increases to a maximum of 60 mg per day (divided into two doses) may be necessary. There should be an interval of at least seven days between increases in dosage. The usual maintenance dose is 20 to 40 mg per day. Timolol can be used concomitantly with other antihypertensive agents, including thiazide diuretics,[47] hydralazine,[49] and methyldopa.

For treatment of survivors of an acute myocardial infarction, the recommended dose is 10 mg given twice daily. The drug should be started seven to 28 days after infarction in patients who have no contraindications to β-adrenergic blockade. It has not been determined whether benefit would ensue if drug administration were started after 28 days, and it is not known how long timolol treatment should be continued after it is initiated.

Unlike those of the longer-acting β-blockers nadolol and atenolol, the pharmacokinetics of timolol are not greatly altered by renal impairment. However, marked hypotensive responses have been seen in patients with marked renal dysfunction who are undergoing hemodialysis after 20-mg doses. Such patients should be treated with caution. Timolol treatment should not be discontinued abruptly but should be gradually and cautiously withdrawn over a one to two-week period. The safety of timolol during pregnancy and lactation and its effectiveness and safety in children have not been established.

Like atenolol and other β-blockers, timolol is contraindicated in cardiovascular conditions in which blockade of adrenergic stimulation may be poorly tolerated.[1,36] The drug may be given cautiously with digitalis and diuretics to patients with compensated congestive heart failure. Oral timolol should not be administered to patients with bronchospastic disease.[1,6]

When switching from moderate daily doses of propranolol, metoprolol, nadolol, or propranolol, it is recommended that timolol therapy be started at 10 mg, given twice daily. If the patient has previously been receiving large daily doses of other β-blockers, then a timolol dose of 10 to 20 mg given twice daily should be used. Further dose adjustment will depend on "titrating" for optimal clinical response.

Side Effects and Precautions

Any serious side effects of timolol are related to its β-adrenergic-blocking activity and are similar to those described with atenolol and other β-adrenergic-blocking drugs.[1,36] The profile of less serious adverse reactions is also similar to that of propranolol and other active oral β-blockers.[4,36,44] Fatigue and dizziness have occurred in about 2 to 4 per cent of patients. Nausea, diarrhea, abdominal discomfort, and constipation are seen in about 1 to 5 per cent of patients. Rarely, skin rashes, pruritus, and bronchial spasm have been reported. Like all other β-blockers, timolol can mask some clinical signs of hypoglycemia or hyperthyroidism, and the drug should be used with caution in diabetes. There have been studies demonstrating an increased incidence of certain tumors in male rats (adrenal pheochromocytomas) and female mice (benign and malignant pulmonary tumors and benign uterine polyps) that received 300 to 500 times the maximal recommended human dose of timolol (1 mg per kilogram of body weight per day). However, there is no evidence for carcinogenicity of timolol in human beings, and the drug appears to be devoid of any mutagenic potential.

Cases of timolol overdosage have not been reported. Treatment of an overdose, if one occurs, should follow that of other β-blockers, as previously described.[41] Timolol has an enormous margin of safety in patients, like all the other available systemically active β-adrenergic blockers.

References

1. Frishman WH. β-Adrenoceptor antagonists: new drugs and new indications. N Engl J Med 1981; 305:500-6.
2. Idem. Nadolol: a new β-adrenoceptor antagonist. N Engl J Med 1981; 305:678-82.
3. Heel RC, Brogden RN, Speight TM, Avery GS. Atenolol: a review of its pharmacological properties and therapeutic efficacy in angina pectoris and hypertension. Drugs 1979; 17:425-60.
4. The Norwegian Multicenter Study Group. Timolol-induced reduction in mortality and reinfarction in patients surviving acute myocardial infarction. N Engl J Med 1981; 304:801-7.
5. Frishman W, Silverman R. Clinical pharmacology of the new beta-adrenergic blocking drugs. Part 3. Comparative clinical experience and new therapeutic applications. Am Heart J 1979; 98:119-31.
6. Koch-Weser J. Metoprolol. N Engl J Med 1979; 301:698-703.
7. Benson MK, Berrill WT, Cruickshank JM, Sterling GS. A comparison of four β-adrenoceptor antagonists in patients with asthma. Br J Clin Pharmacol 1978; 5: 415-9.
8. Douglas-Jones AP, Cruickshank JM. Once-daily dosing with atenolol in patients with mild or moderate hypertension. Br Med J 1976; 1:990-1.
9. Myers MG, Lewis GRJ, Steiner J, Dollery CT. Atenolol in essential hypertension. Clin Pharmacol Ther 1976; 19:502-7.
10. Jeffers TA, Webster J, Petrie JC, Barker NP. Atenolol once-daily in hypertension. Br J Clin Pharmacol 1977; 4:523-7.
11. Ibrahim MM, Mossallam R. Clinical evaluation of atenolol in hypertensive patients. Circulation 1981; 64:368-74.
12. Wilcox RG. Randomised study of six beta-blockers and a thiazide diuretic in essential hypertension. Br Med J 1978; 2:383-5.
13. Waal-Manning HJ. Atenolol and three nonselective β-blockers in hypertension. Clin Pharmacol Ther 1979; 25:8-18.
14. Webster J, Jeffers TA, Galloway DB, Petrie JC, Barker NP. Atenolol, methyldopa, and chlorthalidone on moderate hypertension. Br Med J 1977; 1:76-8.
15. Lund-Johansen P, Ohm OJ. Haemodynamic long-term effects of β-receptor-blocking agents in hypertension: a comparison between alprenolol, atenolol, metoprolol and timolol. Clin Sci Mol Med 1976; 51:Suppl 3:481S-3S.
16. Floras JS, Vann Jones J, Fox P, Hassan MO, Turner KL, Sleight P. Effect of long-term, once-daily administration of atenolol on ambulatory blood pressure of hypertensive patients. J Cardiovasc Pharmacol 1981; 3:958-64.
17. Petrie JC, Galloway DB, Webster J, Simpson WT, Lewis JA. Atenolol and bendrofluazide in hypertension. Br Med J 1975; 4:133-5.
18. Zacharias FJ, Cowen KJ, Cuthbertson PJR, et al. Atenolol in hypertension: a study of long-term therapy. Postgrad Med J 1977; 53: Suppl 3:102-10.
19. Marshall AJ, Barritt DW, Pocock J, Heaton ST. Evaluation of beta-blockade, bendrofluazide, and prazosin in severe hypertension. Lancet 1977; 1:271-4.

20. Frishman W, Silverman R. Clinical pharmacology of the new beta-adrenergic blocking drugs. Part 2. Physiologic and metabolic effects. Am Heart J 1979; 97:797-807.

21. Jackson G, Schwartz J, Kates RE, Winchester M, Harrison DC. Atenolol: once-daily cardioselective beta blockade for angina pectoris. Circulation 1980; 61:555-60.

22. Yusuf S, Ramsdale D, Peto R, et al. Early intravenous atenolol treatment in suspected acute myocardial infarction: preliminary report of a randomised trial. Lancet 1980; 2:273-6.

23. Wilcox RG, Roland JM, Banks DC, Hampton JR, Mitchell JRA. Randomised trial comparing propranolol with atenolol in immediate treatment of suspected myocardial infarction. Br Med J 1980; 280:885-8.

24. Robinson C, Birkhead J, Crook B, Jennings K, Jewitt D. Clinical electrophysiological effects of atenolol — a new cardioselective beta-blocking agent. Br Heart J 1978; 40:14-21.

25. Winchester MA, Jackson G, Meltzer RS, et al. Intravenous atenolol and acebutolol in the treatment of supraventricular arrhythmias. Circulation 1978; 57 & 58: Suppl 2:II-49.

26. Fitzgerald JD, Ruffin R, Smedstad KG, Roberts R, McAinsh J. Studies on the pharmacokinetics and pharmacodynamics of atenolol in man. Eur J Clin Pharmacol 1978; 13:81-9.

27. Reeves PR, McAinsh J, McIntosh DAD, Winrow MJ. Metabolism of atenolol in man. Xenobiotica 1978; 8:313-20.

28. Mason WD, Winer N, Kochak G, Cohen I, Bell R. Kinetics and absolute bioavailability of atenolol. Clin Pharmacol Ther 1979; 25:408-15.

29. Cruickshank JM. The clinical importance of cardioselectivity and lipophilicity in beta-blockers. Am Heart J 1980; 100:160-78.

30. Barber HE, Hawksworth GM, Kitteringham NR, Petersen J, Petrie JC, Swann JM. Protein binding of atenolol and propranolol to human serum albumin and in human plasma. Br J Clin Pharmacol 1978; 6:446P-7P.

31. Melander A, Niklasson B, Ingemarsson I, Liedholm H, Schersten B, Sjöberg NO. Transplacental passage of atenolol in man. Eur J Clin Pharmacol 1978; 14:93-4.

32. Neil-Dwyer G, Bartlett J, McAinsh J, Cruickshank JM. β-Adrenoceptor blockers and the blood-brain barrier. Br J Clin Pharmacol 1981; 11:549-53.

33. McAinsh J, Holmes BF, Smith S, Hood D, Warren D. Atenolol kinetics in renal failure. Clin Pharmacol Ther 1980; 28:302-9.

34. Flouvat B, Decurt S, Aubert P, et al. Pharmacokinetics of atenolol in patients with terminal renal failure and influence of haemodialysis. Br J Clin Pharmacol 1980; 9:379-85.

35. Amery A, De Plaen J-F, Lijnen P, McAinsh J, Reybrouck T. Relationship between blood level of atenolol and pharmacologic effect. Clin Pharmacol Ther 1977; 21:691-9.

36. Frishman W, Silverman R, Strom J, Elkayam U, Sonnenblick E. Clinical pharmacology of the new beta-adrenergic blocking drugs. Part 4. Adverse effects: choosing a β-adrenoreceptor blocker. Am Heart J 1979; 98:256-62.

37. Simpson WT. Nature and incidence of unwanted effects with atenolol. Postgrad Med J 1977; 53: Suppl 3:162-7.

38. Doherty CC, McGeown MG, Donaldson RA. Retroperitoneal fibrosis after treatment with atenolol. Br Med J 1978; 2:1786.

39. Zacharias FJ. Cross-sensitivity between practolol and other beta-blockers? Br Med J 1976; 1:1213.

40. Deacon SP, Karunanayake A, Barnett D. Acebutolol, atenolol, and propranolol and metabolic responses to acute hypoglycaemia in diabetics. Br Med J 1977; 2:1255-7.

41. Frishman W, Jacob H, Eisenberg E, Ribner H. Clinical pharmacology of the new beta-adrenergic blocking drugs. Part 8. Self-poisoning with beta-adrenoceptor blocking agents: recognition and management. Am Heart J 1979; 98:798-811.

42. Bobik A, Jennings GL, Ashley P, Korner PI. Timolol pharmacokinetics and effects on heart rate and blood pressure after acute and chronic administration. Eur J Clin Pharmacol 1979; 16:243-9.

43. Pawlowski GJ. Treatment of essential hypertension with a new beta-blocking drug, timolol: experience with a b.i.d. dosage regimen. Curr Ther Res 1977; 22:846-52.

44. Rofman B, Kulaga S, Gabriel M, Thiyagarajan B, Nancarrow JF, Abrams WB. Multiclinic evaluation of timolol in the treatment of mild-to-moderate essential hypertension. Hypertension 1980; 2:643-8.

45. Aronow WS, Ferlinz S, Del Vicario M, Moorthy K, King J, Cassidy J. Effect of timolol versus propranolol on hypertension and hemodynamics. Circulation 1978; 54:47-51.

46. LeBel M, Belleau LJ, Grose JH. Timolol as additive therapy in essential hypertension: effect on plasma renin activity. Curr Ther Res 1978; 24:591-8.

47. Oparil S. Multiclinic double-blind evaluation of timolol combined with hydrochlorothiazide in essential hypertension. Curr Ther Res 1980; 27:527-37.

48. Roginsky MS. Long-term evaluation of timolol maleate combined with hydrochlorothiazide for the treatment of patients with essential hypertension: a cooperative, multicenter study. Curr Ther Res 1980; 27:374-83.

49. Aronow WS, Var Herick R, Greenfield R, Alimadadian H, Burwell D, Mann D. Effect of timolol plus hydrochlorothiazide plus hydralazine on essential hypertension. Circulation 1978; 57:1017-21.

50. Jennings G, Bobik A, Korner P. Comparison of effectiveness of timolol administered once a day and twice a day in the control of blood pressure in essential hypertension. Med J Aust 1979; 2:263-5.

51. Brailovsky D. Timolol maleate (MK-950): a new beta-blocking agent for the prophylactic management of angina pectoris: a multicenter, multinational, cooperative trial. In: Magnani B, ed. Beta-adrenergic blocking agents in the management of hypertension and angina pectoris. New York: Raven Press, 1974:117-37.

52. Brogden RN, Speight TM, Avery GS. Timolol: a preliminary report of its pharmacological properties and therapeutic efficacy in angina and hypertension. Drugs 1975; 9:164-77.

53. Aronow WS, Turbow M, Van Camp S, Lurie M, Whittaker K. The effect of timolol vs placebo on angina pectoris. Circulation 1980; 61:66-9.

54. Tocco DJ, Duncan AEW, DeLuna FA, Hucker HB, Gruber VF, VandenHeuvel WJA. Physiological disposition and metabolism of timolol in man and laboratory animals. Drug Metab Dispos 1975; 3:361-70.

55. Else OF, Sorenson H, Edwards IR. Plasma timolol levels after oral and intravenous administration. Eur J Clin Pharmacol 1978; 14:431-4.

56. Tocco DS, Clineschmidt BV, Duncan AEW, deLuna FA, Baer JE. Uptake of the beta-adrenergic blocking agents propranolol and timolol by rodent brain: relationship to central pharmacological actions. J Cardiovasc Pharmacol 1980; 2:133-43.

Correspondence

Atenolol and Timolol*

To the Editor:

In a recent review of two β-blockers released for clinical use in the United States (June 17 issue) Frishman discusses the use of atenolol in treating hypertension.[1] One side effect not mentioned in the review is the induction of lipoprotein abnormalities during β-blockade. The general pattern in most studies seems to be an increase in the concentration of very-low-density lipoproteins and a decrease in the concentration of high-density lipoproteins during β-blockade.[2] Hyperlipoproteinemia is common in patients with hypertension, and an incidence of up to 40 per cent — twice as high as in controls — has been reported.[3] Hypertriglyceridemia, low levels of high-density lipoproteins, and concentrations of cholesterol are regarded as risk factors for the development of atherosclerosis. It seems wise in the life-long treatment of hypertension to use a drug that has no adverse long-term effects on serum lipoproteins.

In a study of atenolol we found that a dose of 100 mg per day led to a mean 25 per cent increase in the concentration of very-low-density lipoprotein triglycerides.[4] There was a tendency for patients with initially high concentrations to have further increases during treatment with atenolol. In a subsequent study with 50 mg of atenolol per day, however, no changes in lipoprotein concentrations were found (unpublished data). The concentration of very-low-density lipoprotein triglycerides in this second group of patients was 2.51 ± 2.26 mmol per liter (mean $\pm$S.D.). Thus, by using 50 mg of atenolol per day it seems possible to avoid a risk factor that theoretically could counteract the beneficial effect of reduced blood pressure.

Stephan Rössner, M.D.
King Gustaf V Research Institute, Karolinska Hospital
S-10401 Stockholm, Sweden

Leif Weiner, M.D.
Karlskoga Hospital
S-69181 Karlskoga, Sweden

1. Frishman WH. Atenolol and timolol, two new systemic β-adrenoceptor antagonists. N Engl J Med 1982; 306:1456-62.
2. Rössner S. Serum lipoproteins and ischemic vascular disease: on the interpretation of serum lipid versus serum lipoprotein concentrations. J Cardiovasc Pharmacol 1982; 4:S201-5.
3. Thomas GW, Mann JI, Beilin LJ, Ledingham JG. Hypertension and raised serum lipids. Br Med J 1977; 2:805.
4. Eliasson K, Lins LE, Rössner S. Serum lipoprotein changes during atenolol treatment of essential hypertension. Eur J Clin Pharmacol 1981; 20:335-8.

*Originally published on November 18, 1982 (307:1343-1346).

To the Editor:

Frishman comments on the suggestion that atenolol has fewer central-nervous-system-related side effects than lipid-soluble β-blockers do, and he concludes that this difference remains to be proved.

In a double-blind crossover study I examined the difference between the hydrophilic drug atenolol and the lipophilic drugs metoprolol and propranolol in patients with a history of distinct central-nervous-system-related side effects — nightmares, hallucinations, or both — associated with β-blockers. Nine patients were selected for the study: four men and five women. They ranged in age from 33 to 70 years.

The trial started with an open provocation. Metoprolol or propranolol was given in the same dose that was needed earlier to control high blood pressure (metoprolol, 100 to 200 mg twice a day; propranolol, 80 to 160 mg twice a day). A dose of 100 mg of atenolol, taken at the same time as the second daily dose of metoprolol or propranolol, was chosen for comparison. If central-nervous-system side effects appeared during provocation, a double-blind study with two four-week periods was conducted.

All patients had central-nervous-system side effects after 7 to 30 days of provocation. Two patients found the side effects so unpleasant that they did not want to participate in the double-blind study. One patient withdrew because of a long business trip.

Six patients completed the double-blind study. Thirty-one episodes of nightmares or hallucinations (or both) were reported — 30 during treatment with the lipophilic drugs and 1 during treatment with atenolol. All six patients had fewer side effects with atenolol and preferred it ($P < 0.05$). Blood-pressure control was the same with metoprolol and propranolol.

ANDERS WESTERLUND, M.D.
Västra Frölunda Hospital
42144 Gothenburg, Sweden

To the Editor:

The use of propranolol hydrochloride in treating patients with hyperthyroidism has been widely accepted as the sole or adjunctive agent during diagnosis and treatment of thyrotoxicosis.[1,2] In an earlier article on the long-acting β-adrenergic blocking agents recently introduced in this country[3] and in his review of atenolol and timolol, Frishman failed to comment on the therapeutic value of these drugs in thyrotoxicosis. They have not been approved by the Food and Drug Administration for use in this country in the treatment of hyperthyroidism; however, in Western Europe they have been proved beneficial for the treatment of this condition.[4-7]

Because propranolol has the disadvantage of a shortened half-life in the treatment of thyrotoxicosis,[8] larger and more frequent doses of it are required.

This is a problem particularly in patients undergoing surgery, who require oral doses of propranolol on ,the morning of surgery and early in the postoperative period.[2] Another disadvantage with this shortened half-life is that in our experience the patient with hyperthyroidism is poorly compliant; thus, the need for frequent administration of propranolol results in inadequate clinical response. It appears that the longer-acting β-blocker agents are most suitable for treating such patients.

We have successfully used two of the new β-blocker agents — nadolol and atenolol. The optimal dose was tailored to each patient. Treatment was initiated with a low dose taken once daily, and patients were instructed to increase the dose to twice a day on the basis of symptoms or pulse rate. We found that in most patients the condition was improved with a single daily dose, and only those with more severe thyrotoxicosis required more frequent doses. Doses of nadolol ranged from 40 to 360 mg daily, with a mean of 80 mg; for atenolol the range was 50 to 200 mg daily, with a mean of 75 mg.

The clinical improvement associated with these medications cannot be explained by a reduction of the thyroid hormone; this effect was minimal with propranolol and lacking with atenolol.[4,5] There was no difference between the clinical response to the cardioselective agent atenolol and the response to the nonselective agent nadolol or propranolol. Other workers have reported the same experience.[5-7]

JOEL ZONSZEIN, M.D.
PETER BAYLOR, M.D.
Bronx–Lebanon Hospital Center
Bronx, NY 10456

1. Ingbar SH, Woeber KA. The thyroid gland. In: Williams R, ed. Textbook of endocrinology. 6th ed. Philadelphia: WB Saunders, 1981:192-200.
2. Zonszein J, Santangelo RP, Mackin JF, Lee TC, Coffey RJ, Canary JJ. Propranolol therapy in thyrotoxicosis: a review of 84 patients undergoing surgery. Am J Med 1979; 66:411-6.
3. Frishman WH. Beta-adrenoceptor antagonists: new drugs and new indications. N Engl J Med 1981; 305:500-6.
4. How J, Khir ASM, Bewsher PD. The effect of atenolol on serum thyroid hormones in hyperthyroid patients. Clin Endocrinol (Oxf) 1980; 13:299-302.
5. Nilsson OR, Karlberg BE, Kagedal B, Tegler L, Almqvist S. Non-selective and selective beta-1-adrenoceptor blocking agents in the treatment of hyperthyroidism. Acta Med Scand 1979; 206:21-5.
6. McDevitt DG, Nelson JK. Comparative trial of atenolol and propranolol in hyperthyroidism. Br J Clin Pharmacol 1978; 6:233-7.
7. Nelson JK, McDevitt DG. Beta-blockade in thyrotoxicosis: is the cardioselective drug atenolol as satisfactory as propranolol? Ir J Med Sci 1979; 148:156. abstract.
8. Feely J, Stevenson IH, Crooks J. Increased clearance of propranolol in thyrotoxicosis. Ann Intern Med 1981; 94:472-4.

To the Editor:

We enjoyed reading Frishman's review but think that his statements on the relative cardioselectivity of atenolol and metoprolol need expansion.

When atenolol and propranolol were given acutely to volunteers in similar β_1-blocking doses, the quantity of the β_2 stimulant salbutamol required to increase airway conductance by 50 per cent was about 40 times greater for propranolol than for atenolol.[1] When atenolol and metoprolol were similarly compared, about three times more salbutamol was required with metoprolol than with atenolol, indicating the greater cardioselectivity of atenolol.[2]

Results obtained by administering the drugs acutely to normal subjects cannot necessarily be extrapolated to long-term administration of the drugs to patients with obstructive-airways disease. Therefore, we compared the effects on respiratory function of long-term administration of atenolol and metoprolol in 14 patients with hypertension and asthma. First we observed the acute effects of single doses of propranolol (40 mg), metoprolol (100 mg), and atenolol (100 mg). Compared with propranolol, both metoprolol and atenolol produced a similar and smaller fall in forced expiratory volume in one second. Also, they did not interfere with the bronchodilator action of salbutamol, which was almost completely blocked by propranolol.

In a double-blind, randomized, crossover study, the patients then received atenolol (100 mg once a day), metoprolol (100 mg twice a day), and a placebo, each for three weeks. The doses of atenolol and metoprolol were chosen because they had previously been shown to produce an equivalent degree of β_1 blockade (assessed by suppression of heart rate during exercise) over 24 hours after long-term administration to normal subjects.[3]

Among our patients, there were significantly fewer asthmatic attacks ($P<0.05$) with atenolol than with metoprolol. There were significantly more asthma-free days ($P<0.05$) with atenolol than with metoprolol. The percentage of time that patients felt moderately or severely wheezy was significantly greater ($P<0.05$) with metoprolol than with atenolol. The evening peak flow rate was significantly lower ($P<0.05$) with metoprolol than with atenolol. Atenolol did not differ markedly from the placebo. Blood-pressure control was the same with both treatments.

We conclude that nonselective β-blockers are contraindicated in asthma, but if β-blockade is considered essential, atenolol is the preferred agent. The dose should be kept as low as possible, since cardioselectivity is dose-related, and a β_2 stimulant bronchodilator should also be prescribed.

D. S. Lawrence and J. N. Sahay
Clatterbridge Hospital
Merseyside L63 4JY, England

S. S. Chatterjee
Wythenshawe Hospital
Manchester, England

1. Tattersfield AE, Mackay AD, Gribbin HR, Baldwin CJ. How cardioselective are the new beta-blocking drugs? Presented at the 6th Scientific Meeting of the International Society of Hypertension, Gothenburg, June 1979. abstract.

2. Harrison RN, Tattersfield AE. The cardioselectivity of atenolol and metoprolol at 2 and 24 hours after a single dose. Presented at the 9th Scientific Meeting of the International Society of Hypertension, Mexico, February 1982. abstract.

3. Harry JD, Cruickshank JM, Young J, Barker N. Relative activities of atenolol and metoprolol on the cardiovascular system of man. Eur J Clin Pharmacol 1981; 20:9-15.

To the Editor:

In response to Frishman's review we report a possible adverse interaction between topical epinephrine and timolol ophthalmic therapy. Both timolol — a nonselective β-receptor antagonist — and epinephrine — an α-receptor and β-receptor agonist — are systemically absorbed[1,2] and occasionally have extraocular side effects when applied topically to the eye.[3-5] Each of these drugs is usually prescribed alone, but in combination their adrenergic effects may result in unopposed α-adrenergic-induced hypertension. We describe a patient with hypertension, multiple somatic complaints, and elevated urinary metanephrines, which appeared to be related to ophthalmic therapy combining timolol and epinephrine.

The patient was a 48-year-old man with an eight-year history of primary open-angle glaucoma. Two years ago the following therapy was begun: Timoptic (timolol) (0.5 per cent), one drop in each eye twice a day; Epifrine (epinephrine) (2 per cent), one drop in each eye twice a day; carbachol (3 per cent), one drop in each eye every night at bedtime; and Neptazane (methazolamide), 50 mg orally twice a day. At about this time, the patient noticed episodic sweats occurring several times a day without a specific time pattern or provocative factors. Later he began to have right-frontal headaches, impotence, watery diarrhea, occasional vomiting, and exacerbation of childhood asthma. Approximately six months before evaluation, the patient was discovered to be hypertensive (160/108 mm Hg), and he was hospitalized for evaluation of a possible pheochromocytoma. Physical examination was unremarkable with the exception of hypertension and glaucomatous cupping of the left optic disk. Laboratory data, including routine blood and urine screening, thyroid-function tests, and urinary 5-hydroxyindole-acetic acid, were normal. Basal levels of urinary metanephrine and plasma catecholamines were elevated, but the level of plasma norepinephrine decreased more than 50 per cent after treatment with clonidine (0.3 mg taken orally),[7] and the level of urinary metanephrine returned to normal after epinephrine and timolol were withheld. This therapy was associated with relief of nearly all symptoms and a reduction in blood pressure (Table 1). Reinstitution of therapy resulted in a recurrence of hypertension and diaphoretic episodes. After discharge from the hospital, the patient stopped taking timolol but continued taking epinephrine. His pressure remained normal, and he had no symptoms during the subsequent six months of observation.

TABLE 1. Blood Pressure and Urinary Catecholamine Metabolites with and without Topical Epinephrine and Timolol Ophthalmic Therapy.

Day	Epinephrine and Timolol Therapy	Urinary Metabolites			
		MPB *	Catecholamines	Metanephrine	Vanillyl-mandelic Acid
			$\mu g/day$	mg/day	mg/day
1	+	130	128	1.9	3
2	+	126	106	1.6	3
4	−	82	179	1.0	3
5	−	93	112	0.5	2
7	+	119	118	0.8	3
Normal value			<150	<1.0	<10

*MPB denotes mean blood pressure (diastolic + ⅓ pulse pressure).

Although causality between this patient's ophthalmic therapy and the pheochromocytoma-like presentation cannot be established with certainty, adverse effects of β-blocker therapy in hyperadrenergic states have been reported. β-Blockers produce a hypertensive response when used alone in treating pheochromocytoma,[8] and they have been associated with a hypertensive crisis when administered with phenylephrine eye drops.[9,10] Therefore, close hemodynamic monitoring seems to be warranted when topical ophthalmic therapy is combined with β-blockers and adrenergic agonists.

GEORGE T. GRIFFING, M.D.
CHRISTOPHER E. COAKLEY, M.D.
SIMMONS LESSELL, M.D.
JAMES C. MELBY, M.D.
University Hospital
Boston, MA 02118

1. Ballin N, Becker B, Goldman ML. Systemic effects of epinephrine applied topically to the eye. Invest Ophthal 1966; 5:125-9.
2. Adverse systemic effects from ophthalmic drugs. Med Lett Drugs Ther 1982; 24:53-4.
3. Heel RC, Brogden RN, Speight TM, Avery GS. Timolol: a review of its therapeutic efficacy in the topical treatment of glaucoma. Drugs 1979; 17:38-55.
4. Podos SM, Ritch R. Epinephrine as the initial therapy in selected cases of ocular hypertension. Surv Ophthalmol 1980; 22:188-94.
5. Van Buskirk EM. Adverse reactions from timolol administration. Ophthalmology (Rochester) 1980; 87:447-50.
6. Bravo EL, Tarazi RC, Fouad FM, Vidt DG, Gifford RW Jr. Clonidine-suppression test: a useful aid in the diagnosis of pheochromocytoma. N Engl J Med 1981; 305:623-6.
7. Briggs RSJ, Birtwell AJ, Pohl JEF. Hypertensive response to labetalol in phaeochromocytoma. Lancet 1978; 1:1045-6.

8. Cass E, Kadar D, Stein HA. Hazards of phenylephrine topical medication in persons taking propranolol. Can Med Assoc J 1979; 120:1261-2.
9. Phenylephrine, eye drops and β-blockers. Med Lett Drugs Ther 1982; 24:70.

To the Editor:

In Frishman's review of atenolol the term "dose-dependent pharmacokinetics" is used incorrectly. Drugs with dose-dependent (or nonlinear) pharmacokinetics exhibit a disproportional increase of the serum concentration (or, more precisely, of the area under the serum concentration curve) with increasing doses.* Therefore, the fact that an "increase of the atenolol dose . . . can be expected to cause a proportional increase in the drug concentration . . ." indicates that atenolol pharmacokinetics are not dose-dependent.

S. VOŽEH, M.D.
University Hospital
CH-4031 Basel, Switzerland

The above letters were referred to the author of the article in question, who offers the following reply:

To the Editor:

In response to the letter from Drs. Rössner and Weiner, I agree that the issue of β-adrenergic blockade and plasma lipids is an important one. However, the clinical importance of β-blocker effects on lipids and lipoprotein fractions is far from being resolved. There have been multiple small population studies of the effects of different β-blocking agents on lipids in patients with hypertension, and they have produced a wide spectrum of inconsistent findings.[1] For this reason I avoided mentioning this subject in my review. The findings of Drs. Rössner and Weiner in their small study are of interest; however, the 25 per cent reduction in very-low-density lipoprotein triglycerides that is associated with atenolol may be of no clinical relevance, since this lipoprotein fraction is the least predictive of coronary risk. Also, other investigators have reported a 25 per cent increase in plasma triglycerides with long-term administration of atenolol.[2] In my own experience with metoprolol — a β₁-selective blocker — and labetalol — an α-blocker and β-blocker — I found that neither drug had an effect on plasma lipids.[1,3] Certainly, more work must be done in this area, with larger numbers of patients, more consistent laboratory methods, and controlled study designs.

It has been suggested that there are fewer central-nervous-system side effects with the β-blockers that have less lipid solubility than propranolol and metoprolol do. This clinical observation is based largely on anecdotal reports, and placebo-controlled comparative studies still need to be done to substantiate this claim. The observations reported by Dr. Westerlund are of interest; however, they

*Rowland M, Tozer TN. Clinical pharmacokinetics. Philadelphia: Lea & Febiger, 1980:93.

too are made on the basis of a small group of patients and thus are far from conclusive.

The letter by Drs. Zonszein and Baylor is provocative, but more information on the metabolism of β-blockers in patients with thyrotoxicosis needs to be provided. Their experience in treating thyrotoxicosis with atenolol and nadolol is impressive, but whether these drugs are more useful than short-acting β-blockers has yet to be proved. Also, when initiating treatment of thyrotoxicosis with a β-blocker, it is sometimes prudent to begin with a short-acting agent, since there will be less chance of prolonged toxicity, should it occur.

The letter from Drs. Lawrence, Sahay, and Chatterjee raises the age-old questions the relevance of β_1-adrenergic selectivity with the use of β-blockers in treating obstructive lung diseases and whether two β_1-selective antagonists — atenolol and metoprolol — differ in their effects on pulmonary function. The information they have reported is of interest; however, it is still unclear what part, if any, β_1-selective blockers play in patients with asthma and cardiovascular disease, when so many alternative therapies are now available for the treatment of hypertension, angina pectoris, and arrhythmia. Also, despite the experience reported in their letter, it has not been determined conclusively whether the bronchoprotective activity of atenolol is different from that of metoprolol.

The clinical observation that both epinephrine, an adrenergic agonist, and timolol, a β-adrenergic agonist, are useful as topical ophthalmic treatments for reducing intraocular pressure is one of the great pharmacologic enigmas. A possible explanation for the usefulness of topical timolol in treating increased intraocular pressure is that the drug may work indirectly, through its nonselective β-blocking activity, to potentiate the effects of endogenous circulating epinephrine in the eye. I appreciate the interesting report by Griffing et al., describing a patient who had systemic hypertension with combined epinephrine–timolol ophthalmic therapy. Their findings are consistent with the hemodynamic response to systemic nonselective β-adrenergic blockade and an increased level of circulating epinephrine, which is a potentiation of α-adrenergic activity and peripheral vasoconstriction. As they described, these findings are similar to those observed in patients with pheochromocytoma who received β-blocking drugs. I agree that patients who are receiving combined epinephrine–timolol therapy for treatment of glaucoma should be monitored.

WILLIAM H. FRISHMAN, M.D.
Albert Einstein College of Medicine
Bronx, NY 10461

1. Johnson B. The emerging problem of plasma lipid changes during antihypertensive therapy. J Cardiovasc Pharmacol 1982; 4: Suppl 2:5213-21.

2. Day JL, Simpson N, Metcalfe J, et al. Metabolic consequences of atenolol and propranolol in treatment of essential hypertension. Br Med J 1979; 1:77-80.

3. Frishman W, Michelson E, Johnson B, et al. Effects of beta-adrenergic blockade on plasma lipids: a double-blind randomized placebo-controlled multi-center comparison of labetalol and metaprolol in patients with hypertension. Am J Cardiol 1982; 49:984. abstract.

Thrombolytic Therapy

G. V. R. K. Sharma, M.D.,

Giuseppe Cella, M.D.,

Alfred F. Parisi, M.D.,

and Arthur A. Sasahara, M.D.

IN the continuing search for new and improved methods of treating thrombo-embolic diseases, the concept of an agent to dissolve clots has always been attractive. After the efficacy of heparin in venous thromboembolism was established by Barritt and Jordan,[1] many physicians regarded its use as definitive, but in reality its action was only preventive. What was needed was an agent that would act on the morbid event directly — i.e., that would dissolve thrombo-emboli in pulmonary embolism. By restoring pulmonary vascular space, relieving pulmonary hypertension, and recompensating right ventricular function, such therapy could minimize morbidity and perhaps decrease mortality, particularly in patients with previously compromised cardiopulmonary status or with massive pulmonary embolism. The long search for such an agent resulted in the approval of two plasminogen activators, streptokinase and urokinase, in the United States in 1977.

Streptokinase and Urokinase

Streptokinase and urokinase are compared in Table 1. Streptokinase was discovered in 1933 by Tillett and Garner when they observed that a filtrate of Group C beta-hemolytic streptococci lysed a human plasma clot.[2] Subsequent studies, including those by Sherry,[3] helped to characterize the interaction of this extract with the fibrinolytic system and showed that the activator substance acted on plasminogen to produce an active enzyme plasmin. The activator was named streptokinase. In 1959 Johnson and McCarty successfully lysed thrombi that had been experimentally induced in forearm veins of volunteers.[4]

Urokinase, isolated from human urine by Macfarlane and Pilling in 1946,[5] was given its name by Sobel and his colleagues.[6] Further investigations demon-

From the Medical and Research Services, Veterans Administration Medical Center, West Roxbury, Mass., and the Departments of Medicine, Brigham and Women's Hospital and Harvard Medical School, Boston.

Originally published on May 27, 1982 (306:1268-1276).

strated that urokinase was also a plasminogen activator. Subsequently, Sherry et al. provided important pharmacologic and clinical information[7] that led to the experimental use of urokinase for therapeutic thrombolysis. By 1960, Ploug and Kjeldgaard had developed purification methods for isolating urokinase from urine

TABLE 1. Comparison of the Features of Streptokinase and Urokinase.

Feature	Streptokinase	Urokinase
Source	Group C streptococci	Human fetal kidney tissue culture; human urine
Molecular weight	47,000 daltons	32,000–54,000 daltons
Half-life	10–12 min	11–16 min
Stability	Room temperature	4°C
Antigenicity	Yes	No
Pyrogenicity	Minimal	None
Indications	Pulmonary embolism. Deep-vein thrombosis. Arterial thrombosis. Occluded access shunts. Acute transmural myocardial infarction.	Pulmonary embolism. Occluded access shunts.
Retreatment	Wait 6–12 mo	As needed
Retail price per 100,000 IU (1982)	$8	$50

in a form suitable for clinical investigations.[8] Shortly thereafter, the National Institutes of Health (NIH) formed the Committee on Thrombolytic Agents, which identified urinary urokinase as the most promising agent for use in clinical trials of treatment of thromboembolism. This urokinase possessed high specific activity; it was free of contamination and was also virus-inactivated, nontoxic, and nonpyrogenic. The Committee established a unit dose (CTA unit) that was equivalent to the present international unit (IU).

Mechanism of Action

The exogenous plasminogen activators streptokinase and urokinase produce fibrinolysis by activating the body's natural fibrinolytic system (Fig. 1). In essence, the inactive proenzyme plasminogen is converted to the active enzyme plasmin, which lyses fresh fibrin clots, with generation of fibrin (or fibrinogen) degradation products. Plasminogen is present in human plasma and is not subject to wide swings in concentration. Its concentration tends to be low in infants and in patients with advanced cirrhosis of the liver and disseminated intravascular coagulation, and to be high in patients with conditions associated with increased amounts of acute-phase reactants — e.g., surgery, trauma, infections, and acute myocardial infarction.[9] Plasminogen is synthesized rapidly, and its concentration usually returns to normal within 24 hours after cessation of thrombolytic therapy.

Plasmin, the active enzyme, is a nonspecific proteolytic agent that can digest fibrin, fibrinogen, prothrombin, and factors V and VIII. It is "specific" for

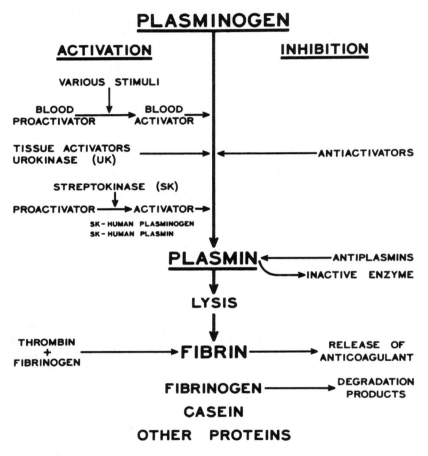

Figure 1. *Fibrinolysis during Thrombolytic Therapy.*
Urokinase and streptokinase activate the fibrinolytic system and convert plasminogen to the active enzyme plasmin, which then lyses a fresh fibrin clot.

dissolving fibrin clots within the thrombus, in which plasmin inhibitor concentration is very low; however, in the circulation the large excess of plasmin inhibitor (antiplasmin) neutralizes its action on other circulating proteins.

Although both streptokinase and urokinase are capable of activating the fibrinolytic system, they do so by different mechanisms. Streptokinase is an indirect activator, converting plasminogen to plasmin by way of a proactivator-activator mechanism. When streptokinase is administered, it combines with plasminogen on an equimolar basis (1:1 ratio) to form the activator complex. This streptokinase–plasminogen complex then activates the fibrinolytic mechanism by converting uncomplexed plasminogen to plasmin. As this process continues, the streptokinase–plasminogen complex is gradually converted to the streptokinase–plasmin form, which can also activate and convert plasminogen. Because this conversion takes place slowly, the initial activator activity is due to the streptokinase–plasminogen complex, whereas later activity is due to the streptokinase-–plasmin form.

One of the major problems with streptokinase is that it is a foreign protein and therefore antigenic. Antibodies to streptococci are present in almost everyone in various amounts, depending on the nature of previous streptococcal infections. When streptokinase is infused, an antigen–antibody complex is formed, neutralizing its activity. Hence, at the beginning of streptokinase therapy a sufficient loading dose must be given to neutralize or inhibit circulating antibodies.

Urokinase, on the other hand, is a direct activator. It is capable of initiating fibrinolysis without forming an activator complex. Since it is a protein secreted by the human kidney, it is also nonantigenic. It can be administered to all patients without concern for neutralizing antibodies; the problem of pyrogenicity is related simply to the purity of the preparation. Because of the high cost of collecting large amounts of human urine and isolating and purifying urokinase, alternative methods of producing the enzyme have been sought. In 1967 Bernik and Kwaan reported their success in producing urokinase from tissue cultures of human embryonic kidney cells.[10] The urokinase produced from these tissue cultures has activities in vitro that are similar to those of urinary urokinase. A pilot trial of the two preparations in acute pulmonary embolism showed no important biochemical and fibrinolytic differences, demonstrating their pharmacologic equivalence.[11] Currently, both urinary and tissue-culture urokinase preparations are available for clinical use.

Clinical Investigations

A number of clinical studies have been carried out in Europe and the United Kingdom, principally in the treatment of deep-vein thrombosis. In the United States, most of the clinical studies using urokinase have been performed in patients with pulmonary embolism in order to determine optimal dosages and blood concentrations.[12-15] These pilot studies demonstrated that urokinase accelerated thrombolysis without significant toxicity; that patients with very recent, massive pulmonary embolism appeared to respond well, whereas patients with pulmonary embolism of a week's duration or more did not; and that there was no relation between the intensity of fibrinolysis established (dose dependent) and the degree of clot resolution as judged by serial pulmonary angiograms, lung scans, and hemodynamic changes.

As a result of these encouraging studies, the National Heart, Lung, and Blood Institute launched the first of two controlled clinical trials comparing urokinase and heparin (Phase I, Urokinase Pulmonary Embolism Trial)[16] and subsequently urokinase and streptokinase (Phase II, Urokinase-Streptokinase Pulmonary Embolism Trial).[17] In essence, these two trials, in which 327 patients with angiographically confirmed pulmonary embolism were studied, showed the following: (1) greater resolution of pulmonary emboli with lytic therapy than with heparin, as assessed by pretreatment and post-treatment pulmonary angiography; (2) greater improvement of the abnormal hemodynamics of the right heart and pulmonary circulation with lytic therapy than with heparin, as assessed by pretreatment and post-treatment measurements of these pressures; (3) greater reperfusion of the original perfusion defects with lytic therapy than with heparin, as assessed by pretreatment and post-treatment perfusion lung scans; (4) maximum clot resolution and general improvement in patients with the largest pulmonary emboli; and (5) lack of differences in mortality between patients given heparin and those given thrombolytics. Since the mortality of patients with pulmonary embolism treated with conventional anticoagulants was relatively low (8 to 10 per cent), it had been anticipated that the number of patients necessary to demonstrate differences in clot resolution would not be sufficient to demonstrate differences in mortality.

Resolution of Emboli in the Pulmonary Microcirculation

Although thrombolytic agents were shown to have much more impressive beneficial effects in acute pulmonary embolism, long-term studies with perfusion lung scans in the Urokinase Pulmonary Embolism Trial showed that comparable resolution could be achieved by heparin therapy in about 85 per cent of the patients. This observation can be misleading, however, since neither the perfusion lung scan nor the pulmonary angiogram is a very sensitive method for evaluation of the status of the pulmonary microcirculation. Therefore, pulmonary capillary blood volume and diffusing capacity were measured in our laboratory to compare the long-term effects of heparin and thrombolytic agents on pulmonary perfusion and diffusion.[18] Measurement was carried out approximately two weeks and one year after therapy. Patients who had clinical cardiopulmonary disease were excluded from the study because the anatomic and functional changes associated with previous disease would have rendered the interpretation of these tests difficult, if not impossible. The results showed that at two weeks, pulmonary capillary blood volume and diffusing capacity were abnormally low in the heparin-treated group but normal in the group receiving lytic therapy. These differences persisted for up to one year, indicating that the thrombolytic agents achieved a more complete resolution of thromboemboli from the pulmonary microcirculation than did heparin treatment, thus improving capillary perfusion and diffusion. The long-term implication of these observations is that thrombolytic agents may prevent or at least minimize the chronic pulmonary hypertension that may develop from incomplete resolution of thromboemboli, particularly in recurrences.

Resolution of Thrombi in the Deep Venous System

During the past several years, there has been a growing appreciation of the importance of deep-vein thrombosis in pulmonary embolism, as originally pointed out by Sevitt and Gallagher, who noted at autopsy that virtually all patients who died of massive pulmonary embolism had deep-vein thrombosis of the lower limbs as the source of the emboli.[19] Kakkar et al. showed that extension of thrombi to the popliteal and the more proximal veins posed a serious threat for pulmonary embolism and noted also that the rapid lysis of thrombi in the deep venous system with streptokinase therapy tended to preserve the anatomy and function of the venous valves much more often than did heparin therapy.[20] Our own findings with impedance plethysmography confirmed the increased rate of resolution of deep-vein thrombi with thrombolytic therapy as compared with heparin therapy.[21] These observations concerning the rapidity and completeness of clearing of deep-vein thrombi and the early preservation of the venous valves with streptokinase therapy may have important long-term implications in the prevention or reduction of chronic venous insufficiency. A final judgment must await the publication of data from studies of valvular function and manifestations of venous stasis present at one year or more after treatment.

Clinical Indications for Thrombolytic Therapy

The clinical indications for thrombolytic therapy have been defined by the Food and Drug Administration. On the basis of results from clinical investigations, streptokinase has been approved for treatment of the following conditions: acute pulmonary embolism and deep-vein thrombosis (within seven days of onset of symptoms), arterial thrombosis, acute myocardial infarction, and occlusion of access shunts and intravascular or cavity catheters. Urokinase may be used in cases of acute pulmonary embolism (within seven days of onset of symptoms) and occlusion of access shunts and intravascular or cavity catheters.

Venous Thromboembolism

Once it has been determined that the thromboembolic process is "fresh," the next consideration should be the patient's safety. The guiding principle should be an awareness that exogenous activation of the body's fibrinolytic system by these agents results in a more profound alteration of the hemostatic status of the patient than occurs with anticoagulant therapy. This awareness should lead to selection of patients in whom the potential for bleeding is minimal.

Who, then, should not receive thrombolytic agents? From the experience of the NIH clinical trials, a list of exclusions (summarized in Table 2) has been compiled.

TABLE 2. Contraindications to Thrombolytic Therapy.

Absolute Contraindications
Active internal bleeding
Cerebrovascular process, disease, or procedure within two months

Relative Contraindications
Conditions requiring fibrin strands and plugs for normal hemostasis or healing (fibrinolysis is usually contraindicated within 10 days of onset of these conditions)
Major surgery, organ biopsy, puncture of noncompressible blood vessel
Postpartum period
Cardiopulmonary resuscitation during presence of rib fractures
Thoracentesis, paracentesis, lumbar puncture
Recent serious trauma
Potentially serious bleeding
Uncontrolled coagulation defects
Uncontrolled severe hypertension
Pregnancy
Other conditions deemed potential bleeding risks

Absolute contraindications include an active internal bleeding state and a recent (within two months) cerebrovascular process or procedure. A more remote (more than two months) cerebrovascular process or procedure should be considered a very strong but relative contraindication, and a decision to use lytic agents must be based on an assessment of the risk-benefit status. Other relative contraindications include surgery in which the immediate use of lytic agents after the procedure would probably dissolve fibrin strands and plugs and thus delay wound healing. Similar reasoning can be applied to recent biopsy of an organ. Patients who have had a recent invasive procedure of a body cavity or vessel that cannot be compressed for a long period should not receive lytic therapy unless the severity of the thromboembolic process overrides the increased risk of bleeding. Each physician must make a risk-benefit assessment of the clinical situation before selecting or excluding thrombolytic therapy. Such a decision should be based on the fact that thrombolytic therapy does not differentiate between "good clots" (part of the normal hemostatic mechanism) and "bad clots" (venous or arterial thromboembolism). This consideration permits the physician to make a rational decision in most clinical situations.

Peripheral Arterial Thrombosis

The use of thrombolytic therapy in acute arterial thrombosis present for less than 10 days has been shown to be effective, and marked improvement has been achieved in the great majority of the patients treated. Although standard systemic doses have been employed in most patients, it has also been reported that a low dose of lytic agents infused through small arterial catheters positioned adjacent to the thrombus has been effective in resolving thrombi.[22-24]

Streptokinase and urokinase seem to be equally effective in acute arterial occlusions, although only streptokinase is officially approved for use in the United States. Dotter et al. used selective catheter administration of 3000 to 10,000 units of streptokinase per hour for 18 to 112 hours in patients with thromboembolism occurring soon after a procedure (four to 20 hours), with excellent results,[22] whereas Katzen and van Breda used 5000 U per hour for five to 16 hours.[23] Fiessinger et al. gave urokinase in a loading dose of 75,000 IU and then a maintenance dose of 37,500 IU per hour for 72 hours, with equally good results.[24]

Although experience is still limited, thrombolytic agents are probably most useful in patients with peripheral arterial thrombosis at the time of an acute episode or after failure of reconstructive surgery, and in patients whose thrombi are inaccessible to surgery.

Chronic Arterial Occlusion

The results of intravenous infusion of thrombolytic agents in chronic arterial occlusion and stenosis have not been encouraging, on the whole. Poliwoda et al. were able to restore arterial blood flow in only 17 of 85 limbs (20 per cent) with chronic arterial occlusion and stenosis.[25] Verstraete et al., using the standard loading dose of 250,000 units of streptokinase and a maintenance dose of 100,000 units per hour for at least 72 hours, reported that chronic arterial occlusion could be lysed only occasionally and that lysis appeared to be influenced by the duration and the length and location of the occlusion.[26] Martin, using a titrated loading dose and a 72-hour infusion of 100,000 units per hour, reported successful treatment in only 8.9 per cent of patients with chronic femoral occlusions, 19.5 per cent of those with chronic iliac occlusions, and 24.4 per cent of those with chronic aortic occlusions.[27] The reocclusion rate was 15 per cent for the early occlusions and between 21 and 29 per cent for the late closures. The rate of reocclusion was highly influenced by the smoking habits of the patients, the use of anticoagulant therapy, and the location of the lesions.

In the most recent study of patients with chronic peripheral arterial disease, Long administered standard doses of streptokinase intravenously for up to 96 hours in 16 patients who had severe arterial insufficiency and no distal pulses, as an alternative to limb amputation.[28] The distal pulses were restored in 13 patients (81 per cent), and amputation was not required. Four patients had good functional results and did not need reconstructive surgery. Seven patients had initial thrombolysis followed by successful arterial bypass grafting, and two had successful lysis two to 10 days after a vascular procedure. It was notable that despite the temporal proximity to vascular surgery and other invasive arterial procedures, only two of the 16 patients had bleeding complications during lytic therapy — one from a very recent femoral arteriotomy, and another from the site of a femoral arteriographic puncture performed on the previous day. Long's approach in combining thrombolytic therapy with peripheral arterial bypass grafting appears very promising and deserves further application.

Acute Transmural Myocardial Infarction

Although the precise mechanism of myocardial infarction remains unclear and post-mortem examinations show a widely varying incidence of occlusive coronary-artery thrombi (20 to 90 per cent), recent surgical and angiographic experiences in acute transmural myocardial infarction have shown a high incidence of occlusive thrombi in the early hours after the onset of symptoms.[29,30]

Systemic Thrombolytic Therapy

Systemic infusion of thrombolytic agents in acute myocardial infarction was introduced by Fletcher et al. in 1959.[31] Since then, some 20 clinical trials have been reported, involving more than 6000 patients. Most of these trials suffered from faulty protocol design, improper selection of patients, and inappropriate data collection that made it difficult to draw conclusions.[32,33]

Streptokinase was used in 15 trials, in most of which a loading dose of 250,000 units was followed by an infusion of 100,000 units per hour for 12 to 24 hours and then anticoagulant therapy. Despite these doses, bleeding complications were not a major problem.[32] There was no consensus, however, concerning the effect on overall mortality, probably because only a few patients were treated within three to six hours of the onset of symptoms. Recently, it was shown that systemic administration of streptokinase or urokinase in acute myocardial infarction (500,000 units infused in 10 to 30 minutes) achieved angiographic resolution of a totally occluded coronary artery in 45 per cent of 22 patients within one hour and in 86 per cent after 24 hours and at three weeks.[34]

Intracoronary Thrombolytic Therapy

The possibility that intracoronary infusion of lytic agents has an important role in the treatment of evolving myocardial infarction by limiting myocardial damage and improving ventricular function has recently been investigated. The first report of intracoronary administration of fibrinolysin appeared 22 years ago, but it offered no direct evidence of resolution of thrombi because coronary angiography was not performed.[35]

The success of intracoronary thrombolysis seems to be greatest when treatment is instituted early. In recent reports the criteria for selection of patients with respect to the onset of symptoms have not been uniform and ranged from less than three hours to up to 18 hours. Streptokinase was the most widely used lytic agent, but there was no consensus about its dosage. (The published results of intracoronary infusion of streptokinase are summarized in Table 3.) Some investigators injected a bolus dose of 10,000 to 20,000 units and infused the drug at a rate of 1000 to 5000 units per minute until thrombus dissolution[36-38,41]; others did not use a loading dose.[39,42] If the obstruction was not reversed within 1½ hours, the infusion was not continued. Urokinase has been used less frequently in these investigations, and the total dose has varied considerably.

Both the European and American studies have shown a high incidence of successful recanalization (about 80 per cent) within one hour of the beginning of

TABLE 3. Studies of Reperfusion of Completely Occluded Coronary Arteries by Intracoronary Infusion of Streptokinase.

Study	No. of Cases	Duration of Symptoms	Streptokinase Dosage		Duration of Infusion before Patency	Outcome	
			Loading Dose	Infusion Rate		Artery Reperfused	No Response
		mean hr ±S.D. Hours	units	units/min	mean min ±S.D.	no. of cases (per cent)	
Rentrop[36]	5		10,000–20,000	1000–2000	15–16	4 (80)	1
Reduto[37]	29	9.2±4.0 (2–18)	10,000	2000	24±13 (7–90)	20 (69)	9
Markis[38]	9	3.5 (2.3–4.3)	20,000	2000–4000	20	9 (100)	0
Gold[39]	25	≤3	None	2000–4000	30–40	17 (68)	8
Ganz[40]	20	≤3	None	1000–2000 (thrombolysin)	8–80	19 (95)	1
Cowley[41]	9	5.5±0.6	20,000	1000–2500	24±7 (8–50)	7 (78)	2
Lee[42]	20	<5–>7	None	2000–5000	60–300	16 (80)	4
West Germany studies[43,44]	160	2.5–4.5	None	2000–4000	35.5±8.4 (30–50)	129 (81)	31

therapy in most instances. In a few patients recanalization was delayed and occurred five hours after streptokinase infusion. In patients with incomplete coronary-artery obstruction, little benefit was gained. When early recanalization was established, ST segments became normal on electrocardiography, regional perfusion quantitatively improved on thallium-201 myocardial scanning, and peak creatine kinase activity appeared earlier. The changes in left ventricular function seem to be highly influenced by the presence of collaterals and the duration of symptoms. In the absence of collaterals, only very early reperfusion may result in preservation of function.[45] It is important, however, to point out that spontaneous improvement of global and regional left ventricular function can take place during the first 24 hours after an acute myocardial infarction.[46]

Since the underlying atherosclerotic lesion is not affected, coronary-artery by-pass grafting may be required in some patients after successful recanalization and in others with reocclusion occurring days or weeks after recanalization. In a few patients with partially obstructive lesions after lysis, percutaneous transluminal coronary angioplasty has been performed successfully. Reocclusion after successful lysis seems to occur more frequently when the left circumflex coronary artery is involved, and neither oral anticoagulants nor antiplatelet agents seem to affect the reocclusion rate.[45] Only heparin seems to be beneficial during the early days after patency has been established.

The incidence of serious systemic hemorrhagic complications requiring blood transfusion seems to be low (3.9 to 7.4 per cent); these complications most often occur when the total dose of streptokinase is greater than 200,000 units and when the fibrinogen level falls to less than 100 mg per deciliter (3 μmol per liter).[43,44] At autopsy some patients have been found to have trans-mural hemorrhagic infarction in the area supplied by the reperfused vessel; however, this reperfusion hemorrhage seems to be a consequence of vascular damage rather than reperfusion itself.[40,47] The incidence of reperfusion arrhythmias ranges from 25 to 94 per cent. Most arrhythmias are easy to control with antiarrhythmic agents, but the reperfusion of an occluded right coronary artery carries a substantial risk of serious arrhythmias or hypotension or both.[42,48] The in-hospital mortality in patients successfully treated in one study was significantly lower than those in whom the occluded vessel could not be reperfused. The reinfarction rate and the recurrence of angina, however, were similar in both groups.[43]

As promising as the current results may seem, we believe that studies to date showing recanalization of fresh coronary thrombi demonstrate only that it is feasible to lyse coronary thrombi by intracoronary administration of thrombolytic agents. Long-term effects on ventricular function and survival of restricting performance of this procedure to institutions with expertise in coronary angiography, of the cost-benefit aspects of this expensive procedure, and the potential impact on the millions of patients with coronary-artery disease can only be determined by a large, multicenter trial. Such a trial should also compare the efficacy of intracoronary administration with that of systemic administration, which has potentially greater applicability.

Other Applications of Thrombolytic Therapy

Thrombolytic therapy has been used in a variety of thromboembolic conditions, but the small number of patients studied does not permit any conclusions to be drawn, and therefore no clinical recommendations can be made. Kwaan et al. reported that in patients with central retinal-vein occlusion, systemic administration of streptokinase produced changes in visual acuity comparable to those produced by administration of heparin.[49]

The application of streptokinase and urokinase to restore the patency of occluded shunts in patients undergoing renal dialysis has been effective in 70 to 90 per cent of cases.[50] In addition, occluded intravascular lines or catheters in body cavities can be successfully opened by local thrombolytic therapy.

The only controlled clinical trial of thrombolysis for acute cerebrovascular occlusion showed poor improvement in patients given streptokinase; their mortality (35 per cent) was greater than that of the heparin-treated control group (11 per cent).[51] Currently, limited experience with selective catheter administration of small doses of urokinase in acute cerebral thrombosis is being obtained in Japan, but definitive data are not yet available. Until it can be shown that acute cerebral thrombosis can be safely and effectively treated, thrombolytic therapy is contraindicated. In fact, thrombolytic agents are contraindicated in all patients who have had a cerebrovascular procedure or evidence of disease within the prior two months. Even when these events have occurred before then, we believe that they constitute a very strong relative contraindication.

Drug Administration for Systemic Fibrinolysis

No schedule for optimal dosage in thrombolytic therapy has been established, particularly for urokinase. Samama and Conard investigated various dosage regimens for urokinase and concluded that a loading dose of 150,000 IU, followed by 2500 IU per kilogram of body weight per hour, was entirely adequate to produce fibrinolysis.[52] However, most investigators recommend the dosage schedule used in the large NIH clinical trials of treatment for pulmonary embolism.

Loading Dose

Both streptokinase and urokinase should be initiated with a loading dose administered through a peripheral line by a constant-infusion pump. The dose of streptokinase should be 250,000 units, given over 20 to 30 minutes, and that of urokinase should be 4400 IU per kilogram, given over 10 minutes.

Because some patients with prior streptococcal infections may have relatively high titers of streptococcal antibodies, it has been recommended that a streptokinase-resistance test should be performed to determine the dosage. However, we have not found it necessary to perform this test, because the loading dose of 250,000 units of streptokinase is sufficient to overcome resistance in over 85 to 90 per cent of patients. Since urokinase is a human protein, no resistance develops and a predictable response can be anticipated.

It is recommended that when streptokinase is used, 100 mg of hydrocortisone should be administered intravenously before the infusion of the streptokinase so that the mild but annoying side reactions that may occur may be prevented. This dose should be repeated every 12 to 24 hours during the infusion.

Maintenance Dose

The following dose schedule, used in the NIH trials, is recommended: 100,000 units of streptokinase per hour, for 24 hours in pulmonary embolism and for 48 to 72 hours in deep-vein thrombosis; and 4400 IU of urokinase per kilogram per hour for 12 to 24 hours in pulmonary embolism.

Although the Phase II Urokinase-Streptokinase Pulmonary Embolism Trial showed no significant differences between 12 and 24 hours of urokinase treatment, it is our belief that 24 hours would be more beneficial for lysis of thrombi in the deep venous system, which invariably accompany pulmonary embolism.

Repeat Administration

Because of its antigenicity, streptokinase should generally not be used for six to 12 months after a course of therapy. However, if a streptokinase-resistance test shows that resistance is not inordinately high but can be overcome by a loading dose of 250,000 units, streptokinase may be given again. Our preference, however, is to use urokinase.

Concurrent Treatment Guidelines

Recommendations for the general treatment of patients receiving thrombolytic therapy are summarized in Table 4. They are intended to promote safety. It is important to discontinue parenteral injections, particularly intramuscular ones, to avoid unnecessary local bleeding. Required venipunctures should be confined to the arms and should be covered with a simple pressure bandage. It is not unusual to observe a slight bluish discoloration of the skin around the needle tracks, but a compression bandage will prevent major extravasation. Arterial punctures and other invasive procedures should be avoided during infusion of lytic agents.

Laboratory Monitoring

In contrast to the practice during heparin therapy, laboratory monitoring for lytic therapy is not used to adjust dosage, which is fixed for both activators. Monitoring is used simply to determine whether some degree of systemic fibrinolysis has

TABLE 4. Clinical Guidelines for Patient Treatment.

1. Minimize physical handling of patient
2. Discontinue parenteral medications
3. Substitute appropriate oral medications
4. Minimize invasive procedures, including needle punctures
5. Apply compression bandages at sites of vessel puncture
6. Avoid concurrent anticoagulation
7. Avoid concurrent use of platelet-active drugs

been established. As long as some degree of lysis is established, vigorous dissolution of clots can be expected, provided that the fibrin clots are fresh. Simple but adequate laboratory monitoring for safe and effective administration of thrombolytic therapy is outlined in Table 5.

The most sensitive test for fibrinolysis is the whole-blood euglobulin lysis time. The next most sensitive is the thrombin time. If they are unavailable, the partial thromboplastin time and prothrombin time or the measurement of fibrin degradation products can be used. Particularly useful if the patient is already

TABLE 5. Laboratory Monitoring for Thrombolytic Therapy.

Tests
Whole-blood euglobulin lysis time, *or*
Thrombin time, *or*
Partial thromboplastin and prothrombin times, *or*
Fibrin(ogen) degradation products

Time of Testing
Before therapy
Detect and correct coagulation defects (by means of thrombin, partial thromboplastin, and prothrombin times)
Determine base line or control for fibrinolysis (any of the above tests; euglobulin lysis time or fibrin(ogen) degradation products if patient has been receiving heparin)
During therapy (3–4 hr after start)
Use same test(s) used for establishing base line or control
After therapy
Use partial thromboplastin time if heparin therapy is to begin

Objective
Ensure establishment of fibrinolytic state:
Determine whether values have marked prolongation over control value
Administer streptokinase:
If values not changed from control at 3–4 hr, give another loading dose (250,000 units) and continue infusion (standard, 100,000 units per hour)
Recheck in another 3–4 hr. If still no change, discontinue streptokinase and switch to urokinase, or begin heparin therapy

receiving heparin is the euglobulin lysis time or the fibrin degradation products. Whichever test is selected, it should be performed during a control period and after three to four hours of lytic treatment. As long as the test values during thrombolytic infusion are prolonged beyond the control value (except the euglobulin lysis time, which should be shortened), it can be assumed that systemic lysis has been established. Monitoring is especially important when streptokinase is used, because an occasional patient may have very high titers of streptococcal antibodies from a previous infection, which will render streptokinase therapy ineffective. Without the lytic and anticoagulant effects, the patient will be at risk for recurrent thromboembolism.

Anticoagulation after Thrombolytic Therapy

After thrombolytic therapy is completed, the partial thromboplastin time should be measured to determine when conventional heparin therapy should be instituted. When this value falls to therapeutic levels (i.e., twice the control value), heparin should be administered by continuous pump infusion, without a loading dose, for the usual period (five to 10 days) and then followed by oral anticoagulants. If the partial thromboplastin time is less than twice control, an appropriate loading dose of heparin should be given, followed by a dose adequate to maintain therapeutic levels.

| Complications of Thrombolytic Therapy

Bleeding

Although bleeding complications occurred frequently in the NIH clinical trials, severe bleeding from sites that were not invaded was infrequent. Early bleeding (within 24 hours) occurred almost as frequently as late bleeding (up to two weeks). The late bleeding occurred during anticoagulant therapy instituted immediately after termination of thrombolytic therapy. The great majority of bleeding events occurred at sites of blood-vessel punctures and cutdowns. When patients are carefully selected and treated with a minimum of invasive procedures, the frequency of bleeding can be markedly reduced. The incidence of severe bleeding (requiring blood replacement) was 4 per cent among more than 100 of our patients and was considerably less — no severe bleeding in over 200 consecutive therapeutic applications —among patients at the Johns Hopkins Medical Institutions (Bell WR: personal communication).

Unlike anticoagulant therapy, in which the frequency of bleeding is related to excessive dose, thrombolytic therapy does not appear to have a correlation between the incidence of bleeding complications and the degree of systemic fibrinolysis, which is dose dependent. Instead, the patients who bleed during thrombolytic therapy are those who have some prior hemostatic defect and who should be identified by careful history taking before therapy.

When bleeding occurs during therapy, its treatment depends on its severity. Generally, light bleeding or oozing occurs from the invaded areas. As long as these vessel punctures are confined to the arms, simple, mechanical compression with a pledget will suffice. Occasionally, stubborn oozing can be stopped with a pledget soaked with aminocaproic acid (Amicar, EACA).

More severe bleeding calls for discontinuation of the lytic agent. Because of the very short half-life of these agents (10 to 15 minutes), lytic activity stops promptly. If blood replacement is indicated, whole blood, preferably fresh, is best. Alternatively, packed red cells and fresh-frozen plasma or cryoprecipitate (several units) may be given and should rapidly reverse the hemostatic alterations. In desperate situations, aminocaproic acid may be administered in 5-g doses, although no investigator in the NIH trials was forced to use this fibrinolytic inhibitor. Aminocaproic acid should not be given for bleeding from the genitourinary tract because a renal-ureteral thrombotic cast may be produced.

Other Complications

Other complications of thrombolytic therapy include fever and allergic reactions. About 25 per cent of the patients in the NIH trials who received streptokinase had temperature elevations of more than 0.9°C (1.5°F), whereas 14 to 15 per cent of the urokinase-treated patients had such elevations — an incidence similar to that in the patients given heparin. Allergic reactions such as skin rashes were infrequent but more common (6 per cent) among the streptokinase-treated patients. Anaphylactic shock did not develop in any patient. Other mild reactions, primarily to streptokinase, include urticaria, nausea, vomiting, flushing, headaches, and muscle pain. None of these were severe enough to require discontinuation of therapy.

Management of Untoward Reactions

These minor adverse reactions may be treated with antihistamines at the time of detection; acetaminophen is very effective in treating temperature elevations. However, it has been our practice to administer 100 mg of hydrocortisone intravenously before beginning streptokinase therapy and to continue giving the same dose orally every 12 to 24 hours for the duration of thrombolytic treatment, thereby eliminating annoying adverse reactions. Such prophylactic therapy is not necessary with urokinase therapy.

| References

1. Barritt DW, Jordan SC. Anticoagulant drugs in the treatment of pulmonary embolism: a controlled trial. Lancet 1960; 1:1309-12.
2. Tillett WS, Garner RL. The fibrinolytic activity of hemolytic streptococci. J Exp Med 1933; 58:485-502.

3. Sherry S. The fibrinolytic activity of streptokinase activated human plasmin. J Clin Invest 1954; 33:1054-63.

4. Johnson AJ, McCarty WR. The lysis of artificially induced intravascular clots in man by intravenous infusions of streptokinase. J Clin Invest 1959; 38:1627-43.

5. Macfarlane RG, Pilling J. Observations on fibrinolysis: plasminogen, plasmin, and antiplasmin content of human blood. Lancet 1946; 2:562-5.

6. Sobel GW, Mohler SR, Jones NW, Dowdy ABC, Guest MM. Urokinase: an activator of plasma profibrinolysin extracted from urine. Am J Physiol 1952; 171:768-9. abstract.

7. Sherry S, Lindemeyer RI, Fletcher AP, Alkjaersig N. Studies on enhanced fibrinolytic activity in man. J Clin Invest 1959; 38:810-22.

8. Ploug J, Kjeldgaard NO. Urokinase: an activator of plasminogen from human urine. I. Isolation and properties. Biochim Biophys Acta 1957; 24:278-82.

9. Lesuk A, Terminiello L, Traver JH. Crystalline human urokinase: some properties. Science 1965; 147:880-2.

10. Bernik MB, Kwaan HC. Origin of fibrinolytic activity in cultures of the human kidney. J Lab Clin Med 1967; 70:650-61.

11. Marder VJ, Donahoe JF, Bell WR, et al. Changes in the plasma fibrinolytic system during urokinase therapy: comparison of tissue culture urokinase with urinary source urokinase in patients with pulmonary embolism. J Lab Clin Med 1978; 92:721-9.

12. Sasahara AA, Cannilla JE, Belko JS, Morse RL, Criss AJ. Urokinase therapy in clinical pulmonary embolism: a new thrombolytic agent. N Engl J Med 1967; 277:1168-73.

13. Tow DE, Wagner HN Jr, Holmes RA. Urokinase in pulmonary embolism. N Engl J Med 1967; 277:1161-7.

14. Sautter RD, Emanuel DA, Fletcher FW, Wenzel FJ, Matson JI. Urokinase for the treatment of acute pulmonary thromboembolism. JAMA 1967; 202:215-8.

15. Genton E, Wolf PS. Urokinase therapy in pulmonary thromboembolism. Am Heart J 1968; 76:628-37.

16. Sasahara AA, Hyers TM, Cole CM, et al., eds. The Urokinase Pulmonary Embolism Trial: A National Cooperative Study. Circulation 1973; 47: Suppl 2:II-1-108.

17. Urokinase-Streptokinase Embolism Trial: phase 2 results: a cooperative study. JAMA 1974; 229:1606-13.

18. Sharma GVRK, Burleson VA, Sasahara AA. Effect of thrombolytic therapy on pulmonary capillary blood volume in patients with pulmonary embolism. N Engl J Med 1980; 303:842-5.

19. Sevitt S, Gallagher N. Venous thrombosis and pulmonary embolism: a clinico-pathologic study in injured and burned patients. Br J Surg 1961; 48:475-89.

20. Kakkar VV, Howe CT, Laws JW, Flanc C. Late results of treatment of deep vein thrombosis. Br Med J 1969; 1:810-1.

21. Sasahara AA, Sharma GVRK, Tow DE, Armenia RJ, Belko JS. Methodology in diagnosis of pulmonary embolization. In: Bergan JJ, Yao JST, eds. Venous problems. Chicago: Year Book, 1978:309-17.

22. Dotter CT, Rösch J, Seaman AJ. Selective clot lysis with low-dose streptokinase. Radiology 1974; 111:31-7.

23. Katzen BT, van Breda A. Low dose streptokinase in treatment of arterial occlusions. AJR 1981; 136:1171-8.

24. Fiessinger JN, Vayssairat M, Juillet Y, et al. Local urokinase in arterial thromboembolism. Angiology 1980; 31:715-20.

25. Poliwoda H, Alexander K, Buhl V, Holsten D, Wagner HH. Treatment of chronic arterial occlusions with streptokinase. N Engl J Med 1969; 280:689-92.

26. Verstraete M, Vermylen J, Donati MB. The effect of streptokinase infusion on chronic arterial occlusion and stenoses. Ann Intern Med 1971; 74:377-82.

27. Martin M. Thrombolytic therapy in arterial thromboembolism. Prog Cardiovasc Dis 1979; 21:351-74.

28. Long D. Thrombolytic therapy in severe arterial insufficiency and absent distal pulses. Angiology. (in press).

29. DeWood MA, Spores J, Notske R, et al. Prevalence of total coronary occlusion during the early hours of transmural myocardial infarction. N Engl J Med 1979; 303:897-902.

30. Phillips SJ, Kongatahworn C, Zeff RH, et al. Emergency coronary artery revascularization: a possible therapy for acute myocardial infarction. Circulation 1979; 60:241-6.

31. Fletcher AP, Sherry S, Alkjaersig N, Smyrniotis FE, Jick S. The maintenance of a sustained thrombolytic state in man. II. Clinical observations on patients with myocardial infarction and other thromboembolic disorders. J Clin Invest 1959; 38:1111-9.

32. Duckert F. Thrombolytic therapy in myocardial infarction. Prog Cardiovasc Dis. 1979; 21:342-50.

33. European Cooperative Study Group for Streptokinase Treatment in Acute Myocardial Infarction. Streptokinase in acute myocardial infarction. N Engl J Med 1979; 301:797-802.

34. Schröder R, Biamino G, von Lietner ER. Intravenous short-time thrombosis in acute myocardial infarction. Circulation 1981; 64: Suppl 4:IV-10. abstract.

35. Boucek RJ, Murphy WP Jr. Segmental perfusion of the coronary arteries with fibrinolysin in man following a myocardial infarction. Am J Cardiol 1960; 6:525-33.

36. Rentrop KP, Blanke H, Karsch KR, et al. Acute myocardial infarction: intracoronary application of nitroglycerin and streptokinase. Clin Cardiol 1979; 2:354-63.

37. Reduto LA, Freund GC, Gaeta JM, Smalling RW, Lewis B, Gould KL. Coronary artery reperfusion in acute myocardial infarction: beneficial effects of intracoronary streptokinase of left ventricular salvage and performance. Am Heart J 1981; 102:1168-77.

38. Markis JE, Malagold M, Parker JA, et al. Myocardial salvage after intracoronary thrombolysis with streptokinase in acute myocardial infarction: assessment by intracoronary thallium-201. N Engl J Med 1981; 305:777-82.

39. Gold HK, Leinbach RC, Buckley MJ, Akins CW, Levine FH, Austen WG. Intracoronary streptokinase in evolving infarction. Hosp Pract 1981; 16(9):105-19.

40. Ganz W, Buchbinder N, Marcus H, et al. Intracoronary thrombolysis in evolving myocardial infarction. Am Heart J 1981; 101:4-13.

41. Cowley MJ, Hastillo A, Vetrovec GW, Hess ML. Effects of intracoronary streptokinase in acute myocardial infarction. Am Heart J 1981; 102:1149-58.

42. Lee G, Amsterdam EA, Low R, et al. Efficacy of percutaneous transmural coronary recanalization utilizing streptokinase in patients with acute myocardial infarction. Am Heart J 1981; 102:1159-67.

43. Merx W, Dörr R, Rentrop P, et al. Evaluation of the effectiveness of intracoronary streptokinase infusion in acute myocardial infarction: postprocedure management and hospital course in 204 patients. Am Heart J 1981; 102:1181-7.

44. Rutsch W, Schartl M, Mathey D, et al. Percutaneous transluminal coronary recanalization: procedure, results, and acute complications. Am Heart J 1981; 102:1178-81.

45. Rentrop P, Blanke H, Karsch RK, et al. Changes in left ventricular function after intracoronary streptokinase infusion in clinically evolving myocardial infarction. Am Heart J 1981; 102:1188-93.

46. Wackers F, Berger H, Zaret B. Spontaneous changes of global and regional left ventricular function during the first 24 hours of acute myocardial infarction: implications for evaluating thrombolytic therapy. Circulation 1981; 64: Suppl 4:IV-196. abstract.

47. Mathey D, Klöppel G, Kuck K-H, Beil U, Schofer J. Transmural, hemorrhagic infarction following intracoronary streptokinase: clinical, angiographic and autoptical findings. Circulation 1981; 64: Suppl 4:IV-194. abstract.

48. van den Brand M, v.d. Smissen H, Seruys PW, Hooghoudt T. Potential risks of intracoronary streptokinase during acute myocardial infarction. Circulation 1981; 64: Suppl 4:IV-246. abstract.

49. Kwaan HC, Dobbie JG, Fetkenhour CL, Levin RD. Thrombolytic therapy of central retinal vein occlusion. In: Martin M, Schoop W, Hirsh J, eds. New concepts in streptokinase dosimetry. Bern: Hans Huber, 1978:221-9.

50. Albert FW. Application of streptokinase treatment in shunt occlusions. In: Martin M, Schoop W, Hirsh J, eds. New concepts in streptokinase dosimetry. Bern: Hans Huber, 1978:203-7.

51. Meyer JS, Gilroy J, Barnhart MI, Johnson JF. Anticoagulants plus streptokinase therapy in progressive stroke. JAMA 1964; 189:373.

52. Samama M, Conard J. Biological results during urokinase therapy at different doses. In: Paoletti R, Sherry S, eds. Thrombosis and urokinase. London: Academic Press, 1977:243-4.

Drug Disposition in Old Age

David J. Greenblatt, M.D.,

Edward M. Sellers, M.D., Ph.D.,

and Richard I. Shader, M.D.

THE appropriate and rational use of drugs by the elderly is a matter of growing medical and social concern. Life expectancy in the Western world currently stands at 69 years for men and 77 years for women and is increasing. [1,2] In 1980 an estimated 11 per cent of the total population was over 65 years old; the proportion is expected to exceed 15 per cent by the year 2040. As compared with the young, elderly persons on the average spend more money and a greater fraction of their income on health care. Old people have more illnesses and hospitalizations than do young people, and their hospitalizations and periods of acute care are longer. The need for long-term institutionalization is also greatly increased among the elderly. An estimated 1.3 million Americans, mostly over the age of 65, currently reside in nursing homes.

It is not surprising that both the frequency of drug therapy and the average number of drugs taken per person progressively increase with age. Most of our scientific understanding of therapeutics, clinical pharmacology, and pharmacokinetics is based on studies in young people, whereas our approach to therapeutics in the elderly patient is often based on anecdotal data, clinical impression, and trial and error. Much of this information is perpetuated as fact in the medical literature. This article reviews the current knowledge of age-related changes in drug absorption, distribution, and clearance and the possible implications of these changes for clinical therapeutics in the geriatric population.

Adverse Drug Reactions in the Elderly

Concern about drugs in the elderly is partly attributable to the development over the past 15 years of systematic epidemiologic surveillance systems for monitoring

From the Division of Clinical Pharmacology, departments of Psychiatry and Medicine, Tufts University School of Medicine and New England Medical Center Hospital, Boston, and the Clinical Institute, Addiction Research Foundation, departments of Pharmacology and Medicine, University of Toronto, Canada.

Supported in part by a grant (MH-34223) from the U.S. Public Health Service and by a Clinical Pharmacology Unit Developmental Grant from the Pharmaceutical Manufacturers' Association Foundation.

Originally published on May 6, 1982 (306:1081-1088).

patterns of drug use and toxicity. These systems are usually hospital based, and they focus on the nature and frequency of untoward drug effects and factors predisposing patients to toxicity. Reports from several monitoring systems demonstrate an overall increased frequency of adverse drug reactions associated with increasing age.[3-6] Studies from the Boston Collaborative Drug Surveillance Program have focused on the relation of age to the frequency of adverse reactions to a number of commonly used agents. A clear relation of age to untoward effects has been demonstrated for the benzodiazepine derivatives chlordiazepoxide,[7] diazepam,[7] flurazepam,[8] and nitrazepam[9] and for the antithrombotic agent heparin.[10] In the case of heparin, the age-related frequency of adverse effects (primarily bleeding) is greater in women than in men. For the cardiac agents lidocaine[11] and propranolol,[12] a relatively weak association of age to clinical toxicity has been reported. For some 90 other drugs in common clinical use, age alone is not a major determinant of clinical toxicity.

Reports from surveillance systems have greatly increased our awareness of problems associated with drug therapy in old age. These systems involve prospective monitoring of drug effects during actual clinical use rather than controlled clinical or scientific trials.[13] Aging itself cannot be isolated as the sole biologic factor explaining the association of toxicity with age. Particularly in the hospital setting, age is closely related to increased severity and duration of disease, which themselves may lead to more frequent toxicity. Administration of the same average daily drug dose to young and elderly persons actually reflects a higher weight-corrected dosage in the elderly because of their lower body weight, and it may increase dose-dependent adverse effects in the elderly. Conversely, a lack of association between age and clinical toxicity in epidemiologic studies does not rule out an important contribution of age as a biologic determinant of toxicity. Increased caution when treating the elderly, as in the use of lower doses or more careful monitoring of drug effects, could offset an actual biologic difference in drug sensitivity in the geriatric population. Intensive monitoring programs have contributed greatly to our awareness of therapeutic problems in the elderly, but the limitations of these data for the identification of underlying biologic mechanisms must be recognized.

Mechanisms of Altered Drug Effects in Old Age

The apparently increased frequency of adverse reactions to certain drugs in the elderly, together with clinical impressions of increased drug sensitivity in old age, has stimulated research focusing on the biologic mechanisms of these effects and on methods of predicting quantitative and qualitative changes in drug sensitivity in the geriatric population. Two principal conceptual approaches to this problem are the pharmacodynamic and the pharmacokinetic.

The pharmacodynamic hypothesis postulates that a given drug concentration at receptor sites yields a greater pharmacodynamic response in an elderly person than in a young one, assuming that all other modifying factors remain constant. Rigorous testing of this hypothesis in vivo is difficult, particularly in human beings, and few studies convincingly demonstrate a true change in drug sensitivity in old age. For example, work involving the benzodiazepine derivatives diazepam[14, 15] and nitrazepam[16] suggests greater depression of the central nervous system at any given plasma drug concentration in the elderly than in the young. Some[17-19] (but not all[20]) studies indicate a greater anticoagulant response (evidenced by greater prolongation of the prothrombin time) at any given dose or plasma concentration of a coumarin anticoagulant in elderly patients than in young patients. In one report, elderly persons appeared to have reduced sensitivity to the effects of beta-adrenergic agonists and antagonists.[21]

The second major conceptual approach to altered drug effects in old age focuses on changes in drug disposition. Even if receptor sensitivity to a drug in an older person is not altered, changes in a drug's pharmacokinetic fate that cause higher concentrations at the site of action will increase the response if the drug's effect is proportional to its concentration at the receptor site. Thus, the ability to understand and predict clinically important age-related changes in drug disposition would help in the design of more effective and less toxic dosage schedules for the elderly. Numerous investigations over the past decade have focused on pharmacokinetic changes in the elderly,[22-26] many of which are logical consequences of age-related changes in body composition and organ-system function. This area of research is not without its methodologic pitfalls and problems, but some meaningful generalizations can be developed.

Drug Clearance and the Function of Clearing Organs

A drug's total-body clearance, expressed in units of volume per unit of time, represents a hypothetical volume of blood from which the drug is completely cleared per unit of time. Total clearance is the best indicator of an organism's ability to remove or eliminate a drug. For most drugs, clearance is accomplished by one or more clearing organs, usually the kidney or liver; total clearance cannot exceed blood flow to the organ or organs responsible for clearance.

Total clearance is a major determinant of the extent of drug accumulation during multiple dosage. If a maintenance dose of any drug is administered at equally spaced time intervals, and if each dose is completely available to the systemic circulation (100 per cent bioavailability), then the mean plasma concentration of the total drug at a steady state (Css) can be expressed as:

$$Css = \frac{\text{dose per interval of time}}{\text{clearance}}. \qquad (Eq.\ 1)$$

Thus, at any given dose rate, Css will increase as clearance decreases. If old age is associated with reduced total clearance of a drug, then Css will increase accordingly. If clinical drug effects are in turn proportional to the plasma concentration, then enhancement of these effects (therapeutic or toxic or both) can be expected. In principle, this change in clinical effect could be reversed if either the size of each dose were appropriately reduced or the interval between doses were lengthened to compensate for the reduction in clearance. A clinician's ability to anticipate the need for such changes is considerably enhanced by an understanding of the major route or routes of clearance for individual drugs and of the likely effect of the aging process on the function of clearing organs.

Renal Clearance

The glomerular filtration rate declines predictably in old age, with a mean 35 per cent reduction in the elderly as compared with the young.[27-31] For drugs whose total clearance is accomplished partly or entirely by renal excretion of the intact drug, the total clearance will predictably decline approximately in proportion to the reduced glomerular filtration rate.[32-36] Examples of such drugs include digoxin, cimetidine, lithium, procainamide, chlorpropamide, and the most commonly used antimicrobial agents. To prevent excessive accumulation of such drugs in elderly persons, a need for downward adjustment of the dosage must be anticipated. Translation of this general principle to any specific patient, however, requires knowledge of that patient's level of renal function, based on measurement or estimation of creatinine clearance. Often overlooked is the decline of muscle mass and lean body mass relative to total body weight that occurs with old age.[37-39] Since the serum creatinine concentration depends on creatinine turnover as well as renal creatinine clearance, the decline in renal function in the elderly may not cause a meaningful elevation in serum creatinine concentration. Thus, reliance on serum creatinine as the sole indicator of renal function in the elderly may be misleading. Creatinine clearance, which is based on 24-hour urinary excretion as well as on serum creatinine concentration, is obviously a far more reliable indicator of renal function. When a complete urine collection is not feasible, creatinine clearance can be estimated from serum creatinine on the basis of nomograms or equations that take into account expected changes associated with age and sex.[40,41]

Hepatic Clearance

The mechanisms controlling hepatic biotransformation of drugs and their alterations with old age are considerably more complex than those involved in renal excretion. Hepatocytes carry out not one but many biotransformation reactions that contribute to the removal of drugs and other foreign chemicals. A traditional and still useful scheme categorizes these reactions as either Phase I (preparative) or Phase II (synthetic) biotransformations. Phase I reactions include the oxidations (hydroxylation, N-dealkylation, and sulfoxidation), the reductions, and the hydrolyses. These preparative reactions generally constitute relatively minor molecular modifications, often making drugs somewhat more polar (water-soluble) and yielding products that may retain part or all of the pharmacologic activity of the parent compound. Phase II reactions involve conjugation or attachment of a drug molecule to a larger substituent, usually glucuronide, sulfate, or acetate. The resulting conjugates are much more polar than the parent compound and are generally excreted in the urine. Although some acetylated metabolites of drugs are pharmacologically active, products of Phase II reactions usually have little or no

TABLE 1. Studies of the Relation of Age to the Clearance of Drugs Cleared by Hepatic Biotransformation.

Drug or Metabolite	Initial Pathway of Biotransformation	References
Evidence suggesting age-related reduction in clearance		
Antipyrine †	Oxidation (OH, DA)	42–46
Diazepam †	Oxidation (DA)	47–51
Chlordiazepoxide	Oxidation (DA)	52, 53
Desmethyldiazepam †	Oxidation (OH)	54–56
Desalkylflurazepam †	Oxidation (OH)	57
Clobazam †	Oxidation (DA)	58
Alprazolam †	Oxidation (OH)	59
Quinidine	Oxidation (OH)	60, 61
Theophylline	Oxidation	62, 63
Propranolol	Oxidation (OH)	64–66
Nortriptyline	Oxidation (OH)	67
Small or negligible age-related change in clearance		
Oxazepam	Glucuronidation	68–70
Lorazepam	Glucuronidation	71, 72
Temazepam	Glucuronidation	73
Warfarin	Oxidation (OH)	18
Lidocaine	Oxidation (DA)	74
Nitrazepam	Nitroreduction	16, 75
Flunitrazepam	Oxidation (DA), nitroreduction	76
Isoniazid	Acetylation	77
Ethanol	Oxidation (alcohol dehydrogenase)	78
Metoprolol	Oxidation	79
Digitoxin	Oxidation	80
Prazosin	Oxidation	81
Data conflicting or not definitive		
Meperidine	Oxidation (DA)	82
Phenylbutazone	Oxidation (OH)	42, 83, 84
Phenytoin	Oxidation (OH)	85, 86
Imipramine	Oxidation (OH, DA)	87
Amitriptyline	Oxidation (OH, DA)	87
Acetaminophen	Glucuronidation, sulfation	83, 88–90
Amobarbital	Oxidation (OH)	91

*OH denotes hydroxylation and DA dealkylation.

†Evidence suggests that the age-related reduction in clearance is greater in men than in women.

pharmacologic activity. For a number of drugs, the overall metabolic pathway can involve a sequence of biotransformation reactions of the Phase I and Phase II types.

With the exception of the plasma albumin concentration, which tends to be lower in the elderly, the usual clinical tests of hepatic function as reported in laboratory screening profiles are not importantly altered in healthy elderly persons. However, the results of such tests do not necessarily reflect drug-metabolizing capacity. The function of the hepatic microsomal enzymes responsible for Phase I oxidative drug metabolism (principally hydroxylation and N-dealkylation) may be importantly impaired in old age, leading to reduced total drug clearance and higher steady-state plasma concentrations during multiple dosage (Table 1). On the other hand, studies of biotransformations of the Phase II glucuronide-conjugation type suggest that aging has a much smaller effect on glucuronide-conjugating capacity (Table 1).

Hepatic blood flow, rather than microsomal-enzyme activity, is the major determinant of total clearance of a number of commonly used drugs.[92] Hepatic blood flow declines with age, partly because of reduced cardiac output. An estimated 40 to 45 per cent reduction in total liver blood flow may be observed in elderly persons, as compared with young adults.[93] Likewise, liver size decreases with age, both in absolute terms and as a percentage of total body weight. One would expect a predictable age-related decline in total clearance of drugs with flow-dependent clearance, but the data are again conflicting. Reduced total clearance in old age has been demonstrated for propranolol but not for lidocaine — two drugs with high and therefore flow-dependent hepatic clearance (Table 1).

Thus, changes in drug clearance in old age are not necessarily predictable consequences of well-understood alterations of hepatic function, and normal values on liver-function tests do not imply normal metabolism of drugs.

Drug Distribution

Body Composition

Changes in body composition with age may influence drug distribution. On the average, lean body mass declines and adipose-tissue mass increases in relation to total body weight in the aging person.[37-39] The fraction of total body weight composed of adipose tissue may increase with age from approximately 18 to 36 per cent in men and from 33 to 48 per cent in women. The effect of these changes on drug distribution within the body depends largely on a drug's aqueous and lipid solubility. Some drugs, such as acetaminophen,[90] antipyrine,[46] and ethanol,[78] are relatively water soluble and lipid insoluble, and their distribution to tissues may decrease in the elderly. Conversely, more lipid-soluble drugs, such as diazepam[47-51] and lidocaine,[74] become more extensively distributed in the elderly (Fig. 1). Differences in body composition between men and women, regardless of age, may be as profound as those between the young and the elderly. Consequently,

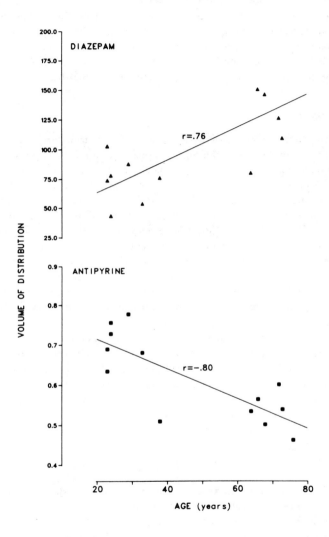

Figure 1. *Relation of Age to Apparent Volume of Distribution (Determined by the Area Method) for Antipyrine and Diazepam among 13 Healthy Male Volunteers Who Received Single Intravenous Doses of Both Drugs on Two Occasions.*[46,49]

The positions of the solid lines were determined by least-squares regression analysis, indicating an age-related decline in the volume of distribution for antipyrine, as opposed to an increase in the volume of distribution with age for diazepam (the volumes of distribution for diazepam were corrected for individual values of protein binding, yielding data for the unbound drug). The units on the ordinate are liters per kilogram of body weight.

women will have more extensive distribution of lipid-soluble drugs[49,54,58] and less extensive distribution of relatively water-soluble drugs.[46,90]

Unless age-related changes in body composition by themselves influence the function of clearing organs, altered drug distribution in old age will not alter steady-state plasma concentrations during multiple dosage, since these levels depend only on the dose rate and the total clearance (Equation 1). However, distribution has an important effect on the elimination half-life.[94]

Protein Binding

The apparent distribution of extensively protein-bound drugs may also be influenced by changes in the extent of binding to plasma protein. Most protein-bound drugs are bound partly or entirely to plasma albumin, and an age-related decline in plasma albumin concentrations has been consistently reported.[30,95] The reduction may be large when elderly subjects are poorly nourished, have advanced illness, or are severely debilitated.[96] Even in well-nourished, healthy elderly persons, however, albumin concentrations are lower than those in young persons, even though they may not fall below the usual normal range. Not surprisingly, the degree of drug binding to protein, particularly for extensively bound drugs, may be reduced in old age, at least in part because of the reduction in the concentration of the major binding protein. However, neither age nor albumin concentration necessarily explains a large proportion of the overall variability between individuals in the protein binding of a given drug.

An understanding of what altered binding does and does not mean in terms of a drug's pharmacokinetic properties or clinical effects is of critical importance. For the great majority of protein-bound drugs, only the unbound fraction of the total amount present in serum or plasma is available for diffusion out of the vascular system to sites of pharmacologic activity and of biotransformation or excretion.[97] Under these conditions, Equation 1, when correctly adjusted for protein binding, is written as follows:

$$\text{CssF} = \frac{\text{dose per interval of time}}{\text{free clearance}} \qquad (Eq.\ 2)$$

where CssF is the mean steady-state concentration of the free drug in plasma and free clearance (sometimes called intrinsic clearance) represents the ability of the clearing organ to remove the unbound drug. It is commonly but incorrectly assumed that an increase in the free fraction of a drug in plasma, which may occur in old age, implies an increased CssF and therefore an increased intensity of clinical action. However, Equation 2 clearly indicates that CssF does not depend on the free fraction. Therefore, a change in drug binding with old age does not itself alter clinical drug effects.

On the other hand, changes in binding may influence the interpretation of serum or plasma drug concentrations used to monitor therapy.[98] Most assay techniques used by clinical laboratories measure total rather than free drug concentrations in plasma. Css depends on CssF and the free fraction as follows:

$$Css = \frac{CssF}{\text{free fraction}}. \qquad (Eq.\ 3)$$

For any given dose rate and free clearance, Css will decline as the free fraction increases, whereas CssF (and therefore the intensity of the clinical effect) will remain the same. For extensively protein-bound drugs whose binding is reduced in old age and whose free fraction is therefore increased, clinicians should expect lower ranges of therapeutic and toxic plasma concentrations of the total drug.

Drug Absorption

Changes in the function of the gastrointestinal tract in old age include a reduction in gastric parietal-cell function, leading to impaired acid secretion and an elevation in gastric pH.[93] A reduced rate of gastric emptying has also been described.[99] Impaired absorption of certain nutrients by active transport suggests that these transport processes may be less functional in the elderly.[100] For most drugs used in clinical practice, however, the rate and extent of absorption are determined by passive diffusion during contact with the vast surface area available for absorption in the proximal small bowel. Despite speculation to the contrary in many review articles and secondary sources, there is essentially no available evidence that drug absorption is impaired in old age.[101-103] Well-controlled studies of the analgesic drug acetaminophen[104] and of the antianxiety agent lorazepam[72,105] suggest that the rate and extent of gastrointestinal absorption are not importantly altered in elderly persons.

Pitfalls in Interpretation of Data

Reading the research literature on age-related changes in pharmacokinetics requires close attention to several methodologic pitfalls that can make data difficult or impossible to interpret.

Half-Life versus Clearance

Many pharmacokinetic studies focus on elimination half-life ($t\frac{1}{2}$) rather than clearance as the most important pharmacokinetic variable. The $t\frac{1}{2}$ is actually a hybrid quantity, depending on both the clearance and the volume of drug distribution (Vd) as follows:

$$t\frac{1}{2} = \frac{0.693 \times Vd}{\text{clearance}}. \qquad (Eq.\ 4)$$

In this equation, $t\frac{1}{2}$ refers to the apparent half-life of drug elimination during the terminal phase of the plasma-concentration curve after distribution equilibrium has been attained, and Vd is the hypothetical volume relating the amount of drug in the body to the plasma concentration at all times after the attainment of distribution equilibrium. Thus, t½ is inversely proportional to clearance, with reductions in clearance reflected in prolongation of t½ only when Vd is not importantly altered in the groups being compared. This is by no means the case in studies comparing young and elderly persons, since the change in body composition associated with old age may lead to substantial alterations in drug distribution. Changes in Vd, therefore, may lead to incorrect conclusions if t½ rather than clearance is used as an index of drug-metabolizing capacity. For example, t½ may be considerably prolonged in the absence of a change in clearance if Vd is increased.[94] Conversely, t½ may change minimally, despite a substantial reduction in clearance, if Vd is reduced to the same extent. In summary, evaluation of clearance rather than t½ must be the primary objective in interpreting studies of drug disposition in old age.

Clearance of Total versus Unbound Drug

For extensively protein-bound drugs, age-related changes in the free fraction may complicate interpretation of studies of clearance of the total drug. The problem is analogous to the influence of alterations in the free fraction on the interpretation of total serum or plasma drug concentrations during therapeutic monitoring.[98] The general pharmacokinetic calculation of clearance relates it to the dose of a drug reaching the systemic circulation as follows:

$$\text{clearance} = \frac{\text{dose}}{\text{AUC}} \qquad (Eq.\ 5)$$

where, after single drug doses, AUC is the total area under the curve of time versus plasma concentration, from the time of drug administration to infinity. Clearance can also be calculated during multiple-dose therapy if the same dose is administered at equal intervals. In this case, clearance is the dose reaching the systemic circulation divided by the AUC over a single dosage interval. However, since only the free drug is available for metabolism and excretion as well as for diffusion to sites of pharmacologic activity, Equation 5 should be corrected for the extent of protein binding as follows:

$$\text{free clearance} = \frac{\text{dose}}{\text{AUC}_{\text{free}}} \qquad (Eq.\ 6)$$

where AUC$_{\text{free}}$ is the total area under the curve of free drug concentration versus time, from the time of drug administration to infinity. Assuming that the extent of binding in a given person is constant over time, then AUC$_{\text{free}}$ is related to AUC for the total drug as follows:

$$\text{AUC}_{\text{free}} = \text{AUC} \times \text{free fraction.} \qquad (Eq.\ 7)$$

Combining Equations 5, 6, and 7 yields the following relation between clearance of the total drug and clearance of the free drug:

$$\text{clearance} = \text{free clearance} \times \text{free fraction.} \qquad (Eq.\ 8)$$

Most pharmacokinetic studies evaluate total rather than free drug clearance, but free clearance is what actually determines steady-state plasma concentrations of the pharmacologically active unbound drug (Equation 2). Total and free clearance remain proportional as long as the free fraction varies little between individuals. However, a clinically important reduction in free clearance associated with age might not be reflected in a similar reduction in total clearance if the free fraction concurrently increased.[49,63] Thus, studies of total drug clearance in old age must be interpreted with great caution unless data on age-related alterations in the free fraction are simultaneously provided.

Different Effects of Age on Men and Women

The effect of age on drug distribution and clearance is not necessarily identical for men and women. Because women in any age group generally have a larger proportion of adipose tissue, drug distribution may differ as a function of sex, regardless of age.[46,49,51,54,55,58,90,94,106] Furthermore, clearance of drugs may be differently influenced by age in the two sexes. Several studies of drugs or drug metabolites that are biotransformed by oxidative mechanisms (antipyrine, diazepam, clobazam, alprazolam, desmethyldiazepam, and desalkylflurazepam) indicate a strong age-related decline in total drug clearance in men, whereas the effect of age in women is far less pronounced (Table 1). Because sex can influence drug distribution and clearance, data on age-related changes in pharmacokinetics in one sex do not necessarily apply to the other.

Cigarette Smoking

Cigarette smoking is known to stimulate hepatic metabolizing capacity for a number of drugs, increasing total metabolic clearance.[107] The effect of exposure to enzyme-inducing agents may be greater in the young than in the elderly.[44,45,64,108] Thus, cigarette smoking may make data from pharmacogeriatric studies difficult to interpret. Smoking is more likely to be prevalent in the young population, since early mortality tends to select against heavy smokers in the geriatric population. Even if smoking were equally prevalent in young and elderly groups, the reduced inducibility in the geriatric population would mean that the effects of this exposure on drug clearance would tend to magnify apparent age-related differences. Closely related to the confounding influence of cigarette smoking is that of marijuana use, which appears to have a greater inducing effect than cigarette smoking.[62]

Alcohol Consumption

Acute ethanol ingestion inhibits oxidative but not conjugative drug metabolism;

the effect lasts as long as ethanol is still present in the body.[109-111] In contrast, chronic ingestion of large amounts of ethanol in the absence of severe liver disease increases the clearance of many drugs, probably by induction of microsomal drug-metabolizing enzymes. Although no studies of these phenomena in the elderly have been reported, differences in the effects of alcohol consumption, like those of cigarette smoking, may complicate the interpretation of pharmacogeriatric research. On the average, alcohol ingestion is lower in the geriatric population than in the young, and the inducing effect of ethanol may be reduced among the elderly.

Therapeutic Implications of Kinetic Changes in the Elderly

The importance of an age-related reduction in total drug clearance depends on the therapeutic index of the particular drug. Compounds such as digoxin, quinidine, and theophylline have reasonably well-defined and relatively narrow ranges of usually effective plasma concentrations, above which the likelihood of clinical toxicity increases. A need to reduce the daily dosage of such drugs in the elderly should be anticipated in order to avoid excessive drug accumulation. Age-related changes in clearance are less likely to be important for such drugs as diazepam, for which a clear relation of plasma concentration to clinical effect has not been established. Although epidemiologic studies suggest that the elderly may be more sensitive to diazepam, this is not a proved consequence of excessive drug accumulation. Conversely, clinicians should not abandon a cautious approach during the use of drugs such as lidocaine in the elderly, even though no clear age-related alteration in kinetics has been demonstrated. Unfortunately, definitive kinetic data are not available for many important drugs commonly prescribed to the elderly.

We are indebted to Marcia Divoll, Dr. Darrell R. Abernethy, Jerold S. Harmatz, Dr. H. G. Giles, Dr. Hermann R. Ochs, Dr. Hershel Jick, Dr. Dean S. MacLaughlin, and the staff of the Clinical Study Unit, New England Medical Center Hospital (supported by a grant [RR 24040] from the U.S. Public Health Service) for their assistance and collaboration.

References

1. Fries JF. Aging, natural death, and the compression of morbidity. N Engl J Med 1980; 303:130-5.
2. Rowe JW. Clinical research on aging: strategies and directions. N Engl J Med 1977; 297:1332-6.
3. Seidl LG, Thornton GF, Smith JW, Cluff LE. Studies on the epidemiology of adverse drug reactions. III. Reactions in patients on a general medical service. Bull Johns Hopkins Hosp 1966; 119:299-315.
4. Steel K, Gertman PM, Crescenzi C, Anderson J. Iatrogenic illness on a general medical service at a university hospital. N Engl J Med 1981; 304:638-42.
5. Hurwitz N. Predisposing factors in adverse reactions to drugs. Br Med J 1969; 1:536-9.

6. Miller RR. Drug surveillance utilizing epidemiologic methods: a report from the Boston Collaborative Drug Surveillance Program. Am J Hosp Pharm 1973; 30:584-92.

7. Clinical depression of the central nervous system due to diazepam and chlordiazepoxide in relation to cigarette smoking and age: a report from the Boston Collaborative Drug Surveillance Program, Boston University Medical Center. N Engl J Med 1973; 288:277-80.

8. Greenblatt DJ, Allen MD, Shader RI. Toxicity of high-dose flurazepam in the elderly. Clin Pharmacol Ther 1977; 21:355-61.

9. Greenblatt DJ, Allen MD. Toxicity of nitrazepam in the elderly: a report from the Boston Collaborative Drug Surveillance Program. Br J Clin Pharmacol 1978; 5:407-13.

10. Jick H, Slone D, Borda IT, Shapiro S. Efficacy and toxicity of heparin in relation to age and sex. N Engl J Med 1968; 279:284-6.

11. Pfeifer HJ, Greenblatt DJ, Koch-Weser J. Clinical use and toxicity of intravenous lidocaine: a report from the Boston Collaborative Drug Surveillance Program. Am Heart J 1976; 92:168-73.

12. Greenblatt DJ, Koch-Weser J. Adverse reactions to propranolol in hospitalized medical patients: a report from the Boston Collaborative Drug Surveillance Program. Am Heart J 1973; 86:478-84.

13. Jick H. Drugs — remarkably nontoxic. N Engl J Med 1974; 291:824-8.

14. Reidenberg MM, Levy M, Warner H, et al. Relationship between diazepam dose, plasma level, age, and central nervous system depression. Clin Pharmacol Ther 1978; 23:371-4.

15. Giles HG, MacLeod SM, Wright JR, Sellers EM. Influence of age and previous use on diazepam dosage required for endoscopy. Can Med Assoc J 1978; 118:513-4.

16. Castleden CM, George CF, Marcer D, Hallett C. Increased sensitivity to nitrazepam in old age. Br Med J 1977; 1:10-2.

17. Husted S, Andreasen F. The influence of age on the response to anticoagulants. Br J Clin Pharmacol 1977; 4:559-65.

18. Shepherd AMM, Hewick DS, Moreland TA, Stevenson IH. Age as a determinant of sensitivity to warfarin. Br J Clin Pharmacol 1977; 4:315-20.

19. Hotraphinyo K, Triggs EJ, Maybloom B, Maclaine-Cross A. Warfarin sodium: steady-state plasma levels and patient age. Clin Exp Pharmacol Physiol 1978; 5:143-9.

20. Jones BR, Baran A, Reidenberg MM. Evaluating patients' warfarin requirements. J Am Geriatr Soc 1980; 28:10-2.

21. Vestal RE, Wood AJJ, Shand DG. Reduced β-adrenoreceptor sensitivity in the elderly. Clin Pharmacol Ther 1979; 26:181-6.

22. Triggs EJ, Nation RL. Pharmacokinetics in the aged: a review. J Pharmacokinet Biopharm 1975; 3:387-418.

23. Richey DP, Bender AD. Pharmacokinetic consequences of aging. Annu Rev Pharmacol Toxicol 1977; 17:49-65.

24. Vestal RE. Drug use in the elderly: a review of problems and special considerations. Drugs 1978; 16:358-82.

25. Crooks J, O'Malley K, Stevenson IH. Pharmacokinetics in the elderly. Clin Pharmacokinet 1976; 1:280-96.

26. Greenblatt DJ, Shader RI. Pharmacokinetics in old age: principles and problems of assessment. In: Jarvik LF, Greenblatt DJ, Harman D, eds. Clinical pharmacology and the aged patient. New York: Raven Press, 1981:27-46.

27. Friedman SA, Raizner AE, Rosen H, Solomon NA, Sy W. Functional defects in the aging kidney. Ann Intern Med 1972; 76:41-5.

28. Rowe JW, Andres R, Tobin JD, Norris AH, Shock NW. The effects of age on creatinine clearance in man: a cross-sectional and longitudinal study. J Gerontol 1976; 31:155-63.

29. Ochs HR, Greenblatt DJ, Harmatz JS, Bodem G, Dengler HJ. Clinical implications of serum digoxin concentrations. Klin Wochenschr 1981; 59:501-7.

30. Dybkaer R, Lauritzen M, Krakauer R. Relative reference values for clinical chemical and haematological quantities in 'healthy' elderly people. Acta Med Scand 1981; 209:1-9.

31. Rowe JW, Andres R, Tobin JD, Norris AH, Shock NW. Age-adjusted standards for creatinine clearance. Ann Intern Med 1976; 84:567-9.

32. Ewy GA, Kapadia GG, Yao L, Lullin M, Marcus FI. Digoxin metabolism in the elderly. Circulation 1969; 39:449-53.

33. Cusack B, Kelly J, O'Malley K, Noel J, Lavan J, Horgan J. Digoxin in the elderly: pharmacokinetic consequences of old age. Clin Pharmacol Ther 1979; 25:772-6.

34. Redolfi A, Borgogelli E, Lodola E. Blood level of cimetidine in relation to age. Eur J Clin Pharmacol 1979; 15:257-61.

35. Reidenberg MM, Camacho M, Kluger J, Drayer DE. Aging and renal clearance of procainamide and acetylprocainamide. Clin Pharmacol Ther 1980; 28:732-5.

36. Drayer DE, Romankiewicz J, Lorenzo B, Reidenberg MM. Age and renal clearance of cimetidine. Clin Pharmacol Ther 1982; 31:45-50.

37. Bruce A, Andersson M, Arvidsson B, Isaksson B. Body composition. Prediction of normal body potassium, body water and body fat in adults on the basis of body height, body weight and age. Scand J Clin Lab Invest 1980; 40:461-73.

38. Novak LP. Aging, total body potassium, fat-free mass, and cell mass in males and females between ages 18 and 35 years. J Gerontol 1972; 27:438-43.

39. Forbes GB, Reina JC. Adult lean body mass declines with age: some longitudinal observations. Metabolism 1970; 19:653-63.

40. Siersbaek-Nielsen K, Hansen JM, Kampmann J, Kristensen M. Rapid evaluation of creatinine clearance. Lancet 1971; 1:1133-4.

41. Cockcroft DW, Gault MH. Prediction of creatinine clearance from serum creatinine. Nephron 1976; 16:31-41.

42. O'Malley K, Crooks J, Duke E, Stevenson IH. Effect of age and sex on human drug metabolism. Br Med J 1971; 3:607-9.

43. Liddell DE, Williams FM, Briant RH. Phenazone (antipyrine) metabolism and distribution in young and elderly adults. Clin Exp Pharmacol Physiol 1975; 2:481-7.

44. Wood AJJ, Vestal RE, Wilkinson GR, Branch RA, Shand DG. Effect of aging and cigarette smoking on antipyrine and indocyanine green elimination. Clin Pharmacol Ther 1979; 26:16-20.

45. Vestal RE, Norris AH, Tobin JD, Cohen BH, Shock NW, Andres R. Antipyrine metabolism in man: influence of age, alcohol, caffeine, and smoking. Clin Pharmacol Ther 1975; 18:425-32.

46. Greenblatt DJ, Divoll M, Abernethy DR, Harmatz JS, Shader RI. Antipyrine kinetics in the elderly: prediction of age-related changes in benzodiazepine oxidizing capacity. J Pharmacol Exp Ther 1982; 220:120-6.

47. Kanto J, Mäenpää M, Mäntylä R, Sellman R, Valovirta E. Effect of age on the pharmacokinetics of diazepam given in conjunction with spinal anesthesia. Anesthesiology 1979; 51:154-9.

48. Macklon AF, Barton M, James O, Rawlins MD. The effect of age on the pharmacokinetics of diazepam. Clin Sci 1980; 59:479-83.

49. Greenblatt DJ, Allen MD, Harmatz JS, Shader RI. Diazepam disposition determinants. Clin Pharmacol Ther 1980; 27:301-12.

50. Klotz U, Avant GR, Hoyumpa A, Schenker S, Wilkinson GR. The effects of age and liver disease on the disposition and elimination of diazepam in adult man. J Clin Invest 1975; 55:347-59.

51. Ochs HR, Greenblatt DJ, Divoll M, Abernethy DR, Feyerabend H, Dengler HJ. Diazepam kinetics in relation to age and sex. Pharmacology 1981; 23:24-30.

52. Roberts RK, Wilkinson GR, Branch RA, Schenker S. Effect of age and parenchymal liver disease on the disposition and elimination of chlordiazepoxide (Librium). Gastroenterology 1978; 75:479-85.

53. Shader RI, Greenblatt DJ, Harmatz JS, Franke K, Koch-Weser J. Absorption and disposition of chlordiazepoxide in young and elderly male volunteers. J Clin Pharmacol 1977; 17:709-18.

54. Allen MD, Greenblatt DJ, Harmatz JS, Shader RI. Desmethyldiazepam kinetics in the elderly after oral prazepam. Clin Pharmacol Ther 1980; 28:196-202.

55. Shader RI, Greenblatt DJ, Ciraulo DA, Divoll M, Harmatz JS, Georgotas A. Effect of age and sex on disposition of desmethyldiazepam formed from its precursor clorazepate. Psychopharmacology (Berlin) 1981; 75:193-7.

56. Klotz U, Müller-Seydlitz P. Altered elimination of desmethyldiazepam in the elderly. Br J Clin Pharmacol 1979; 7:119-20.

57. Greenblatt DJ, Divoll M, Harmatz JS, Maclaughlin DS, Shader RI. Kinetics and clinical effects of flurazepam in young and elderly noninsomniacs. Clin Pharmacol Ther 1981; 30:475-86.

58. Greenblatt DJ, Divoll M, Puri SK, Ho I, Zinny MA, Shader RI. Clobazam kinetics in the elderly. Br J Clin Pharmacol 1981; 12:631-6.

59. Greenblatt DJ, Divoll M, Abernethy DR, Moschitto LJ, Smith RB, Shader RI. Alprazolam kinetics in the elderly: relation to antipyrine disposition. Arch Gen Psychiatry. (in press).

60. Ochs HR, Greenblatt DJ, Woo E, Smith TW. Reduced quinidine clearance in elderly persons. Am J Cardiol 1978; 42:481-5.

61. Drayer DE, Hughes M, Lorenzo B, Reidenberg MM. Prevalence of high (3S)-3-hydroxyquinidine/quinidine ratios in serum, and clearance of quinidine in cardiac patients with age. Clin Pharmacol Ther 1980; 27:72-5.

62. Jusko WJ, Gardner MJ, Mangione A, Schentag JJ, Koup JR, Vance JW. Factors affecting theophylline clearance: age, tobacco, marijuana, cirrhosis, congestive heart failure, obesity, oral contraceptives, benzodiazepines, barbiturates, and ethanol. J Pharm Sci 1979; 68:1358-66.

63. Antal EJ, Kramer PA, Mercik SA, Chapron DJ, Lawson IR. Theophylline pharmacokinetics in advanced age. Br J Clin Pharmacol 1981; 12:637-45.

64. Vestal RE, Wood AJJ, Branch RA, Shand DG, Wilkinson GR. Effects of age and cigarette smoking on propranolol disposition. Clin Pharmacol Ther 1979; 26:8-15.

65. Castleden CM, George CF. The effect of ageing on the hepatic clearance of propranolol. Br J Clin Pharmacol 1979; 7:49-54.

66. Feely J, Crooks J, Stevenson IH. The influence of age, smoking, and hyperthyroidism on plasma propranolol steady state concentration. Br J Clin Pharmacol 1981; 12:73-8.

67. Dawling S, Crome P, Braithwaite R. Pharmacokinetics of single oral doses of nortriptyline in depressed elderly hospital patients and young healthy volunteers. Clin Pharmacokinet 1980; 5:394-401.

68. Greenblatt DJ, Divoll M, Harmatz JS, Shader RI. Oxazepam kinetics: effects of age and sex. J Pharmacol Exp Ther 1980; 215:86-91.

69. Shull HJ Jr, Wilkinson GR, Johnson R, Schenker S. Normal disposition of oxazepam in acute viral hepatitis and cirrhosis. Ann Intern Med 1976; 84:420-5.

70. Ochs HR, Greenblatt DJ, Otten H. Disposition of oxazepam in relation to age, sex, and cigarette smoking. Klin Wochenschr 1981; 59:899-903.

71. Kraus JW, Desmond PV, Marshall JP, Johnson RF, Schenker S, Wilkinson GR. Effects of aging and liver disease on disposition of lorazepam. Clin Pharmacol Ther 1978; 24:411-9.

72. Greenblatt DJ, Allen MD, Locniskar A, Harmatz JS, Shader RI. Lorazepam kinetics in the elderly. Clin Pharmacol Ther 1979; 26:103-13.

73. Divoll M, Greenblatt DJ, Harmatz JS, Shader RI. Effect of age and gender on disposition of temazepam. J Pharm Sci 1981; 70:1104-7.

74. Nation RL, Triggs EJ, Selig M. Lignocaine kinetics in cardiac patients and aged subjects. Br J Clin Pharmacol 1977; 4:439-48.

75. Kangas L, Iisalo E, Kanto J, et al. Human pharmacokinetics of nitrazepam: effect of age and diseases. Eur J Clin Pharmacol 1979; 15:163-70.

76. Kanto J, Kangas L, Aaltonen L, Hilke H. Effect of age on the pharmacokinetics and sedative effect of flunitrazepam. Int J Clin Pharmacol 1981; 19:400-4.

77. Farah F, Taylor W, Rawlins MD, James O. Hepatic drug acetylation and oxidation: effects of aging in man. Br Med J 1977; 2:155-6.

78. Vestal RE, McGuire EA, Tobin JD, Andres R, Norris AH, Mezey E. Aging and ethanol metabolism. Clin Pharmacol Ther 1977; 21:343-54.

79. Quarterman CP, Kendall MJ, Jack DB. The effect of age on the pharmacokinetics of metoprolol and its metabolites. Br J Clin Pharmacol 1981; 11:287-94.

80. Donovan MA, Castleden CM, Pohl JEF, Kraft CA. The effect of age on digitoxin pharmacokinetics. Br J Clin Pharmacol 1981; 11:401-2.

81. Rubin PC, Scott PJW, Reid JL. Prazosin disposition in young and elderly subjects. Br J Clin Pharmacol 1981; 12:401-4.

82. Mather LE, Tucker GT, Pflug AE, Lindop MJ, Wilkerson C. Meperidine kinetics in man: intravenous injection in surgical patients and volunteers. Clin Pharmacol Ther 1975; 17:21-30.

83. Triggs EJ, Nation RL, Long A, Ashley JJ. Pharmacokinetics in the elderly. Eur J Clin Pharmacol 1975; 8:55-62.

84. Whittaker JA, Evans DAP. Genetic control of phenylbutazone metabolism in man. Br Med J 1970; 4:323-8.

85. Hayes MJ, Langman MJS, Short AH. Changes in drug metabolism with increasing age. 2. Phenytoin clearance and protein binding. Br J Clin Pharmacol 1975; 2:73-9.

86. Sherwin AL, Loynd JS, Bock GW, Sokolowski CD. Effects of age, sex, obesity, and pregnancy on plasma diphenylhydantoin levels. Epilepsia 1974; 15:507-21.

87. Nies A, Robinson DS, Friedman MJ, et al. Relationship between age and tricyclic antidepressant plasma levels. Am J Psychiatry 1977; 134:790-3.

88. Briant RH, Dorrington RE, Cleal J, Williams FM. The rate of acetaminophen metabolism in the elderly and the young. J Am Geriatr Soc 1976; 24:359-61.
89. Fulton B, James O, Rawlins MD. The influence of age on the pharmacokinetics of paracetamol. Br J Clin Pharmacol 1979; 7:418P.
90. Divoll M, Abernethy DR, Ameer B, Greenblatt DJ. Acetaminophen kinetics in the elderly. Clin Pharmacol Ther 1982; 31:151-6.
91. Irvine RE, Grove J, Toseland PA, Trounce JR. The effect of age on the hydroxylation of amylobarbitone sodium in man. Br J Clin Pharmacol 1974; 1:41-3.
92. Wilkinson GR, Shand DG. A physiological approach to hepatic drug clearance. Clin Pharmacol Ther 1975; 18:377-90.
93. Geokas MC, Haverback BJ. The aging gastrointestinal tract. Am J Surg 1969; 117:881-92.
94. Abernethy DR, Greenblatt DJ, Divoll M, Harmatz JS, Shader RI. Alterations in drug distribution and clearance due to obesity. J Pharmacol Exp Ther 1981; 217:681-5.
95. Greenblatt DJ. Reduced serum albumin concentration in the elderly: a report from the Boston Collaborative Drug Surveillance Program. J Am Geriatr Soc 1979; 27:20-2.
96. MacLennan WJ, Martin P, Mason BJ. Protein intake and serum albumin levels in the elderly. Gerontology 1977; 23:360-7.
97. Koch-Weser J, Sellers EM. Binding of drugs to serum albumin. N Engl J Med 1976; 294:311-6, 526-31.
98. Greenblatt DJ, Sellers EM, Koch-Weser J. Importance of protein binding for the interpretation of serum or plasma drug concentrations. J Clin Pharmacol. (in press).
99. Evans MA, Triggs EJ, Cheung M, Broe GA, Creasey H. Gastric emptying rate in the elderly: implications for drug therapy. J Am Geriatr Soc 1981; 29:201-5.
100. Montgomery R, Haeney MR, Ross IN, et al. The ageing gut: a study of intestinal absorption in relation to nutrition in the elderly. Q J Med 1978; 47:197-211.
101. Kramer PA, Chapron DJ, Benson J, Mercik SA. Tetracycline absorption in elderly patients with achlorhydria. Clin Pharmacol Ther 1978; 23:467-72.
102. Ochs HR, Greenblatt DJ, Allen MD, Harmatz JS, Shader RI, Bodem G. Effect of age and Billroth gastrectomy on absorption of desmethyldiazepam from clorazepate. Clin Pharmacol Ther 1979; 26:449-56.
103. Ochs HR, Otten H, Greenblatt DJ, Dengler HJ. Diazepam absorption: effects of age, sex, and Billroth gastrectomy. Dig Dis Sci 1982; 27:225-30.
104. Divoll M, Ameer B, Abernethy DR, Greenblatt DJ. Age does not alter acetaminophen absorption. J Am Geriatr Soc 1982; 30:240-4.
105. Greenblatt DJ, Shader RI, Franke K, et al. Pharmacokinetics and bioavailability of intravenous, intramuscular, and oral lorazepam in humans. J Pharm Sci 1979; 68:57-63.
106. Greenblatt DJ, Shader RI, Franke K, MacLaughlin DS, Ransil BJ, Koch-Weser J. Kinetics of intravenous chlordiazepoxide: sex differences in drug distribution. Clin Pharmacol Ther 1977; 22:893-903.
107. Jusko WJ. Role of tobacco smoking in pharmacokinetics. J Pharmacokinet Biopharm 1978; 6:7-39.
108. Salem SAM, Rajjayabun P, Shepherd AMM, Stevenson IH. Reduced induction of drug metabolism in the elderly. Age Ageing 1978; 7:68-73.

109. Sellers EM, Holloway MR. Drug kinetics and alcohol ingestion. Clin Pharmacokinet 1978; 3:440-52.
110. Sellers EM, Giles HG, Greenblatt DJ, Naranjo CA. Differential effects on benzodiazepine disposition by disulfiram and ethanol. Arzneim Forsch 1980; 30:882-6.
111. Sandor P, Sellers EM, Dumbrell M, Khouw V. Effect of short- and long-term alcohol use on phenytoin kinetics in chronic alcoholics. Clin Pharmacol Ther 1981; 30:390-7.

Correspondence

Drug Disposition in Old Age*

To the Editor:

Greenblatt and his co-workers (May 6 issue)[1] have indicated an important role for reduced organ blood flow in the pharmacokinetic handling of drugs by the elderly patient; these authors have made a major contribution to these investigations. But when all is said and done, most drug therapy in old people, with few exceptions, can be started at the lower recommended dose (or with longer intervals between doses). This practice would be subject to clinical surveillance and titration or, if available, to drug assays.[2] The watchword in prescribing for the elderly could be: Be thrifty with periodic short-term reexamination.

The exceptions chiefly involve drugs with a narrow range of effective, nontoxic plasma concentrations (low therapeutic index), for which drug monitoring should be made available.[2] The premise is that therapeutic and toxic levels of total plasma concentrations of the drug are set lower in those who are elderly than in those under 50. In addition to digoxin, quinidine, and theophylline, it may be advisable to include other drugs with a narrow therapeutic index — e.g., opiate analgesics, chlorpromazine, propranolol, lithium, thyroxine, and gentamicin.

Just as age–weight dosimetry has become mandatory for children, so a renal and hepatic function nomogram, based on a decreasing organ blood flow of up to 30 to 40 per cent in advanced age, could be used with advantage in patients over 50, despite such patients' greater physiologic and metabolic heterogeneity.

Although Greenblatt et al. and other reviewers[3-5] regard altered pharmacodynamics with age as a minor influence, reassessment seems warranted. Apart from alterations in receptor activity[6,7] and active membrane transport, the reduction in the number and metabolic action of pharmacologically sensitive cells (neurons, hepatocytes, renal tubules, muscle fibers, thyroid, and other endocrine elements) can be appreciable with advancing age. Drugs acting on the central nervous system (hypnotics, opioids, antipsychotics, antidepressants, and anticonvulsants) illustrate this point. Standard doses of all these drugs in the elderly produce higher blood levels that last longer. This results from a decreasing volume of drug distribution because of progressive diminution in hepatic blood flow and

*Originally published on October 21, 1982 (307:1087-1089).

biotransformation, renal blood flow and active transport, and lean body mass. But the progressive reduction in cerebral blood flow with age would theoretically deliver an equivalent amount of drug to central-nervous-system cells as in younger persons. The reduction in the number of neurons in old age is insufficient to explain the exquisite and untoward sensitivity of the central nervous system to these drugs.[3] Further consideration and analysis of the pharmacodynamics are required for this and other organ systems.

RALPH E. BERNSTEIN
University of Witwatersrand Medical School
Johannesburg, South Africa

1. Greenblatt DJ, Sellers EM, Shader RI. Drug disposition in old age. N Engl J Med 1982; 306:1081-8.
2. de Wolff FA, Mattie H, Breimer DD. Therapeutic relevance of drug assays. Leiden: Leiden University Press, 1979.
3. Vestal RE. Drug use in the elderly: a review of problems and special considerations. Drugs 1978; 16:358-82.
4. Chapron D, Lawson I. Drug prescribing and care of the elderly. In: Reichel W, ed. Clinical aspects of aging. Baltimore: Williams & Wilkins, 1978:13-32.
5. O'Malley K, Judge T, Crooks J. Geriatric clinical pharmacology and therapeutics. In: Avery GS, ed. Drug treatment. Sydney: Adis Press, 1979:123-42.
6. Smythies JR, Bradley RJ, eds. Receptors in pharmacology. New York: Marcel Dekker, 1978.
7. Mautner HG. Receptor theories and dose-response relationships. In: Wolff ME, ed. Burger's medicinal chemistry. 4th ed. Part 1. New York: Wiley Interscience, 1980:271-84.

To the Editor:

In their review of pharmacogeriatrics Greenblatt et al. note the effects of cigarette smoking and ethanol ingestion on drug disposition. Diet is another environmental variable that may affect drug metabolism[1] and may have particular importance in the elderly.

Kappas et al. have demonstrated that increasing the proportion of protein in the diets of normal volunteers decreased the half-life of theophylline from 8.1 to 5.2 hours.[2] This difference is thought to result from changes in the oxidative transformation of this drug.

Riboflavin is a cofactor involved in the cytochrome P_{450}-dependent mixed-function oxidase system, and a deficiency of this vitamin has been shown to alter drug metabolism in laboratory animals,[3] leading Roe to speculate that such a deficiency of this micronutrient might have a similar effect in human beings.[4]

The elderly, as Greenblatt and his colleagues note, have a diminution in absorptive efficiency of certain micronutrients because of age-related lessening of active transport processes. In addition, the elderly are at an increased risk for protein-calorie malnutrition,[6] as well as vitamin malnutrition,[7] which may be secondary to poor intake resulting from many factors, including poverty, edentulousness, chronic disease, and institutionalization. It therefore seems reasonable to regard nutritional status as another environmental variable affecting drug disposition in the elderly.

BARNETT G. MENNEN, M.D.
5 East 67th St.
New York, NY 10021

1. Campbell TC, Hayes JR. Role of nutrition in the drug-metabolizing enzyme system. Pharmacol Rev 1974; 26:171-97.
2. Kappas A, Anderson KE, Conney AH, Alvares AP. Influence of dietary protein and carbohydrate on antipyrine and theophylline metabolism in man. Clin Pharm Ther 1976; 20:643-53.
3. Patel JM, Pawrr SS. Riboflavin and drug metabolism in adult male and female rats. Biochem Pharmacol 1974; 23:1467-77.
4. Roe DA. Drug-induced nutritional deficiencies. Westport, Conn.: Avi Publishing, 1976:24.
5. Montgomery R, Haeney MR, Ross IN, et al. The ageing gut: a study of intestinal absorption in relation to nutrition in the elderly. Q J Med 1978; 47:197-211.
6. United States Department of Health, Education, and Welfare, Health Services, Mental Health Administration. Ten state nutrition survey, 1968-1970. Washington, D.C.: Government Printing Office, 1972. (DHEW publication no. 72-8132, 72-8133).
7. Brin M, Bauernfeind JC. Vitamin needs of the elderly. Postgrad Med 1978; 63:155-63.

To the Editor:

The review of drug disposition in old age by Greenblatt et al. dispenses the traditional teaching that the removal of drugs from the circulation proceeds at rates proportional to the plasma concentration of the free or unbound species. A number of recent studies[1-3] (and Forker EL, et al.: unpublished data) belie this idea, at least insofar as the liver is concerned, and I believe that readers of the *Journal* should be aware of them.

Many drugs and endogenous products extensively bound to albumin are metabolized or excreted by the liver. A number of such solutes — indeed, all those examined so far — have a steady-state extraction fraction much higher than can be accounted for by the conventional view that hepatic uptake is governed by the plasma concentration of free material. This phenomenon is not attributable simply to the fact that the sinusoidal endothelium is freely permeable to protein (although this undoubtedly has a permissive role), nor can it be accounted for by spontaneous dissociation of the albumin–ligand complex (although this certainly occurs as a free ligand is removed along the length of the sinusoids). Instead, it appears to depend on the capacity of the liver-cell surface to reduce the affinity of the ligand for albumin to well below the value observable in free solution.

It is not known whether this surface-mediated dissociation should be attributed to specific membrane receptors for albumin or whether it represents a transient conformational change in albumin incidental to nonspecific collisions with the cell surface. The following features must be accounted for, however. The mediated dissociation displays saturation kinetics in the sense that uncomplexed albumin inhibits ligand removal. Surface debinding is not a necessary intermediate in the transport sequence, because free ligand is removed even faster than that bound to albumin. Finally, the phenomenon is not species-specific, since bovine albumin engages the dissociation mechanism in both rats and elasmobranchs.

The concept that is emerging from these observations envisions a limited number of sites on the liver-cell surface that, when occupied by an albumin–ligand complex, generate high local concentrations of the free ligand, presumably at a location favorable for ultimate transport of the ligand into the cell. These sites may also be occupied by albumin alone, however, so that as the molar ratio of total albumin to total ligand increases, the chances that sites will be available to liberate bound ligand are reduced, and accordingly, so is the ligand-extraction fraction. The capacity of excess albumin to reduce the ligand-extraction fraction is qualitatively in accord with the conventional wisdom, and this may explain why the quantitative predictions of the traditional teaching have not been challenged heretofore.

E. L. FORKER, M.D.
University of Missouri
Columbia, MO 65212

1. Forker EL, Luxon BA. Albumin helps mediate removal of taurocholate by rat liver. J Clin Invest 1981; 67:1517-22.
2. Weisiger R, Gollan J, Ockner R. Receptor for albumin on the liver cell surface may mediate uptake of fatty acids and other albumin-bound substances. Science 1981; 211:1048-51.
3. Weisiger R, Zacks C, Smith N, Boyer J. Hepatic uptake of ^{35}-S-sulfobromophtalein (BSP) from albumin solutions in elasmobranchs. Gastroenterology 1982; 82:1249. abstract.

The above letters were referred to the authors of the article in question, who offer the following reply:

To the Editor:
Dr. Bernstein's general recommendation for cautious and carefully titrated drug therapy in the elderly is well taken and one that we fully support. Yet, a rational scientific basis for pharmacogeriatrics requires biomedical science to broaden its research data base on the biologic mechanisms of changes in response to drugs in the aging person. Although altered pharmacodynamics was not the specific focus of our article, it was hardly dismissed as having "a minor influence." We attempted principally to outline physiologic changes associated with aging and their possible relation to alterations in drug disposition. Bernstein's formulation of the same subject unfortunately contains important inaccuracies. Centrally acting

drugs by no means always or even usually produce higher blood levels that last longer in the elderly. The extent of drug distribution is as likely to be increased in the elderly as decreased; neither change is necessarily related to hepatic or renal blood flow, drug biotransformation, or active transport. A reduction in cerebral blood flow could theoretically increase, decrease, or cause no change in drug delivery to the brain. There is no evidence that use of a nomogram based on organ blood flow would improve drug therapy in the elderly; it might well make matters worse.

Dr. Mennen correctly points out that diet can influence drug-metabolizing capacity. Nutritional deficiencies could accentuate the impaired drug-oxidizing capacity observed for some drugs in some elderly persons. Unfortunately, a "state of nutrition" is notoriously difficult to quantitate, and its influence on the outcome of pharmacogeriatric studies is usually unknown except in cases of overt dysnutrition. In our own studies, reduced oxidizing capacity has been observed among most elderly men, despite their apparently "normal" nutritional status (see references 46, 49, 53 through 55, and 57 through 60 in our article).

The discussion on interpretation of total and unbound drug clearance of protein-bound drugs assumed that only the unbound drug in serum or plasma is available for biotransformation. This assumption is valid for the majority of drugs used in clinical practice. However, for some exceptional compounds, as pointed out by Dr. Forker, both the free and the bound drug fractions are extracted by the liver. With such compounds total clearance is more important than free clearance. Lidocaine and propranolol are examples of drugs that may fall into this category.

DAVID J. GREENBLATT, M.D.
Tufts–New England Medical Center
Boston, MA 02111

EDWARD M. SELLERS, M.D., PH.D.
Addiction Research Foundation
University of Toronto
Toronto, ON M5S 2S1, Canada

RICHARD I. SHADER, M.D.
Tufts–New England Medical Center
Boston, MA 02111

Captopril

Donald G. Vidt, M.D.,

Emannuel L. Bravo, M.D.,

and Fetnat M. Fouad, M.D.

CAPTOPRIL (d-3-mercapto-2-methylpropranoyl-l-proline [SQ 14,225, Capoten]) is the first orally active inhibitor of angiotensin-converting enzyme, the enzyme responsible for conversion of inactive angiotensin I to the potent pressor peptide angiotensin II. It is a potent, relatively specific competitive inhibitor of angiotensin-converting enzyme (kininase II), as well as an effective antihypertensive agent. Prior experience with the nonapeptide inhibitor of angiotensin-converting enzyme, teprotide (SQ 20,881), demonstrated that this parenterally administered agent was effective in the treatment of most patients with hypertension.[1,2] The search for an orally effective inhibitor led to the development of captopril (Fig. 1),[3] which has since undergone intensive clinical investigation for the treatment of hypertension with high, normal, or low plasma renin. Since not all patients respond to available therapies, the development of this new class of antihypertensive drugs is welcome.

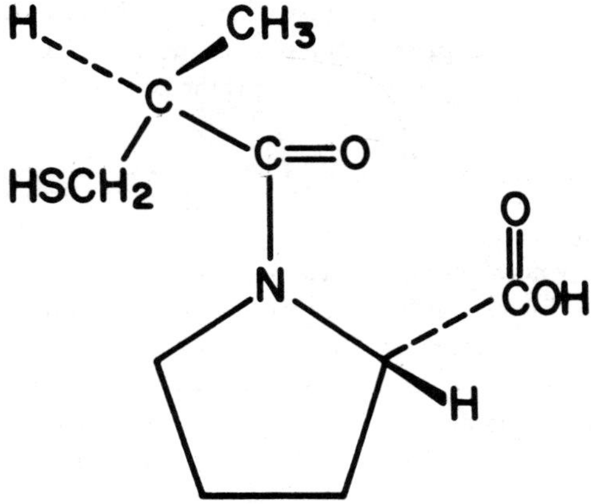

Figure 1. Structural Formula of Captopril (Capoten).

From the Department of Hypertension and Nephrology and the Department of Clinical Science, Division of Research, The Cleveland Clinic Foundation.

Originally published on January 28, 1982 (306:214-219).

Pharmacokinetics

Absorption, Metabolism, and Excretion

Limited information is available on captopril's disposition in human beings. After oral administration, captopril is rapidly absorbed, with peak blood levels reached in 30 to 90 minutes. Approximately 75 per cent of the administered dose is absorbed during fasting, but food in the gastrointestinal tract reduces absorption by 30 to 40 per cent. Although captopril is about 30 per cent protein-bound in blood, it is distributed rapidly to most tissues, except in the central nervous system.

The drug is rapidly metabolized, and although the half-life of unchanged captopril is difficult to determine accurately, it is probably less than two hours.[4]

Renal excretion of the drug is rapid: about 50 per cent appears in the urine within four hours of administration, rising to 66 per cent within 24 hours.[5] During the first 24 hours 38 per cent of the drug is excreted unchanged in the urine. The elimination of captopril and its metabolites correlates closely with endogenous creatinine clearance, and patients with renal insufficiency have much higher peak plasma concentrations than patients with normal renal function. The dose must be reduced when renal function is impaired.[5]

Hormonal Changes

Treatment with captopril results in a marked increase in plasma renin activity, probably because of the absence of a negative feedback normally exerted by angiotensin II on renin release. Despite this increase in renin, aldosterone production is reduced considerably, which also reflects the blockade of angiotensin II production.[6-8] Circulating plasma norepinephrine is unchanged and responds appropriately when a patient assumes an upright posture.[6,9,10]

Mechanism of Action

The interpretation of blood-pressure responses to inhibitors of angiotensin-converting enzyme may be adversely affected by several factors. Because angiotensin-converting enzyme is responsible for inactivating bradykinin,[11] its inhibition would lead to concomitant increases in vasodilator substances (bradykinin) and to decreases in vasoconstrictor substances (such as angiotensin II). In addition to exerting its direct vascular effect, bradykinin releases vasoactive prostaglandins from various organs.[12] Therefore, inhibition of angiotensin-converting enzyme, which is present in most organs, would allow large amounts of bradykinin to release prostaglandins; this could enhance the hypotensive effects of bradykinin. It has been demonstrated that inhibition of angiotensin-converting enzyme potentiates the magnitude and duration of the vasodepressor responses elicited by bradykinin, and this enhanced bradykinin-induced hypotension is markedly attenuated by indomethacin, an inhibitor of prostaglandin.[13]

Although the hypotensive action of captopril involves enhanced production of vasodilators, there is evidence that its vasodepressor action is largely the result of inhibition of angiotensin II generation. Responses to various vasoconstrictors are unaltered by captopril; we have found that it normalizes blood pressure without affecting urinary excretion of prostaglandin E_2 in patients with renovascular hypertension. Also, cardiac output and heart rate are unchanged in hypertensive patients responding to captopril.[14] These hemodynamic features contrast markedly with those of bradykinin, which causes increased cardiac output and heart rate and tends to produce orthostatic hypotension.[15]

It has recently been reported that captopril markedly inhibits pressor responses to sympathetic-nerve stimulation in pithed, spontaneously hypertensive rats, but that cardiac responses are unaffected. Pressor responses to angiotensin I are abolished, but those to angiotensin II and norepinephrine are not markedly altered, suggesting that this effect has a prejunctional component.[16] Since the inhibition can be reversed by angiotensin II, Antonaccio and Kerwin have suggested that captopril may act at the vascular level to decrease local angiotensin II formation. If correct, these studies may explain some perplexing situations in which specific antagonists of angiotensin II do not reduce blood pressure but captopril is still highly effective. Presumably, these intracellular vascular sites are accessible to captopril but not to angiotensin II antagonists, which act at receptor sites on vascular membranes.

Systemic Hemodynamic Effects

Captopril lowers total peripheral resistance and causes little change in cardiac output, heart rate, or pulmonary wedge pressure.[14,17,18] Early hemodynamic changes occurring 30 to 60 minutes after administration are similar to those observed with the angiotension II antagonist, (Sar^1-Thr^8)-angiotensin II. The effects are independent of pretreatment cardiac output or blood pressure.[17] Reduction of blood pressure is relatively greater with captopril, suggesting that some mechanism other than angiotensin-converting enzyme inhibition contributes to the drug's acute effects.[19,20]

During long-term therapy, a spectrum of cardiac output responses may occur without any correlation with changes in mean arterial pressure.[21,22] A correlation between cardiac output and blood volume suggests that the effect of captopril on venous tone varies. Other studies have also supported venodilation after converting enzyme inhibition.[23-28]

In patients with congestive heart failure due to primary myocardial disease or coronary-artery disease, captopril produces both hemodynamic and clinical improvement. The most prominent hemodynamic findings are increased cardiac output and reduced mean transit time; the latter is more common in patients with moderate to excellent clinical improvement.

Baroreceptor Reflexes

The failure of the heart rate to change despite reductions in blood pressure has raised questions regarding the integrity of the autonomic nervous system after inhibition of angiotensin-converting enzyme.[29,30] Our experience has demonstrated that patients given captopril have a normal response to head-up tilt and to norepinephrine infusions, even during associated diuretic therapy, suggesting that captopril does not interfere with the homeostatic cardiovascular responses to posture. This finding is clinically important in view of the frequent need for diuretics in captopril-treated patients.[31,32] There are other possible explanations for the observation that the heart rate does not respond to captopril. Studies of saralasin and (Sar[1]-Thr[8])-angiotensin II have suggested that these antagonists may interfere with the activity of the parasympathetic nervous system, and one might speculate that angiotensin-converting enzyme inhibitors have a similar effect. It is also possible that the effect is analogous to that of vasodilators, which affect veins as well as arterioles. It seems likely that this feature is common to agents that interfere with the renin-angiotensin system, including those like captopril, which are not known to cross the blood-brain barrier.

Relation to the Renin Angiotensin System

Numerous reports have confirmed the relation of the acute response of blood pressure to initial plasma renin activity.[10,18,19] When therapy is continued, this correlation tends to be lost, and the long-term response does not appear to be dependent on or related to a high level of renin activity before treatment.[8,18] No definite explanation for this phenomenon has been established. Moreover, the delayed increase in blood pressure in patients who responded initially cannot be explained by known counteracting mechanisms. Neither an increase in cardiac output nor an expansion of blood volume appears to be of major importance in this respect, but a subtle alteration in sodium metabolism may play a part, as suggested by the restoration of blood-pressure response after these patients are given a diuretic.[23]

Clinical Use

Hypertension

Captopril effectively lowers blood pressure in patients with severe or resistant hypertension or renovascular hypertension, and in selected patients with hypertension associated with renal failure or scleroderma.[6,10,33] Because of the adverse effects reported during clinical trials, captopril should be considered only when patients do not have a satisfactory response or when they have unacceptable side effects during multiple-drug regimens. Such regimens may include a diuretic, an adrenergic blocking agent, and a vasodilator. Data from numerous studies indicate that diastolic blood pressures are reduced in most patients treated with captopril, and that the antipressor effects are enhanced by concomitant administration of a natriuretic agent.[6-8,10,15,34] Patients with malignant hypertension or renovascular hypertension and high levels of plasma renin activity respond extremely well to the effect of angiotensin-converting enzyme inhibition by captopril. The initial fall in pressure is proportional to the level of renin activity before treatment, whereas continued therapy does not show a direct correlation, and many patients with normal or even low levels of renin activity have considerable reductions in blood pressure.[6,8,35] The finding that patients with suppressed renin activity respond to captopril suggests that extremely small amounts of circulating angiotensin II participate in maintaining blood pressure, or that bradykinin becomes physiologically important when its degradation is inhibited.[36]

Some patients with resistant hypertension do not respond to a diuretic-captopril combination, and the addition of other agents such as a beta-blocker will be required to control this disorder. During therapy, patients retain potassium and serum potassium levels rise, probably because of aldosterone suppression. The addition of captopril to thiazide therapy can correct thiazide-induced hypokalemia and obviate the need for potassium supplements. Captopril is well tolerated, and delayed tolerance or resistance does not appear to be a problem, particularly when the drug is taken with a diuretic. Abrupt discontinuation of captopril is not associated with rebound hypertension; blood pressure returns to normal within several days.[6] Plasma renin activity returns slowly to pretreatment levels, and plasma catecholamines are not influenced. Most investigations of captopril have involved high doses (200 to 600 mg per day), and most of the major side effects have also been observed at these doses.

The role of captopril in the treatment of patients with mild to moderate, uncomplicated hypertension must be defined. Possibly, this drug has fewer side effects when it is administered in lower doses, but the relevant data are not yet available.

Congestive Heart Failure

Results of preliminary studies suggest that captopril is useful in patients with congestive heart failure. Beneficial acute hemodynamic changes include increased cardiac output, decreased left ventricular end-diastolic pressure, and decreased peripheral and pulmonary vascular resistance.[37] Sustained improvement and increased performance on exercise tests have lasted for as long as six months in several patients given repeated doses.[22]

Other Indications

Alterations in the response of the renin-angiotensin-aldosterone system have a role in the postural retention of sodium and water in women with idiopathic edema; one brief report suggests that captopril therapy can decrease the difference between weight in the morning and in the evening, and can increase sodium and water excretion in this peculiar syndrome.[38,39]

Several patients with scleroderma crisis have had dramatic improvement with rapid lowering of blood pressure after the initiation of captopril. Of particular interest was renal function and rapid healing of digital ulcers.[40,41] Further evaluation of captopril in this life-threatening condition will be important.

Adverse Effects

Clinical trials with captopril have shown a very low incidence of many of the adverse effects commonly reported with other antihypertensive drugs. Reports of sexual dysfunction, bronchospasm, tachycardia, fatigue, or orthostatic hypotension have been infrequent. There have been no reports of cardiac depression, glucose intolerance, severe bradycardia, mental depression, sleep disturbances, nasal congestion, or hypokalemia. Unlike some other antihypertensive agents for which particular cautions or contraindications exist, captopril can be used to treat hypertension in patients with cardiac arrhythmias, asthma or chronic obstructive pulmonary disease, congestive heart failure, diabetes mellitus, or hepatic disease.

Severe or potentially serious adverse effects have been reported and are responsible for the limitations recommended in the use of this agent. In some instances, an association with captopril has been suggested but an absolute casual relation has not been established.

Hematologic Effects

Neutropenia has been reported in approximately 0.3 per cent of patients; it develops within the first three to 12 weeks of treatment and has been associated with myeloid hypoplasia of the bone marrow.[42,43] Agranulocytosis has been observed in several cases, and two patients have died of septicemia. It should be noted that almost all patients had complex medical problems, including immune complex disorders, metastatic disease, and advanced renal failure, and many were concomitantly receiving other medications capable of bone-marrow suppression. Blood counts should be obtained frequently during the first three months of therapy and periodically thereafter.

Renal Effects

Unpublished data from clinical trials suggest that proteinuria (>1.0 g per day) occurs in about 1.2 per cent of patients placed on a regimen of captopril, and the nephrotic syndrome occurs in one fourth of these patients. Like the data concerning hematologic side effects, the data in these cases are difficult to interpret, since most of the affected patients have evidence of renal disease. Proteinuria may subside despite continued treatment with captopril, but heavy proteinuria and a clinical nephrotic syndrome may also be associated.[44] Findings of membranous glomerulonephritis with epimembranous electron-dense deposits on renal biopsy indicate the possibility of an immune-complex glomerulopathy. The membranous glomerulopathy that may accompany captopril therapy is similar clinically and histologically to other drug-induced nephropathies, such as those caused by trimethadione, gold, mercury, and penicillamine. Clinical interpretation of these observations is difficult because the results of pretreatment biopsies were not available and the incidence of preexisting renal disease was high.

Acute reversible renal failure has been noted during captopril therapy, and serum creatinine levels may increase within several days of instituting treatment, usually in patients with preexistent renal impairment.[45,46] Transient elevations in serum creatinine levels have also been observed during therapy.

Cutaneous and Mucous-Membrane Effects

Rashes, occasionally accompanied by pruritus, fever, and eosinophilia, have been observed in about 10 per cent of patients. These symptoms usually occur during the first several weeks of therapy, and in some cases they appear to be dose-related. A generalized morbilliform eruption with fever or a transient pruritic, maculopapular rash may occur. Angioedema of the face or mucous membranes has been observed rarely, and one case of severe aphthous ulcers has been reported.

Disturbances of Taste

Temporary ageusia has been noted in approximately 6 per cent of patients. The symptoms appear to be drug-related and are usually transient.

Drug Interactions

Although orthostatic symptoms have not been a problem with captopril, hypotension may be observed when the drug is administered with other antihypertensive agents, particularly to patients who are volume-depleted by diuretics.[10,47,48] Merely reducing the dosage of captopril will not prevent episodes of hypotension, since even small doses can inhibit angiotensin conversion.

Since captopril is associated with increases in serum potassium levels, the risk of hyperkalemia may be increased with concomitant administration of potassium supplements or potassium-sparing agents such as spironolactone, triamterene, or amiloride. Neurologic dysfunction has been reported in two patients receiving captopril and cimetidine,[49] although a causal relation has not been established. Indomethacin has been shown to attenuate the reduction of blood pressure and the increases in plasma renin activity in captopril-treated patients.[50]

| Dosage and Administration

Captopril should be taken at least one hour before meals, and the dosage should be titrated according to the patient's clinical response. The manufacturer (Squibb) recommends an initial dose of 25 mg three times daily, with stepwise increases to a maximal dosage of 150 mg three times daily. The risk of an acute hypotensive response to initiation of captopril can be minimized by discontinuing other antihypertensive agents for several days to a week before starting captopril. Since elimination of the drug is markedly reduced in patients with renal failure, careful adjustments in dosage along the guidelines recommended by the manufacturer are required. Doses as low as 12.5 mg twice daily have been given to patients who are undergoing dialysis because of chronic renal failure and whose blood levels of captopril are maintained for a prolonged period.

References

1. Gavras H, Brunner HR, Laragh JH, Sealey JE, Gavras I, Vukovich RA. An angiotensin converting-enzyme inhibitor to identify and treat vasoconstrictor and volume factors in hypertensive patients. N Engl J Med 1974; 291:817-21.
2. Case DB, Wallace JM, Keim HJ, Weber MA, Sealey JE, Laragh JH. Possible role of renin in hypertension as suggested by renin-sodium profiling and inhibition of converting enzyme. N Engl J Med 1977; 296:641-6.
3. Ondetti MA, Rubin B, Cushman DW. Design of specific inhibitors of angiotensin-converting enzyme: new class of orally active antihypertensive agents. Science 1977; 196:441-4.
4. Kripalani KJ, McKinstry DN, Singhvi SM, Willard DA, Vukovich RA, Migdalof BM. Disposition of captopril in normal subjects. Clin Pharmacol Ther 1980; 27:636-41.
5. Rommel AJ, Pierides AM, Heald A. Captopril elimination in chronic renal failure. Clin Pharmacol Ther 1980; 27:282. abstract.
6. Bravo EL, Tarazi RC. Converting enzyme inhibition with an orally active compound in hypertensive man. Hypertension 1979; 1:39-46.
7. Brunner HR, Gavras H, Waeber B, et al. Oral angiotensin-converting enzyme inhibitor in long-term treatment of hypertensive patients. Ann Intern Med 1979; 90:19-23.
8. Gavras H, Brunner HR, Turini GA, et al. Antihypertensive effect of the oral angiotensin converting-enzyme inhibitor SQ 14225 in man. N Engl J Med 1978; 298:991-5.
9. Case DB, Atlas SA, Laragh JH, Sealey JE, Sullivan PA, McKinstry DN. Clinical experience with blockade of the renin-angiotensin-aldosterone system by an oral converting-enzyme inhibitor (SQ 14,225, captopril) in hypertensive patients. Prog Cardiovasc Dis 1978; 21:195-206.
10. MacGregor GA, Markandu ND, Roulston JE, Jones JC. Essential hypertension: effect of an oral inhibitor of angiotensin-converting enzyme. Br Med J 1979; 2:1106-9.
11. Ferreira SH. A bradykinin-potentiating factor (BPF) present in the venom of *Bothrops Jararaca*. Br J Pharmacol Chemother 1965; 24:163-9.
12. McGiff JC, Terragno NA, Malik KU, Lonigro AJ. Release of a prostaglandin E-like substance from canine kidney by bradykinin: comparison with eledoisin. Circ Res 1972; 31:36-43.

13. Murthy VS, Waldron TL, Goldberg ME. The mechanism of bradykinin potentiation after inhibition of angiotensin-converting enzyme by SQ 14,225 in conscious rabbits. Circ Res 1978; 43: Part 2:I-40-5.

14. Cody RJ Jr, Tarazi RC, Bravo EL, Fouad FM. Haemodynamics of orally-active enzyme inhibitor (SQ 14225) in hypertensive patients. Clin Sci Mol Med 1978; 55:453-9.

15. Streeten DHP, Kerr LP, Kerr CB, Prior JC, Dalakos TG. Hyperbradykinism: a new orthostatic syndrome. Lancet 1972; 2:1048-53.

16. Antonaccio MH, Kerwin L. Pre- and post-junctional inhibition of vascular sympathetic function by captopril in SHR: implications of vascular angiotensin II in hypertension and antihypertensive actions of captopril. Hypertension 1981; 3:I-54-62.

17. Fouad FM, Ceimo JMK, Tarazi RC, Bravo EL. Contrasts and similarities of acute hemodynamic responses to specific antagonism of angiotensin II ([Sar^1 Thr^8]A$_{II}$) and to inhibition of converting enzyme (captopril). Circulation 1980; 61:163-9.

18. Sullivan JM, Ginsburg BA, Ratts TE, et al. Hemodynamic and antihypertensive effects of captopril, an orally active angiotensin converting enzyme inhibitor. Hypertension 1979; 1:397-401.

19. Thurston H, Swales JD. Converting enzyme inhibitor and saralasin infusion in rats: evidence for an additional vasodepressor property of converting enzyme inhibitor. Circ Res 1978; 42:588-92.

20. Antonaccio MH, Asaad M, Rubin B, Horovitz ZP. Captopril: factors involved in its mechanism of action. In: Horovitz ZP, ed. Angiotensin converting enzyme inhibitors. Baltimore: Urban & Schwarzenberg, 1981:161-80.

21. Bravo EL. Hemodynamic effects of long-term captopril therapy in hypertensive man. In: Horovitz ZP, ed. Angiotensin converting enzyme inhibitors. Baltimore: Urban & Schwarzenberg, 1981:263-72.

22. Fouad FM, Tarazi RC, Bravo EL, Hart NJ, Castle L, Salcedo EE. Long-term control of congestive heart failure with captopril. Am J Cardiol. (in press).

23. Tarazi RC, Bravo EL, Fouad FM, Omvik P, Cody RJ Jr. Hemodynamic and volume changes associated with captopril. Hypertension 1980; 2:576-85.

24. Tarazi RC, Dustan HP, Bravo EL, Niarchos AP. Vasodilating drugs contrasting haemodynamic effects. Clin Sci Mol Med 1976; 51: Suppl 3:575s-8s.

25. Lund-Johansen P. Hemodynamic changes at rest and during exercise in long-term prazosin therapy for essential hypertension. Postgrad Med 1975; 58: Suppl:45-52.

26. Collier JG, Robinson BF. Comparison of effects of locally infused angiotensin I and II on hand veins and forearm arteries in man: evidence for converting enzyme activity in limb vessels. Clin Sci Mol Med 1974; 47:189-92.

27. Johns DW, Baker KM, Ayers CR, Carey RM, Peach MJ. Dilatation of forearm vasculature following angiotensin converting enzyme inhibition by captopril (SQ 14225) in severe hypertension. Circulation 1979; 59 & 60: Suppl 2:II-227. abstract.

28. Tarazi RC, Fouad FM, Ceimo JK, Bravo EL. Renin, aldosterone and cardiac decompensation: studies with an oral converting enzyme inhibitor in heart failure. Am J Cardiol 1979; 44:1013-8.

29. Heavey DJ, Reid JL. The effect of SQ 14225 on baroreceptor reflex sensitivity in conscious normotensive rabbits. Br J Pharmacol 1978; 64:389P-40P.

30. Sancho J, Re R, Burton J, Barger AC, Haber E. The role of the renin-angiotensin-aldosterone system in cardiovascular homeostasis in normal human subjects. Circulation 1976; 53:400-5.
31. Swartz SL, Crantz FR, Williams GH, et al. Diuretic enhancement of the hypotensive effect of captopril (SQ 14,225). Presented at the 61st annual meeting of the Endocrine Society, Anaheim, California, June 13-15, 1979. abstract.
32. Wallace JM, Keim HJ, Case DB, Lopez J, Laragh JH. Reduction of cardiac output with angiotensin blockade in hypertension. Clin Res 1976; 24:244A. abstract.
33. Atkinson AB, Brown JJ, Davies DL, et al. Hyponatraemic hypertensive syndrome with renal-artery occlusion corrected by captopril. Lancet 1979; 2:606-8.
34. Jenkins AC, McKinstry DN. Review of clinical studies of hypertensive patients treated with captopril. Med J Aust 1979; 2: Suppl 2:32-7.
35. Atkinson AB, Robertson JIS. Captopril in the treatment of clinical hypertension and cardiac failure. Lancet 1979; 2:836-9.
36. Swartz SL, Williams GH, Hollenberg NK, Moore TJ, Dluhy RG. Converting enzyme inhibition in essential hypertension: the hypotensive response does not reflect only reduced angiotensin II formation. Hypertension 1979; 1:106-11.
37. Turini GA, Brunner HR, Gribic M, Waeber B, Gavras H. Improvement of chronic congestive heart-failure by oral captopril. Lancet 1979; 1:1213-5.
38. Streeten DHP, Louis LH, Con JW. Secondary aldosteronism in "idiopathic edema." Trans Assoc Am Physicians 1960; 73:227-90.
39. Mimran A, Targhetta R. Captopril treatment of idiopathic edema. N Engl J Med 1979; 301:1289-90.
40. D'Angelo WA, Lopez-Ovejero JA, Saal SD, Laragh JH. Early versus late treatment of scleroderma renal crisis and malignant hypertension with captopril. Arthritis Rheum 1980; 23:664. abstract.
41. Lopez-Ovejero JA, Saal SD, D'Angelo WA, Cheigh JS, Stenzel KH, Laragh JH. Reversal of vascular and renal crisis of scleroderma by oral angiotensin-converting enzyme blockade. N Engl J Med 1979; 300:1417-9.
42. Amann FW, Bühler FR, Conen D, Brunner F, Ritz R, Speck B. Captopril-associated agranulocytosis. Lancet 1980; 1:150.
43. Van Brummelen P, Willemze R, Tan WD, Thompson J. Captopril-associated agranulocytosis. Lancet 1980; 1:150.
44. Case DB, Atlas SA, Mouradian JA, Fishman RA, Sherman RL, Laragh JH. Proteinuria during long-term captopril therapy. JAMA 1980; 244:346-9.
45. Grossman A, Eckland D, Price P, Edwards CRW. Captopril: reversible renal failure with severe hyperkalaemia. Lancet 1980; 1:712.
46. Woodhouse K, Farrow PR, Wilkinson R. Reversible renal failure during treatment with captopril. Br Med J 1979; 2:1146-7.
47. Morganti A, Pickering TG, Lopez-Ovejero JA, Laragh JH. Endocrine and cardiovascular influences of converting enzyme inhibition with SQ 14225 in hypertensive patients in the supine position and during head-up tilt before and after sodium depletion. J Clin Endocrinol Metab 1980; 50:748-54.
48. Brunner HR, Waeber B, Gavras H. Rational use of captopril. Lancet 1979; 1:832.
49. Atkinson AB, Brown JJ, Lever AF, et al. Neurological dysfunction in two patients receiving captopril and cimetidine. Lancet 1980; 2:36-7.
50. Crantz FR, Swartz SL, Hollenberg NK, et al. Role of prostaglandins in the hypotensive response to captopril in essential hypertension. Clin Res 1979; 27:592A. abstract.

Correspondence

Captopril*

To the Editor:

According to the article in the January 28 issue by Vidt et al.,[1] the risk of a hypotensive response to the initiation of captopril therapy can be minimized by discontinuing other antihypertensive agents for "several days." This statement is purely theoretical, given the current indications for the clinical use of captopril, which is recommended for severe drug-resistant hypertension or complicated forms of hypertension — situations in which the discontinuation of previous therapy for "several days" is hardly justifiable and, frankly, impractical except in a hospital setting. The authors have not commented on this paradox.

We have administered captopril in low doses while the previous therapy was being tapered off. Although adverse effects (specifically, hypotension) were not encountered, such action should be undertaken only with close follow-up of the patients.

The authors have alluded to the beneficial hemodynamic effects of captopril in congestive heart failure. It is our understanding that in the reported studies,[2-4] including the one quoted by the authors,[5] captopril was added to preexisting therapy (such as digitalis and diuretics) and was not used alone in congestive heart failure. This point was not made in the review, and readers may draw unwarranted conclusions.

C. Venkata S. Ram, M.D.
University of Texas Health Science Center
Dallas, TX 75235

1. Vidt DG, Bravo EL, Fouad FM. Captopril. N Engl J Med 1982; 306:214-9.
2. Dzau VJ, Colucci WS, Williams GM, Curfman G, Meggs L, Hollenberg NK. Sustained effectiveness of converting-enzyme inhibition in patients with severe congestive heart failure. N Engl J Med 1980; 302:1373-9.
3. Faxon DP, Halperin JL, Creager MA, et al. Angiotensin inhibition in severe heart failure: acute central and limb hemodynamic effects of captopril with observations on sustained oral therapy. Am Heart J 1981; 101:548-56.
4. Ader R, Chatterjee K, Ports T, et al. Immediate and sustained hemodynamic and clinical improvement in chronic heart failure by an oral angiotensin converting enzyme inhibitor. Circulation 1980; 61:931-7.
5. Turini GA, Brunner HR, Gribic M, Waeber B, Gavras H. Improvement of chronic congestive heart-failure by oral captopril. Lancet 1979; 1:1213-5.
6. Linjen P, Farard R, Staessen J, et al. Dose response in captopril therapy of hypertension. Clin Pharmacol Ther 1980; 28:310-5.
7. Brunner HR, Gavras H, Waeber B, et al. Oral angiotensin-converting enzyme inhibitor in long-term treatment of hypertensive patients. Ann Intern Med 1979; 90:19-23.

*Originally published on July 1, 1982 (307:58-60).

To the Editor:

In their well-balanced article on captopril, Vidt and his associates did not elaborate on the fate of aldosterone. The impression generated is that aldosterone remains suppressed throughout the period of enzyme blockade. Although aldosterone is suppressed initially, this response does not persist, and other factors seem to override the suppressive effect of enzyme blockade. Both short-term and long-term studies have shown an increase in aldosterone levels despite enzyme blockade with captopril. Gavras et al.[1] noticed an increase of up to 400 per cent in aldosterone levels in the erect position during converting-enzyme blockade. Long-term studies have shown an increase in aldosterone levels despite suppression of angiotensin II during captopril therapy.[2] The trend toward an increase in aldosterone levels was evident by the third month, and the levels continued to increase throughout the study period of one year. The antihypertensive effect of captopril was not compromised, however, despite the increment in aldosterone.

Only a few speculations can be made with regard to the increase in aldosterone during enzyme blockade. The increment in potassium levels that occurs during captopril therapy may conceivably stimulate aldosterone secretion, since potassium is capable of regulating aldosterone secretion independently of sodium and angiotensin, and since it also sensitizes the adrenal response to the aldosterone-stimulatory properties of ACTH.[3] Natriuresis and resultant sodium depletion may be another consideration, since sodium depletion makes the adrenal more responsive to angiotensin.[4] In addition, the number of angiotensin II-receptor sites per adrenocortical cell has been shown to increase during sodium depletion and potassium loading.[5]

Other factors, such as serotonin, ammonium, and magnesium ions, may have a role in this process, and studies may have to be aimed in this direction to identify the cause of the rise in aldosterone during long-term enzyme blockade. Finally, β-lipotropin may have a role as well, since it is a known aldosterone stimulator.[6]

ROMESH KHARDORI, M.B., M.D.
NANCY KHARDORI, M.B., M.D.
Southern Illinois University School of Medicine
Springfield, IL 62708

1. Gavras H, Gavras I, Texter S, Volicer L, Brunner HR, Rucinska EJ. Effect of angiotensin converting enzyme inhibition on blood pressure, plasma renin activity and plasma aldosterone in essential hypertension. J Clin Endocrinol Metab 1978; 46:220-6.
2. Staessen J, Lijnen P, Fagard R, Verschueren LJ, Amery A. Rise in plasma concentration of aldosterone during long term angiotensin II suppression. J Endocrinol 1981; 91:457-65.
3. Williams GH, Dluhy RG, Underwood RH. The relationship of dietary potassium intake to the aldosterone stimulating properties of ACTH. Clin Sci 1970; 39:489-96.
4. Oelkers W, Brown JJ, Fraser R, Lever AF, Morton JJ, Robertson JIS. Sensitization of adrenal cortex to angiotensin II in sodium deplete man. Circ Res 1974; 34:69-77.

5. Douglas J, Catt KJ. Regulation of angiotensin II receptors in the rat adrenal cortex by dietary electrolytes. J Clin Invest 1976; 58:834-43.
6. Matsuoka H, Mulrow PJ, Li CH. β-lipotropin: a new aldosterone-stimulating factor. Science 1980; 209:307-8.

To the Editor:

The recent review of captopril once again raises the question of the correct dosage of the drug for hypertensive patients with renal impairment. The current recommendations are based on the increased half-life (decreased elimination) of ^{14}C-labeled captopril plus its metabolites in patients with reduced creatinine clearance who were given a single dose of captopril.[1] Most reported clinical experience in

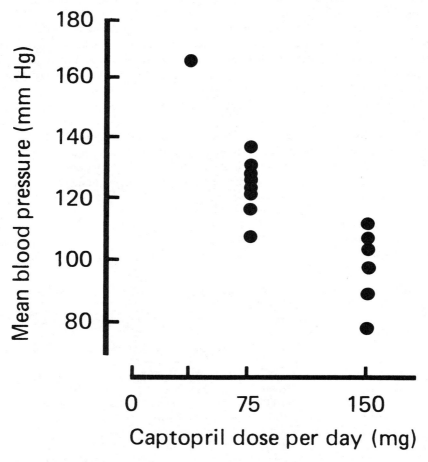

Figure 1. Relation of Blood Pressure to Dosage of Captopril in Patients with Renal Failure.

such patients,[2-4] however, has been gained with doses of 200 to 600 mg daily, which are higher than those now advised.[5] We have administered captopril to 15 patients with renal impairment that was resistant to optimal conventional triple therapy. The supine systolic and diastolic blood pressures during conventional treatment were 218 ± 26 and 131 ± 16 mm Hg, respectively (mean $\pm$S.D.); 10 of the patients had accelerated hypertension. They were stabilized with graded doses of captopril, according to their renal function[5]: patients with creatinine clearance of 10 ml per minute or lower received 37.5 mg of captopril per day; 11 to 34 ml per minute, 75 mg per day; and 35 to 75 ml per minute, 150 mg per day. The drug was administered every eight hours in reduced dosage rather than at extended intervals; 13 patients also received diuretics, and five also received beta blockers. Mean supine blood pressures during captopril therapy were 156 ± 30 and 96 ± 18 mm Hg ($P < 0.0005$ as compared with systolic and diastolic pressures during conventional therapy).

When individual mean pressures (diastolic pressure plus one third of pulse pressure) were plotted against captopril dosage, a clear inverse relation was observed (Fig. 1). This suggests that the present dose recommendations are inadequate for optimal therapeutic activity; further evidence of this is provided by the further falls in blood pressure seen in three patients whose "appropriate" dosage was doubled from 75 to 150 mg daily, with other drugs remaining unchanged.

It seems likely that at least the hematologic toxicity of captopril is in part dose-related.[6] Although the recent development of assays for total and free captopril in blood[7,8] may allow calculation of the safe dosage for such patients in the future, it appears from our results that the current dosage recommendation for patients with renal impairment may be too low.

P. L. Drury, M.R.C.P.
St. Bartholomew's Hospital
London EC1A 7BE, U.K.

1. Rommel AJ, Pierides AM, Heald A. Captopril elimination in chronic renal failure. Clin Pharmacol Ther 1980; 27:282.
2. Bravo EL, Tarazi RD. Converting enzyme inhibition with an orally active compound in hypertensive man. Hypertension 1979; 1:39-46.
3. Atkinson AB, Brown JJ, Lever AF, Robertson JIS. Combined treatment of severe intractable hypertension with captopril and diuretic. Lancet 1980; 2:105-8.
4. White NJ, Rajagopalan B, Yahaya H, Ledingham JGG. Captopril and furosemide in severe drug-resistant hypertension. Lancet 1980; 2:108-10.
5. Heel RC, Brogden RN, Speight TM, Avery GS. Captopril: a preliminary review of its pharmacological properties and therapeutic activity. Drugs 1980; 20:409-52.
6. Captopril: benefits and risks in severe hypertension. Lancet 1980; 2:129-30.
7. Funke PT, Ivashkiv E, Malley MF, Cohen AI. Gas chromatography/selected ion monitoring mass spectrometric determination of captopril in human blood. Anal Chem 1980; 52:1086-9.

8. Perrett D, Drury PL. The determination of captopril in physiological fluids using high performance liquid chromatography with electrochemical detection. J Liq Chromatogr 1982; 5:97-110.

To the Editor:

We wish to report some recent results that support Dr. Vidt and his colleagues' speculation that the absence of reflex tachycardia during captopril-induced reduction of blood pressure is due to increased parasympathetic activity. Fifteen patients with mild to moderate essential hypertension were studied. After an initial washout period of two weeks and one week of placebo treatment, captopril was administered in stepwise weekly dose increments of 75 mg per day, from an initial dose of 25 mg three times a day to a maximum of 450 mg per day or until the diastolic blood pressure was below 95 mm Hg. Parasympathetic tone was assessed before and after three weeks of treatment by measurement of the resting heart rate and the response of the heart rate to the "diving test" — apneic facial immersion in water at 18°C for at least 13 seconds. [1,2] After one hour of supine rest, the blood pressure (with an Arteriosonde Roche) and the heart rate (by electrocardiography) were recorded. The mean of 10 recordings was used in data analysis. After assuming the sitting position, each patient performed the diving test. The heart rate was monitored continuously before and during the test, which was repeated three times at five-minute intervals. The minimum heart rate during apneic facial immersion was measured.

The results are shown in Table 1. Treatment with captopril for three weeks produced a significant reduction in the resting heart rate, despite a significant

TABLE 1. Effect of Captopril Treatment on Resting Systolic and Diastolic Blood Pressures, Heart Rate, and the Change in Heart Rate during the Diving Test in 15 Patients with Essential Hypertension.*

Measurement	Systolic Blood Pressure	Diastolic Blood Pressure	Heart Rate	Change in Heart Rate
	mm Hg		beats/min	
At rest	170.5±3.8	110.6±2.3	75.6±2.5	−25.2±3.2
After captopril	159.8±6.1	99.4±2.8	70.9±2.2	−31.9±2.7
P Value †	<0.05	<0.01	<0.05	<0.01

*Values are means ±S.E.M.

†Estimated with the Wilcoxon signed rank test.

decrease in blood pressure, as reported by previous workers. [3,4] Moreover, after captopril treatment, all patients had a greater slowing of the heart rate during the diving test, despite the decrease in the resting heart rate.

Heart rate is a function of both parasympathetic and sympathetic tone. However, parasympathetic tone is the major factor determining the resting heart rate.[5,6] Hence, a reduction in the resting heart rate during treatment with captopril is itself consistent with an enhancement of vagal activity in our patients.

The diving test is an oxygen-conserving reflex extensively studied in human beings.[1,2] The combination of apnea and facial immersion leads to several physiologic responses, including marked bradycardia.[7] This reflex does not involve baroreceptor reflexes[8]; the immediate reflex bradycardia is mediated by vagal efferents.[1,2] Thus, the diving test is a safe and simple test of parasympathetic function. Our findings of greater bradycardia on apneic facial immersion during treatment with captopril further support the suggestion that captopril alters vagal tone.

Angiotensin II has both central[9] and peripheral[10] inhibitory effects on the vagus nerve. It is therefore possible that captopril enhances vagal activity by decreasing levels of angiotensin II at various neuroeffector sites.

ALESSANDRA STURANI, M.D., CARLA CHIARINI, M.D.,
EZIO DEGLI ESPOSTI, M.D., ANTONIO SANTORO, M.D.,
ALESSANDRO ZUCCALÀ, M.D., AND PIETRO ZUCCHELLI, M.D.,
M. Malpighi Hospital
40138 Bologna, Italy

JOHN A. MILLAR, PH.D., M.R.C.P.
Stobhill General Hospital
Glasgow, Scotland 621 3UW

1. Heistad DD, Abboud FM, Eckstein JW. Vasoconstrictor response to simulated diving in man. J Appl Physiol 1968; 25:542-9.
2. Finley JP, Bonet JF, Waxman MB. Autonomic pathways responsible for bradycardia on facial immersion. J Appl Physiol 1979; 47:1218-22.
3. Friedlander DH. Captopril and propranolol in mild and moderate essential hypertension: preliminary report. NZ Med J 1979; 90:146-9.
4. MacGregor GA, Markandu ND, Roulston JE, Jones JC. Essential hypertension: effect of an oral inhibitor of angiotensin-converting enzyme. Br Med J 1979; 2:1106-9.
5. Kent KM, Cooper T. The denervated heart: a model for studying autonomic control of the heart. N Engl J Med 1974; 291:1017-21.
6. Hager DW, Pieniaszek HJ, Perrier D, Mayersohn M, Goldberger V. Assessment of beta blockade with propranolol. Clin Pharmacol Ther 1981; 30:283-90.
7. Brick I. Circulatory responses to immersing the face in water. J Appl Physiol 1966; 21:33-6.
8. Bennett T, Hasking DJ, Hampton JR. Cardiovascular reflexes responses to apnoeic face immersion and mental stress in diabetic subjects. Cardiovasc Res 1976; 10:192-9.
9. Lee WB, Ishay MJ, Lumbers ER. Mechanisms by which Angiotensin II affects the heart rate of the conscious sheep. Circ Res 1980; 47:286-92.
10. Potter EK. Angiotensin inhibits action of vagus nerve of the heart. Br J Pharmacol 1982; 75:9-11.

The above letters were referred to the authors of the article in question, who offer the following reply:

To the Editor:

We appreciate the interest in our recent review of captopril.

In response to Dr. Ram's letter, the dosage recommendations were not theoretical but were based on the manufacturer's recommendations. We did not consider it prudent to suggest that clinicians consider captopril an "add-on" medication, since early trials have suggested that the risk of hypotension is considerable when captopril is added to concomitant medications, particularly diuretics. The addition of captopril to other medications requires extreme caution, and it should be done only by experienced physicians and only in a hospital setting. The use of captopril for congestive heart failure often represents a different clinical situation, since blood pressure may be normal or even low and small doses may be effective. In this situation, the agent may be added to concomitant medication such as digitalis and diuretics, but again this is best accomplished in a hospital setting. Khardori and Khardori have correctly noted that plasma aldosterone levels may increase fourfold with upright posture during captopril administration, although supine plasma aldosterone levels are persistently suppressed. Unpublished data from our laboratory do suggest, however, that 24-hour aldosterone-excretion rates remain chronically suppressed during captopril administration.[1] We agree that the renin-angiotensin system is not the only stimulus to aldosterone secretion, particularly with upright posture, but there are few in vivo data to suggest other potent stimuli of aldosterone.

Further clinical experience and the availability of an accurate serum assay for captopril will surely allow more accurate calculation of safe dosages for patients with renal failure, as suggested by Drury. However, the determination of a safe daily dosage must also take into consideration variable absorption and the patient's volume status. Experience from our laboratory and others suggests that hypertensive patients with renal failure that is resistant to a given dosage of captopril become responsive after ultrafiltration and weight reduction.[2]

We certainly agree with the observations of Sturani and her colleagues supporting our suggestion that the absence of reflex tachycardia during captopril-induced reduction of blood pressure may be due in part to increased parasympathetic tone.

DONALD G. VIDT, M.D.
EMMANUEL L. BRAVO, M.D.
FETNAT M. FOUAD, M.D.
The Cleveland Clinic Foundation
Cleveland, OH 44106

1. Textor SC, Bravo EL, Fouad FM, Tarazi RC. Hyperkalemia in azotemic patients during angiotensin-converting enzyme inhibition and aldosterone reduction in captopril. Kidney Int 1981; 19:175. abstract.
2. Textor SC, Gavras H, Tifft CP, Bernard DB, Idelson B, Brunner HR. Norepinephrine and renin activity in chronic renal failure: evidence of interacting roles in hemodialysis hypertension. Hypertension 1981; 3:294-9.

Cerebral Vasodilators

(In Two Parts)

Peter Cook, M.B., B.Sc.,

and Ian James, M.B., Ph.D.

M ANY drugs described as cerebral vasodilators have been in use for over 20 years. Most were originally developed as peripheral vasodilators and were then used to improve cerebral blood flow in patients with cerebrovascular disease or dementia. These disorders were assumed to be due to progressive cerebral arteriosclerosis and ischemia, and it was logical to suppose that effective cerebral vasodilators would be of clinical value.

Unfortunately, this basic assumption has been shown to be incorrect. Dementia is not primarily due to cerebral ischemia. Previous reviews have criticized the use of these drugs, for this and other reasons.[1-3] Cerebral blood flow has proved quite resistant to drug-induced change, and there is little evidence that most of the drugs can cause appreciable and sustained increases in flow. Finally, many of the early clinical trials that reported therapeutic benefit were poorly designed and unconvincing.

In spite of these negative results, there is now considerable evidence from double-blind clinical trials that some of the drugs produce mental improvement in patients with dementia. This review summarizes the pathophysiology of cerebrovascular disease and dementia and the pharmacology of cerebral vasodilating drugs, including their use in these disorders. We have excluded studies that failed to use reasonably validated and reliable methods for measurement of cerebral blood flow.[4]

Physiology of Cerebral Blood Flow

The brain consumes about a quarter of the total oxygen used by the body at rest. This large oxygen demand is met by a high rate of perfusion amounting to 50 ml per 100 g of brain tissue per minute. The distribution of flow at rest is not uniform but is 5 to 20 per cent higher over the frontal lobes. Intellectual, sensory,

From the Section of Clinical Pharmacology, Medical Unit, Royal Free Hospital, London.

Originally published in two parts on December 17, 1981 (305:1508-1513) and December 24, 1981 (305:1560-1564).

or motor stimulation is associated with a characteristic pattern of increased flow.[5] The increase in neuronal metabolism raises the production of carbon dioxide and its metabolites. These are potent vasodilators, and an increase in flow results. If for any reason flow cannot increase, the increase in carbon dioxide tension leads to a fall in glucose metabolism and in oxygen use.[6]

Changes in systemic blood pressure result in changes in cerebrovascular resistance, so that flow remains constant. In normal subjects, blood flow remains unchanged over a wide range of induced change in blood pressure.[7] Blood-gas changes also provoke changes in the brain circulation that maintain the constancy of the metabolic environment of brain tissue. Hypercapnia or hypoxia causes an increase in flow, and hypocapnia or high oxygen tension causes a decrease.[8,9]

Until recently, the cerebral vasculature was thought to be almost entirely regulated by local chemical changes. This hypothesis proposed that changes in flow would lead to changes in local tissue carbon dioxide and hydrogen-ion concentration that would offset the changes in flow by causing vasodilation or vasoconstriction.[8] There is now evidence to suggest that cerebral vessels are at least in part reflexively controlled, and that the carotid-body chemoreceptors and carotid-sinus baroreceptors may initiate many of the cerebrovascular responses to hypoxia, hypercapnia, and hypotension.[10-12] An adrenergic pathway that originates in the superior cervical ganglion and is constrictor in nature has been demonstrated. There is also evidence of a dilator pathway that is probably cholinergic and is carried by the seventh cranial nerve.[13] The relative importance of metabolic and neurogenic control is a subject of continuing controversy. It has been suggested that neurogenic control of the proximal arterioles acts as a crude adjustment system, whereas metabolic control of the distal vessels is important for fine regulation.[14]

If this dual-control hypothesis is correct, a cerebral vasodilator could alter cerebral metabolism without an apparent change in flow. For example, if inappropriate proximal vasoconstriction occurred, it would lead to distal acidosis and compensatory distal vasodilation. Reversal of the proximal vasoconstriction would lead to reduced distal acidosis, improved metabolism, and distal vasoconstriction, with little change in flow.

Changes in Physiology with Aging

Cerebral blood flow and metabolism decrease with age. Blood flow drops by about 25 per cent between the ages of 20 and 70.[15,16] However, the degree of change appears to depend on the criteria used for selecting healthy elderly subjects.[17] Initially it was thought that there was a similar drop in cerebral neuron density that would explain the decreased metabolic requirements,[15] but these changes have not been confirmed.[18] It seems reasonable to assume that neuronal metabolism decreases with age and that changes in flow are secondary to this effect.

Pathophysiology of Cerebrovascular Disease and Dementia

Acute Stroke

Acute cerebral infarction is usually due to thrombosis or embolism originating in extracerebral vessels rather than to progressive cerebral arteriosclerosis.[19,20] A number of investigators using radioactive tracer gases such as xenon-133 have shown that the resulting stroke is associated with a decrease in cerebral blood flow in the affected area, with a surrounding zone of hyperperfusion.[21-24] During infarction, oxygen extraction within the area of low blood flow rises and then falls profoundly as tissue death occurs.[25]

These changes are nearly always associated with some impairment of the vascular response, within the affected hemisphere, to changes in carbon dioxide tension and systemic blood pressure. When this "vasoparalysis" is marked, the normal homeostatic mechanisms are lost, and flow in the affected area passively follows changes in perfusion pressure. Hypercapnia may then lead to a local decrease in flow, whereas flow in the normal areas of the brain increases in the usual fashion.[21-24] This redistribution of blood away from an ischemic area is usually called an "intracerebral steal" phenomenon.

The same phenomenon is often seen after the parenteral administration of vasodilators within a few days of an occlusive stroke. Intravenous hexobendine, papaverine, and vincamine and inhaled halothane may all produce it.[26-29] Regional decreases in flow may also occur after oral betahistine therapy.[30] The phenomenon has been regarded as uncommon,[31] but it has been recorded in up to 40 to 50 per cent of patients in some series.[28] It may also occur after nonocclusive stroke.[22]

A "reverse steal" phenomenon has also been described with hyperventilation and after the use of cerebral vasoconstrictors such as aminophylline.[29,32] Vasoconstriction in healthy areas of the brain results in the diversion of blood to ischemic areas. Hyperventilation before cerebral-artery occlusion reduces the area of infarction in laboratory animals.[33] It has been suggested as a rational treatment in patients, but unfortunately it does not appear to be effective after a stroke.[34]

Chronic Stroke

After acute infarction, cerebral blood flow and vasoreactivity gradually improve in the affected hemisphere, although some focal impairment often persists.[22,23] The surrounding zone of hyperperfusion resolves within a few days, but some cerebral ischemia may still be present more than six weeks after the event.[20] This residual ischemia can be improved acutely by parenteral administration of papaverine or hexobendine.[35-37] However, there is only limited evidence that either cerebral metabolism or clinical progress can be substantially improved.[35-37]

Transient Ischemic Attacks

The majority of these episodes are due to emboli from the heart and great vessels.[38,39] Focal ischemia is followed by hyperemia, which usually resolves in a few hours but may persist for several days. In some cases there is also a focal loss of carbon dioxide-induced vasodilatation.[38] There is no evidence that vasodilators can prevent attacks. Treatment with drugs that inhibit platelet aggregation is more rational.

Subarachnoid Hemorrhage

Subarachnoid hemorrhage after rupture of a berry aneurysm or after head trauma is associated with widespread spasm of cerebral arterioles and a fall in brain blood flow.[23] The vasospasm may be very intense. Its cause is unknown, and it is generally resistant to vasodilator therapy. Treatment with phenoxybenzamine or dopamine appears to help some patients, but potent drugs such as papaverine can cause a steal effect.[40]

Dementia

The majority of cases of dementia fall into one of two clearly defined clinicopathological groups.[19] In the first type, known as primary senile, primary neuronal degenerative, or Alzheimer's dementia, the disease tends to be slowly progressive, and the patient usually lacks insight into the condition. At post-mortem study, the brain is smaller than normal and shows a marked reduction in the density of neurons. Characteristic degenerative changes are seen, with neurofibrillar tangles, senile plaques, and lipofuscin deposits. Alzheimer's dementia accounts for 50 to 75 per cent of the cases in post-mortem series.[18,19]

The second type is known as multi-infarct or vascular dementia. These patients typically have an abrupt onset, a stepwise deterioration, and a fluctuating course, with episodes of acute confusion. They often have periods of insight into their mental deterioration and are more often depressed, with emotional lability. A history of hypertension, stroke, or diabetes is common. Focal neurologic abnormalities and evidence of associated arteriosclerosis are frequently seen. Post-mortem examination usually reveals a small brain with multiple areas of cerebral softening and healed infarcts. Over 50 per cent of the neocortical neurons may be lost — an amount similar to that found in advanced Alzheimer's disease. Vascular dementia accounts for 10 to 20 per cent of the cases in reported series.[18,19]

Patients with Alzheimer's dementia tend to have moderately reduced levels of cerbral blood flow and have a normal vasodilator response to carbon dioxide, as compared with normal elderly controls.[41,42] On the other hand, patients with multi-infarct dementia tend to have markedly reduced mean levels of cerebral blood flow and have impaired vasodilator responses to carbon dioxide.[41-43]

A selective loss of brain cholinergic neurons, which tends to be more marked in patients with Alzheimer's dementia, has also been demonstrated.[18] This may explain the loss of short-term memory, since anticholinergic drugs impair short-term memory in young volunteers.[44] However, as mentioned earlier, disturbance of the cholinergic system may also impair the normal cerebral vasodilator response.[45]

Assessment of Clinical Trials of Vasodilating Drugs

Clinical trials in elderly patients with cerebrovascular disease or dementia are fraught with problems. Results may be influenced by the personality of the tester, the attitude of the attendant staff, or changes in the patient's environment.[46] The presence of intercurrent illness and changes in associated drug therapy are also important variables. Spontaneous fluctuations in performance that may far exceed any drug effect are common. It is therefore particularly important for these trials to be completely double-blind. Groups of patients should be homogeneous and should contain only patients with the same disease. However, many trials have failed to distinguish between patients without dementia who have had a stroke and patients with multi-infarct or Alzheimer's dementia.

Evaluation of studies has been further complicated by the bewildering variety of methods used to assess changes in brain function. Comparison is easier and more reliable when well-established clinical rating scales such as the Crichton Royal Behaviour Rating Scale[47] or the Sandoz Clinical Assessment Geriatric (SCAG) Scale[48] are used, particularly when they are combined with established psychometric tests that are sensitive to drug effects. The SCAG Scale is the less useful of the two because it does not include an adequate asseessment of daily activities.

Direct-Acting Vasodilators

Papaverine

Pharmacology
Papaverine is an alkaloid originally derived from crude opium but with no narcotic properties. Dioxyline phosphate and ethaverine are closely related drugs with similar vasodilating properties. The drug is a potent nonspecific smooth-muscle relaxant that causes generalized arteriolar dilatation and smooth-muscle relaxation. Increased levels of intracellular cyclic AMP secondary to inhibition of phosphodiesterase may contribute to this effect.[49] Large doses may cause hypotension and tachycardia. The drug suppresses myocardial excitability and prolongs the refractory period. In fact, it has been used in the past for the treatment of ventricular arrhythmias, but these can be produced by the drug itself when it is taken in high dosage.[50]

Effect on Cerebral Blood Flow
The drug has consistently been found capable of increasing cerebral flow after intravenous injection in patients with cerebrovascular disease.[27,35,36,51-53] The effect tends to be short-lived and can also be offset by the hypotensive effect on systemic blood pressure.[53] Like certain other cerebral vasodilators, papaverine can decrease flow in ischemic areas,[26,28] particularly when used shortly after an occlusive stroke or subarachnoid hemorrhage.[40] Oral therapy has also been shown to produce small increases in flow in healthy volunteers.[54]

Effect on Cerebrovascular Disease and Dementia

Six of nine controlled, double-blind studies have reported some improvment in scores on psychological tests, but only one of these reports claimed practical clinical benefit.[39,55]

Pharmacokinetics

The oral bioavailability of papaverine is about 54 per cent. Peak plasma levels occur one to two hours after an oral dose, and the elimination half-life has been estimated at 0.5 to two hours.[56,57] However, these values may be underestimates, since plasma levels continue to rise for four days with regular administration every six hours, suggesting a true half-life of 24 hours. Sustained-release preparations of the drug are poorly absorbed, and it is doubtful that they have any advantages over conventional preparations.[57] The drug is metabolized by hepatic microsomal oxidation to phenolic metabolites, which are excreted unchanged or as glucuronide conjugates.

Recommended Dosage

Papaverine is commonly given as sustained-release capsules in a dose of 150 mg every 12 hours, increased if necessary to the same amount every eight hours or to 300 mg every 12 hours. It may also be given by injection in a dose of 30 to 100 mg.

Adverse Reactions

The most common symptoms are drowsiness, vertigo, and constipation.[58] On rare occasions the drug can cause a mild hepatitis with eosinophilia, which is reversible on withdrawal.[50] Papaverine interferes with the action of l-dopa in patients with Parkinson's disease, but the mechanism of this interaction is unclear.[59]

Cyclandelate

Pharmacology and Effect on Cerebral Blood Flow

Cyclandelate is a derivative of mandelic acid with some structural similarities to papaverine. In in vitro experiments and in vivo studies in animals, the drug is a direct-acting smooth-muscle relaxant with three times the potency of papaverine.[60] In human beings it appears to be a relatively weak general vasodilator, and in conventionally employed doses it does not produce hypotension or tachycardia. Large doses in rats have been shown to increase cerebral glucose uptake and slightly enhance resistance to cerebral hypoxia, as measured by electroencephalographic extinction time and survival.[61] Studies of cerebral blood flow in human beings have given conflicting results. Two studies have shown improved cerebral blood flow,[52,62] whereas a third has shown a decrease of similar magnitude in patients with cerebrovascular disease.[29]

Effect on Cerebrovascular Disease and Dementia

At least six double-blind, controlled clinical trials have shown some improvements in results of psychomotor tests, and in three trials practical benefit was claimed.[39,55] However, in all these studies the response was incomplete, and there was some inconsistency in the pattern of improvement.[63] Three other well-conducted studies have failed to show any improvement.[63-65] One drug and placebo crossover study that lasted 12 months concluded that the drug appeared to arrest the decline in mental performance with time instead of causing any obvious improvement in performance over that period.[66]

Recommended Dosage
The usual initial dose is 1.2 to 1.6 g daily, given as 400-mg tablets, capsules, or a suspension in divided doses.

Adverse Reactions
The drug is well tolerated, and adverse reactions are uncommon. Epigastric pain and heartburn, flushing, headache, weakness, and tachycardia can occur. These may be avoided by taking the drug with meals.

Nafronyl

Pharmacology
Nafronyl (naftidrofuryl) is a complex acid ester of diethylaminoethanol. It is a direct-acting, papaverine-like vasodilator that also has antinicotinic and antibradykinin effects. Although the drug is a potent vasodilator when given by direct intra-arterial injection to animals, it does not cause hypotension or tachycardia when given by mouth in therapeutic doses in human beings, and it appears to be a relatively weak vasodilator under these conditions.[67,68] Very high doses in animals alter cerebral glycolysis, with a decreased cerebral glucose uptake and an increased pyruvate:lactate ratio. Intracellular ATP levels are increased.[69] These changes appear to give some protection against the acute effects of hypoxia, and regular doses in rats abolish the hypoxia-induced deterioration of conditioned avoidance responses.[70] Therapeutic doses produce improvement in muscle glycolysis after exercise in normal volunteers[71] and at rest in patients with peripheral vascular disease.[72]

All these studies have shown a consistent change in glucose metabolism. A recent small study in patients with mild dementia[73] showed that administration of 400 mg per day also produced an increase in the pyruvate:lactate ratio in cerebrospinal fluid. No changes were seen in the levels of biogenic amine metabolites. The changes in lactate and pyruvate levels were correlated with an increase in fast activity on the electroencephalogram and improvements on certain psychometric tests and behavioral scales.

Effect on Cerebral Blood Flow
Intravenous nafronyl, given in a dose of 80 to 400 mg to patients with cerebrovascular disease, appears to produce an acute drop in cerebral blood flow of up to 12 per cent when measured by repeat xenon-133 clearance.[27,29] Such a decrease can

be artifactual in origin. It is similar to the degree of decrease that is seen with repeated measurements in control subjects and that is due to increasing saturation of slowly clearing brain tissue.[29,52,74] In another study, an intravenous infusion of 120 mg had no effect on blood flow in elderly subjects with cerebrovascular disease or dementia or both, but attenuated the vasodilator response to inhalation of 5 per cent carbon dioxide.[75] Oral nafronyl, 200 mg given three times a day, also had no effect.

Effect on Cerebrovascular Disease and Dementia

Seven double-blind, controlled clinical trials in patients with cerebrovascular disease or dementia have reported an overall pattern of improvement in mental function while the patients were taking the drug, but there was much variability among subjects. All these studies also reported improvement in the general clinical condition of the patients.[39,55] These unanimous results, though encouraging, cannot be entirely accepted, since most of the studies used nonstandardized clinical rating scales whose reproducibility and sensitivity is unknown. Furthermore, improvement in daily activities was demonstrated in only one of the seven studies.[39]

Pharmacokinetics

The drug is well absorbed after oral administration to healthy volunteers. Peak plasma concentrations occur about one hour after dosing.[76] The elimination half-life of the parent drug is about 40 minutes. Further studies are required to confirm the pharmacokinetics in elderly subjects, including the routes of elimination, and to determine whether the drug has active metabolites.

Recommended Dosage

The usual dose is one 100-mg capsule taken by mouth three times daily. An injectable formulation is also available.

Adverse Reactions

The drug appears to be well tolerated, and the incidence of adverse effects is low. Nausea, epigastric pain, diarrhea, headaches, dizziness, and insomnia have all been reported. Gastric irritation occurred in three of 12 elderly subjects taking 800 mg per day.[75]

Hexobendine

Pharmacology

This synthetic derivative of polymethylenediamine was first developed as a coronary vasodilator for the treatment of angina pectoris,[50] but it has not been widely accepted.

Effect on Cerebral Blood Flow

Although the drug has received little attention, a number of studies have demonstrated that 10 to 40 mg given intravenously increases the average cerebral blood flow in patients with cerebrovascular disease, with only a small fall in blood pressure.[27,29,37,77] Oral administration of 400 to 600 mg appears to be much less effective, presumably because of poor bioavailability.[29,77]

Effect on Cerebrovascular Disease

In one controlled pilot study, the drug improved the neurologic recovery of patients who had had a stroke, but the degree of improvement was clinically inconsequential.[77]

Recommended Dosage

The usual dose for angina pectoris is 60 to 180 mg daily, but much larger doses have been used in trials of its value as a cerebral vasodilator.

Adverse Reactions

Little is known about the adverse effects of hexobendine.

Drugs Acting on Adrenoreceptors

Isoxsuprine

Pharmacology

Isoxsuprine is a phenylethylamine derivative of epinephrine. The compound is said to be an alpha-adrenoreceptor antagonist with beta-adrenoreceptor-stimulating properties, but the vasodilator effects on muscle blood flow are not prevented by beta-adrenoreceptor blockade.[78] The drug also lowers blood viscosity and inhibits platelet aggregation when given in high doses.[79]

Effect on Cerebral Blood Flow

Intravenous isoxsuprine produces both cerebral and peripheral vasodilatation. A fall in blood pressure occurs and is not fully compensated by the decrease in cerebrovascular resistance; a small reduction in cerebral blood flow results.[29,51,80]

Effect on Cerebrovascular Disease and Dementia

Three double-blind, controlled studies have been reported. Two found some improvement in cognitive function, and one showed no change.[39,55] Neither of the two positive studies demonstrated any practical benefit.

Pharmacokinetics

Isoxsuprine is absorbed after oral or intramuscular administration, and peak blood levels are reached about one hour after administration by either route. Blood levels become low within three hours.[50]

Recommended Dosage

Isoxsuprine may be given in oral tablets, 20 mg four times daily after meals, or in sustained-release capsules, 40 mg twice per day. An injectable form is also available.

Adverse Reactions
Minor facial flushing is common. High doses may cause tachycardia and hypotension.[50,79]

Nylidrin

Pharmacology
Nylidrin is a water-soluble compound that is struturally similar to isoxsuprine. The drug increases muscle blood flow when administered parenterally or orally.[81] It acts predominantly by stimulation of the beta-adrenoreceptors, but since its action is only partially blocked by propranolol, it probably also has a direct action on vascular smooth muscle.[77] It does not appear to affect skin blood flow. The effects on heart rate and blood pressure are variable, but an increase in cardiac output and a decrease in peripheral vascular resistance usually occur.

Effect on Cerebral Blood Flow
Although the drug may cause cerebral vasodilatation, this is offset by a fall in blood pressure. Most studies have found either no change or a decrease in cerebral blood flow after short-term administration of the drug.[29,51,82] One interesting (though uncontrolled) study showed a considerable increase in cerebral blood flow and oxygen consumption in patients with cerebrovascular disease who were given oral therapy for two to six weeks.[83]

Effect on Cerebrovascular Disease and Dementia
No adequately controlled clinical trials have been reported.

Pharmacokinetics
Nylidrin hydrochloride is readily absorbed from the gastrointestinal tract. Its effect begins in about 10 minutes, reaches a maximum in about 30 minutes, and lasts for about two hours.[50]

Recommended Dosage
The usual oral dose is 18 to 48 mg daily, given as tablets in divided doses. An injectable form is also available.

Adverse Reactions
The drug may cause nausea and vomiting, tremulousness, nervousness, weakness, giddiness, palpitations, and postural hypotension. It is contraindicated in patients with cardiac infarction, hypothyroidism, paroxysmal arrhythmias, or severe angina of effort.[50]

Ergoloid Mesylates

Pharmacology
Dihydroergotoxine mesylate, designated as ergoloid mesylates in the United States and marketed under the trade name of Hydergine, is an equal mixture of

the methane sulfonates of the dihydrogenated derivatives of the three ergotoxine alkaloids ergocornine, ergocristine, and ergocryptine. Dihydrogenation eliminates the vasoconstrictor properties of ergotoxine and enhances its alpha-adrenoreceptor-blocking activity. The compound also has weak dopaminergic activity and retains the emetic properties of the other ergot alkaloids.[48] The mixture is a potent alpha-blocking agent, but like most drugs of this kind, its use as a vasodilator is limited because of the side effects that occur at effective doses. Vasodilatation is accompanied by a fall in blood pressure and postural hypotension. The compounds are potent inhibitors of catecholamine-induced changes in ATP metabolism in vitro.[48] Norepinephrine stimulation of cerebral cyclic AMP synthesis is inhibited at very low concentrations. Norepinephrine stimulation of membrane-bound sodium-potassium ATPase is also counteracted. Such an effect might be expected to alter norepinephrine-induced changes in neuronal membrane potential, but this requires confirmation. The compounds also inhibit one of the brain-specific phosphodiesterase enzymes responsible for cyclic AMP breakdown.[48,84] In spite of this inhibition, experiments with long-term administration in animals indicate that the drug produces a net reduction in intracellular levels of cyclic AMP in the brain.

The relation of these metabolic changes to the mode of action of the drug is not clear. The compound alters the sleep-wakefulness cycle in rats, as measured by continuous electroencephalographic recording.[85] The drug decreases both total sleep time and rapid-eye-movement sleep. A number of double-blind, controlled studies have shown that the drug tends to increase the fast components of the electroencephalogram in elderly subjects for up to eight hours after administration.[48] The proportion of fast-wave activity in the electroencephalogram decreases with age, and some workers have found that this change is more pronounced in demented subjects. Thus, the drug-induced changes have been interpreted as evidence of improvement.

Effect on Cerebral Blood Flow

Most short-term studies using clearance techniques have found either no change or a small drop in cerebral blood flow after intravenous or intracarotid infusion.[27,51,86,86] No studies of oral therapy have been reported.

Effect on Cerebrovascular Disease and Dementia

Over 20 double-blind, controlled clinical trials have now been carried out, and all have reported improvement in scores on at least one psychomotor-test scale.[39,55] A detailed critical review of 12 comparable studies found that the degree of improvement in the subtest variables was usually less than one point on a seven-point scale.[88] Improvement was seen most often in the subjective cognition (including confusion) and affect variables, whereas scores on the mental-status checklist (one of the most objective subtests) and the physical-symptom list were usually unchanged. Six of the studies included some assessment of daily activities, and only walking improved often. At least three weeks is usually required before any improvement is seen, and benefits tend to increase for up to three months. No treatment period has exceeded 12 weeks.

Pharmacokinetics
Studies with tritium-labeled ergoloid mesylates have shown that the compound is poorly absorbed and undergoes extensive first-pass metabolism. Oral bioavailability was about 25 per cent, and peak plasma levels occurred at two to three hours. The absorption and distribution half-life was four hours, and the mean elimination of half-life 13 hours.[48] If the long half-life and duration of action are confirmed, then administration twice daily should be satisfactory.

Recommended Dosage
The recommended dose is 4.5 mg per day, taken by mouth in divided doses or as a single dose.

Adverse Reactions
Adverse effects include sublingual irritation, nausea and vomiting, blurred vision, skin rashes, nasal stuffiness, and postural hypotension. These effects appear to be uncommon.

Drugs Acting on Histamine Receptors

Betahistine

Pharmacology
Betahistine is a beta-2-pyridyl alkylamine, an analogue of histamine that acts as a relatively pure histamine-1-receptor agonist and has no effect on gastric acid secretion.[89] Increases in peripheral blood flow, flushing, and headaches occur at infusion rates of 1 mg per minute. These effects are blocked by the antihistamine diphenhydramine.

Effect on Cerebral Blood Flow
The drug appears to be an effective cerebral vasodilator after intravenous injections of high doses in anesthetized animals.[90] Two studies of the effect of one week of oral therapy with 20 to 32 mg per day in human beings have been reported. In one uncontrolled study in patients with cerebrovascular disease, average cerebral blood flow was increased by 20 per cent.[30] In some cases, focal decreases in flow were seen, demonstrating that minor cerebral-steal effects can also occur. In another investigation, a controlled study in normal young volunteers, a small increase in mean cerebral blood flow was found.[91]

Effect on Cerebrovascular Disease and Dementia
Three double-blind, controlled studies in patients with cerebrovascular disease have been described.[39] Two of them reported improvement in some test scores but

failed to show a clear-cut practical benefit. A fourth study was confined to patients with vertebrobasilar insufficiency and dementia.[92] Most of these patients probably had multi-infarct dementia. Although changes in the neurologic estimation were only minor, statistically significant changes were seen in the scores on psychological tests. These results show that the drug can improve some psychometric-test scores, but whether practical benefit follows these changes has not been established.

Pharmacokinetics
Betahistine is readily absorbed from the gastrointestinal tract but appears to be converted rapidly into two metabolites.[50] Peak concentrations of the two metabolites occur within three to five hours, and they are eliminated in the urine within three days. Their pharmacologic properties are unknown.

Recommended Dosage
The usual oral dose is 8 mg three times daily, and the maximum dose is 16 mg three times daily, given as betahistine hydrochloride or mesylate.

Adverse Reactions
Oral therapy with 8 mg four times daily produces little change in reclining or standing blood pressure.[91] The commonest side effect is probably gastric irritation. Nausea and exacerbation of peptic ulcers may occur. Headache, flushing, and faintness have also been reported.

| Miscellaneous Vasodilators

Vincamine

Pharmacology
Vincamine is an alkaloid derived from the plant *Vinca minor*. (It should not be confused with the cytotoxic alkaloids obtained from *Vinca rosea*.) It has some structural and pharmacologic similarities to reserpine. Ethyl apovincaminate is the closely related synthetic ethyl ester of vincaminic acid. The two drugs have been used extensively as cerebral vasodilators in Europe, but little has been published on them in English-language journals. Both drugs have been shown to lower blood pressure and increase the heart rate in animals. They also appear to have metabolic actions, and high doses have been found to inhibit phosphodiesterase and to alter the cerebral concentration of biogenic amines in animals.[93,94]

Effect on Cerebral Blood Flow
Three open studies have reported an increase in mean cerebral blood flow after intravenous infusion of 30 to 40 mg in patients with cerebrovascular disease.[28,29,95] One of these studies demonstrated an intracerebral-steal effect, with

decreased cerebral blood flow in an area of cerebral infarction in four of six patients.[28] In all these patients, proximal occlusion was demonstrated angiographically. Another study found no effect after intravenous administration of 30 mg but demonstrated a slight increase in blood flow in patients given 40 mg of vincamine or 20 mg of ethyl apovincaminate in a double-blind, controlled crossover study with normal volunteers.[73] The circulatory effects of the drugs are usually transient. No reliable studies of blood flow after oral medication appear to have been published.

Effect on Cerebrovascular Disease and Dementia

A review of seven double-blind studies with vincamine in the German-language literature[96] found that all seven had improved scores on some psychometric tests in treated patients. Once again, no clear-cut practical benefit was demonstrated.

Pharmacokinetics

Vincamine appears to be absorbed rapidly, but its bioavailability is unknown. An aqueous solution of 15 mg gives detectable blood levels of more than 5 ng of unchanged drug per milliliter for six hours, whereas 30 mg given as a slow-release preparation gives similar levels for over 12 hours. The elimination half-life appears to be about 40 minutes in healthy volunteers.

Recommended Dosage

The recommended oral dosage is 40 to 80 mg daily for vincamine and 15 to 30 mg daily for ethyl apovincaminate, given in divided doses. The parenteral dosage is about half the oral dosage.

Adverse Reactions

The drugs have a sedative effect in animals, but the incidence of this or other adverse reactions in human beings is not clear.

Niacin Derivatives

Pharmacology

Niacin (nicotinic acid) is a water-soluble vitamin that is now prepared synthetically. Numerous derivatives are available, including compounds containing inositol, fructose, tartaric acid, xanthine, and methyl alcohol. The vitamin acts as a source of the physiologically active amide nicotinamide before incorporation in the essential nucleotide coenzymes nicotinamide-adenine dinucleotide and nicotinamide-adenine dinucleotide phosphate. Niacin is a potent vasodilator, but nicotinamide does not share these properties. The vasodilation is seen principally in the skin of the face and upper trunk. The drug may be effective for the treatment of cutaneous vasospasm, but it does not produce consistent increases in muscle blood flow.[81] High doses decrease plasma cholesterol, free fatty acids, and fibrinogen and have been used for many years in the treatment of lipid disorders.[97]

Effect on Cerebral Blood Flow

Studies of cerebral blood flow that have used clearance techniques have found either no change[98] or a decrease[27,51] in cerebral blood flow after short-term intravenous administration to patients with cerebrovascular disease. Oral treatment for six weeks with the alcohol tartrate derivative is also ineffective.[99] Use of the xanthinol derivative seems particularly inappropriate, since xanthines are cerebral vasoconstrictors.[27,29,51]

Effect on Cerebrovascular Disease and Dementia

Although a number of open, uncontrolled studies have reported beneficial effects of the drug,[39] we have been unable to find any acceptable double-blind studies.

Pharmacokinetics

Niacin is well absorbed from the gastrointestinal tract and is widely distributed in the body tissues.

Recommended Dosage

When niacin is used in the treatment of hypercholesterolemia, the maximal tolerated doses range from 1 to 6 g daily, given in divided doses.

Adverse Reactions

Facial flushing, a sensation of heat, pounding in the head, gastric irritation, and diarrhea are the most common effects seen after oral doses of niacin. These effects are more common with sustained-release preparations of the parent drug and may be less common if derivatives are used. Other adverse effects include pruritus, skin lesions, abdominal pain and activation of peptic ulcer, blurring of vision, jaundice and impairment of liver function, decreased glucose tolerance, and hyperuricemia.[50,100]

Cinnarizine

Pharmacology and Effect on Cerebral Blood Flow

Cinnarizine is 1-cinnamyl-4-benzhydrylpiperazine. In addition to its well-established antihistaminic properties, the compound is a potent antagonist of numerous vasoactive substances, including angiotensin, serotonin, acetylcholine, epinephrine, norepinephrine, barium chloride, and potassium chloride.[101] It probably acts by selective blockade of calcium influx into depolarized smooth-muscle cells in arterial walls. Although it is a potent inhibitor of induced vasoconstriction, it probably has relatively little effect on resting blood vessels. No studies of cerebral blood flow, using clearance techniques, have been reported in human beings.

Effect on Cerebrovascular Disease and Dementia

Of three apparently adequately controlled, double-blind studies in Europe, two claimed practical benefit.[55] However, three double-blind studies conducted in the United Kingdom failed to show any beneficial effect from the drug.[39]

Recommended Dosage
The recommended oral dosage is 30 mg three times daily.

Adverse Reactions
The drug appears to be well tolerated, and sedative effects are uncommon. Allergic skin reactions have been reported.

| Conclusions

Papaverine, hexobendine, betahistine, and possibly vincamine and cyclandelate are effective cerebral vasodilators when given in single parenteral doses, but their efficacy with regular oral administration is not well established (Table 1). Cerebral-vasodilator therapy might seem logical after acute cerebral infarction, since the rate of resolution of the surrounding cerebral ischemia could help to determine the extent of the recovery. A few reports suggest that the drugs may be capable of producing minor clinical improvement in patients with strokes and multi-infarct dementia, and there are no reports of obvious drug-induced clinical deterioration. However, there is no doubt that all of them can cause localized decreases in flow in ischemic areas.

This intracerebral-steal effect may be an inevitable result of a mixture of vasodilatation and ischemic vasoparalysis. It most often occurs early after occlusive strokes, but it also occurs after nonocclusive strokes, and small decreases in flow are often seen in patients with cerebrovascular disease or multi-infarct dementia. Any flow measurement is derived from the average clearance of tracer gases within the volume of tissue being scanned. A marked but localized decrease may be lost in an area of generalized increase in flow. Some investigators appear to have ignored the fact that even small decreases in average flow could be clinically important. In view of the risk of intracerebral steal, cerebral vasodilator therapy must be regarded as contraindicated in all patients with acute stroke. It is still of unproved value, and it may sometimes be harmful in patients with chronic cerebrovascular disease.

Despite the lack of substantial benefit in cerebrovascular disease, two of the drugs, ergoloid mesylates and nafronyl, have been consistently found to improve mental performance in patients with senile (Alzheimer's) dementia. Neither of the drugs increases cerebral blood flow, but both appear to have metabolic effects in addition to their peripheral vasodilator activity. Cyclandelate and vincamine have not been clearly shown to be of value, and there is insufficient evidence to justify the use of the other drugs for this condition.

Although the results with ergoloid mesylates and nafronyl are encouraging, there are still a number of reservations about their use. In both cases, the overall degree of improvement is usually small. Neither drug has been clearly shown to

TABLE 1.   Summary of the Effect of Cerebral Vasodilators on Cerebral Blood Flow.

Drug	Effect	
	parenteral administration	oral administration
Direct-acting vasodilators		
Papaverine *	Increase	Small increase †
Cyclandelate	Increase or decrease	Small increase †
Nafronyl ‡	Increase or no effect	No effect
Hexobendine *‡	Increase	No effect
Drugs acting on adrenoreceptors		
Isoxsuprine	Decrease	—
Nylidrin *	Decrease or no effect	Large increase †
Ergoloid mesylates (dihydroergotoxine)	Decrease or no effect	—
Drugs acting on histamine receptors		
Betahistine ‡	Increase	Small increase
Miscellaneous vasodilators		
Vincamine *‡	Increase or no effect	—
Niacin (nicotinic acid)	Decrease or no effect	No effect
Cinnarizine ‡	—	—

*Not available in the United Kingdom.

†Unconfirmed reports.

‡Not available in the United States.

improve practical behavior (such as self-care, dressing, and prevention of inconti-
nence) or to reduce hostile behavior. It is these factors, rather than changes in
mood or affect, that largely determine whether patients can remain independent.
The prospective monitoring of side effects has been inadequate, and the long-term
safety of the drugs is still unknown. For instance, no studies have monitored the
incidence of postural hypotension, yet this is an important potential complication
of peripheral vasodilatation. Further studies designed to provide this information
are required. In the meantime, the two drugs can be only cautiously recommended for the treatment of senile dementia.

References

1. Vasodilators in senile dementia. Br Med J 1979; 2:511-2.
2. Drugs for improvement of cerebral function in the elderly. Med Lett Drugs Ther 1976; 18:38-9.
3. Drugs for dementia. Drug Ther Bull 1975; 13:85-7.
4. James IM. Methods for assessment of the effect of drugs on cerebral blood flow in man. Br J Clin Pharmacol 1979; 7:3-12.

5. Ingvar DH. Functional landscapes in the brain studied with regional blood flow measurements. Br J Radiol 1978; 51:657-64.

6. Alexander SC, Cohen PJ, Wollman H, Smith TC, Reivich M, Vander Molen RA. Cerebral carbohydrate metabolism during hypocarbia in man: studies during nitrous oxide anesthesia. Anesthesiology 1965; 26:624-32.

7. Olesen J. Quantitative evaluation of normal and pathologic cerebral blood flow regulation to perfusion pressure: changes in man. Arch Neurol 1973; 28:143-9.

8. Purves MJ. The physiology of the cerebral circulation. London: Cambridge University Press, 1972:173-99. (Monographs of the Physiology Society no. 28).

9. Harper AM. Regulation of cerebral circulation. In: Scientific Basis of Medicine Annual Review: British Post Graduate Medical Federation. London: Athlone Press, 1969:60-81.

10. Purves MJ. The physiology of the cerebral circulation. London: Cambridge University Press, 1972:282-333. (Monographs of the Physiological Society no. 28).

11. Ponte J, Purves MJ. The role of the carotid body chemoreceptors and carotid sinus baroreceptors in the control of cerebral blood vessels. J Physiol (Lond) 1974; 237:315-40.

12. James IM, MacDonell LA. The role of baroreceptors and chemoreceptors in the regulation of the cerebral circulation. Clin Sci Mol Med 1975; 49:465-71.

13. Mchedlishvili GI, Nikolaishvili LS. Evidence of a cholinergic nervous mechanism in mediating the autoregulatory dilatation of the cerebral blood vessels. Pfluegers Arch 1970; 315:27-37.

14. Harper AM, Deshmukh VD, Rowan JO, Jennett WB. The influence of sympathetic nervous activity on cerebral blood flow. Arch Neurol 1972; 27:1-6.

15. Kety SS. Human cerebral blood flow and oxygen consumption as related to ageing. J Chronic Dis 1956; 3:478-86.

16. Naritomi H, Meyer JS, Sakai F, Yamaguchi F, Shaw T. Effects of advancing age on regional cerebral blood flow: studies in normal subjects and subjects with risk factors for atherothrombotic stroke. Arch Neurol 1979; 36:410-6.

17. Dastur DK, Lane MH, Hansen PB, et al. Effects of aging on cerebral circulation and metabolism in man. In: Birren JE, Butler RN, Greenhouse SW, Sokoloff L, Yarrow MR, eds. Human aging. Washington, D.C.: Government Printing Office, 1963; 986:57-76.

18. Davison AN. Biochemical aspects of the ageing brain. Age Ageing 1978; 7: Suppl:4-11.

19. Hachinski VC, Lassen NA, Marshall J. Multi-infarct dementia: a cause of mental deterioration in the elderly. Lancet 1974; 2:207-10.

20. Meyer JS, Ericsson AD. Cerebral circulation and metabolism in neurological disorders. In: Carpi A, ed. Pharmacology of the cerebral circulation. Oxford: Pergamon Press, 1972:280-96.

21. Paulson OB. Regional cerebral blood flow in apoplexy due to occlusion of the middle cerebral artery. Neurology (Minneap) 1970; 20:63-77.

22. Paulson OB, Lassen NA, Skinhøj E. Regional cerebral blood flow in apoplexy without arterial occlusion. Neurology (Minneap) 1970; 20:125-38.

23. Olesen J. Cerebral blood flow: methods for measurement, regulation, effects of drugs and changes in disease. Copenhagen: FADLs, 1974:68.

24. Fieschi C, Agnoli A, Battistini N, Bozzao L, Prencipe M. Derangement of regional cerebral blood flow and its regulatory mechanisms in acute cerebrovascular lesions. Neurology (Minneap) 1968; 18:1166-79.

25. Frackowiak RSJ, Jones T, Lenzi GL. Regional cerebral blood flow and oxygen consumption in acute hemispheric stroke measured with $^{15}O_2$ and positron emission tomography. Clin Sci Mol Med 1981; 60:15P.

26. Olesen J, Paulson OB. The effect of intra-arterial papaverine on the regional cerebral blood flow in patients with stroke or intracranial tumor. Stroke 1971; 2:148-59.

27. Herrschaft H. The efficacy and course of action of vaso- and metabolic-active substances on regional cerebral blood flow in patients with cerebrovascular insufficiency. In: Harper AM, Jennett WB, Miller JD, Rowan JO, eds. Blood flow and metabolism in the brain. Edinburgh: Churchill Livingstone, 1975:11.24-11.28.

28. Capon A, de Rood M, Verbist A, Fruhling J. Action of vasodilators on regional cerebral blood flow in subacute or chronic cerebral ischemia. Stroke 1977; 8:25-9.

29. Heiss W-D, Podreka I. Assessment of pharmacological agents on cerebral blood flow. Eur Neurol 1978; 17: Suppl 1:135-43.

30. Meyer JS, Mathew NT, Hartmann A, Rivera VM. Orally administered betahistine and regional cerebral blood flow in cerebrovascular disease. J Clin Pharmacol 1974; 14:280-9.

31. McHenry LC Jr. Cerebral vasodilator therapy in stroke. Stroke 1972; 3:686-91.

32. Pistolese GR, Faraglia V, Agnoli A, et al. Cerebral hemispheric "counter-steal" phenomenon during hyperventilation in cerebrovascular diseases. Stroke 1972; 3:456-61.

33. Battistini N, Casacchia JL, Bartolini A, Bava G, Fieschi C. Effects of hyperventilation on focal brain damage following middle cerebral artery occlusion. In: Brock M, Fieschi C, Ingvar DH, Lassen NA, Schürmann K, eds. Cerebral blood flow: clinical and experimental results. Berlin: Springer, 1969:249-53.

34. Christensen MS, Paulson OB, Olesen J, et al. Cerebral apoplexy (stroke) treated with or without prolonged artificial hyperventilation. I. Cerebral circulation, clinical course, and cause of death. Stroke 1973; 4:568-631.

35. Meyer Js, Gotoh F, Gilroy J, Nara N. Improvement in brain oxygenation and clinical improvement in patients with strokes treated with papaverine hydrochloride. JAMA 1965; 194:957-61.

36. McHenry LC Jr, Jaffe ME, Kawamura J, Goldberg HI. Effect of papaverine on regional blood flow in focal vascular disease of the brain. N Engl J Med 1970; 282:1167-70.

37. Mchenry LC Jr, Jaffe ME, West JW, et al. Regional cerebral blood flow and cardiovascular effects of hexobendine in stroke patients. Neurology (Minneap) 1972; 22:217-23.

38. Skinhøj E, Høedt-Rasmussen K, Paulson OB, Lassen NA. Regional cerebral blood flow and its autoregulation in patients with transient focal cerebral ischemic attacks. Neurology (Minneap) 1970; 20:485-93.

39. Hyams DE. Cerebral function and drug therapy. In: Brocklehurst JC, ed. Textbook of geriatric medicine and gerontology. 2d ed. Edinburgh: Chruchill Livingstone, 1978:670-711.

40. Mohan J. The neurosurgeon's view. In: Boullin DJ, ed. Cerebral vasospasm. New York: John Wiley, 1980:15-35.

41. Hachinski VC, Iliff LD, Zilhka E, et al. Cerebral blood flow in dementia. Arch Neurol 1975; 32:632-7.

42. Schieve JF, Wilson WP. The influence of age, anesthesia and cerebral arteriosclerosis on cerebral vascular activity to CO_2. Am J Med 1953; 15:171-4.

43. Yamaguchi F, Meyer JS, Yamamoto M, Sakai F, Shaw T. Noninvasive regional cerebral blood flow measurements in dementia. Arch Neurol 1980; 37:410-8.

44. Wetherell A. Some effects of atropine on short-term memory. Br J Clin Pharmacol 1980; 10:627-8.

45. James IM, Millar RA, Purves MJ. Observations on the extrinsic neural control of cerebral blood flow in the baboon. Circ Res 1969; 25:77-93.

46. Gabrynowicz JW, Dumbrill M. A clinical trial of leptazole with nicotinic acid in the management of psycho-geriatric patients. Med J Aust 1968; 1:799-802.

47. Robinson RA. Some problems of clinical trials in elderly people. Gerontol Clin (Basel) 1961; 3:247-54.

48. Berde B, Schild HO, eds. Ergot alkaloids and related compounds. New York: Springer-Verlag, 1978.

49. Poch G, Kukovetz WR. Papaverine-induced inhibition of phosphodiesterase activity in various mammalian tissues. Life Sci 1971; 10:133-44.

50. Martindale W. The extra pharmacopoeia. 27th ed. London: Pharmaceutical Press, 1977.

51. Gottstein U. Pharmacological studies of total cerebral blood flow in man with comments on the possibility of improving regional cerebral blood flow by drugs. Acta Neurol Scand [Suppl] 1965; 14:136-41.

52. Yoshida K, Ishijima Y, Matsuda M. Effect of cyclandelate on regional cerebral blood flow measured by intracarotid injection of Xe^{133}. Arch Jpn Chir (Kyoto) 1968; 37:842-53.

53. Carpi A, Giardini V. Drugs acting on muscular receptors. In: Carpi A, ed. Pharmacology of the cerebral circulation. Oxford: Pergamon Press, 1972:130-1.

54. Wang HS, Obrist WD. Effect of oral papaverine on cerebral blood flow in normals: evaluation by the xenon-133 inhalation method. Biol Psychiatry 1976; 11:217-25.

55. Yesavage JA, Tinklenberg JR, Hollister LE, Berger PA. Vasodilators in senile dementias: a review of the literature. Arch Gen Psychiatry 1979; 36:220-3.

56. Axelrod J, Shofer R, Inscoe JK, King WM, Sjoerdsma A. The fate of papaverine in man and other mammals. J Pharmacol Exp Ther 1958; 124:9-15.

57. Arnold JD, Baldridge J, Riley B, Brody G. Papaverine hydrochloride: the evaluation of two new dosage forms. Int J Clin Pharmacol Biopharm 1977; 15:230-3.

58. Stern FH. Management of chronic brain syndrome secondary to cerebral arteriosclerosis, with special reference to papaverine hydrochloride. J Am Geriatr Soc 1970; 18:507-12.

59. Duvoisin RC. Antagonism of levodopa by papaverine. JAMA 1975; 231:845.

60. Bijlsma UG, Funcke ABH, Tersteege M, Rekker RF, Ernsting MJE, Nauta WT. The pharmacology of Cyclospasmol. Arch Int Pharmacodyn Ther 1956; 105:145-74.

61. Funcke ABH, van Beek MC, Nijland K. Protective action of cyclandelate in hypoxia. Curr Med Res Opin 1974; 2:37-42.

62. O'Brien MD, Veall N. Effect of cyclandelate on cerebral cortex perfusion-rates in cerebrovascular disease. Lancet 1966; 2:729-30.

63. Westreich G, Alter M, Lundgren S. Effect of cyclandelate on dementia. Stroke 1975; 6:535-8.

64. Rogers WF, Shaikh VAR, Clark ANG. Cyclandelate in long standing cerebral arteriosclerosis. Gerontol Clin (Basel) 1970; 12:88-93.

65. Horden A, Wheatley D. Psychotropic drugs in the elderly: cerebral vasodialtors. In: Wheatley D, ed. Stress and the heart. New York: Raven Press, 1981:395-7.

66. Young J, Hall P, Blakemore C. Treatment of the cerebral manifestations of arteriosclerosis with cyclandelate. Br J Psychiatry 1974; 124:177-80.

67. Fontaine L, Grand M, Chabert J, Szarvasi E, Bayssat M. General pharmacology of a new vasodilator substance — naftidrofuryl. Bull Chim Ther 1968; 6:463-75.

68. Cox JR. Double-blind evaluation of naftidrofuryl in treating elderly confused hospitalised patients. Gerontol Clin 1975; 17:160-7.

69. Meynaud A, Grand M, Fontaine L. Effect of naftidrofuryl upon energy metabolism of the brain. Arzneimittelforsch 1973; 23:1431-6.

70. Boismare F, Le Poncin-Lafitte M, Saligaut C, Moore N. Effets de l'hypoxie hypobare sur le conditionnement et les taux cérébraux d'ADP, d'AMP, de dopamine et de noradrénaline chez le rat traité ou non par le naftidrofuryl. J Pharmacol 1981; 12:51-7.

71. Shaw SWJ, Johnson RH. The effect of naftidrofuryl on the metabolic response to exercise in man. Acta Neurol Scand 1975; 52:231-7.

72. Elert C, Niebel W, Karuse E, Satter P. The effect of naftidrofuryl on energy metabolism in the musculature of limbs with impaired blood flow. Therapiewoche 1976; 23:3947-50.

73. Yesavage JA, Tinklenberg JR, Hollister LE, Berger PA. Naftidrofuryl in senile dementia. J Am Geriatr. (in press).

74. Lim CC, Cook PJ, James IM. The effect of an acute infusion of vincamine and ethyl apovincaminate on cerebral blood flow in healthy volunteers. Br J Clin Pharmacol 1980; 9:100-1.

75. James IM, Newbury P, Woollard ML. The effect of naftidrofuryl oxalate on cerebral blood flow in elderly patients. Br J Clin Pharmacol 1978; 6:545-6.

76. Lartique-Mattei C, D'Athis P, Lhoste F, Tillement JP. Etude de la pharmacocinétique du naftidrofuryl et de sa biodisponibilité sous forme de gélule chez l'homme. Int J Clin Pharmacol Biopharm 1978; 16:536-9.

77. Meyer JS, Kanda T, Shinohara Y, et al. Effect of hexobendine on cerebral hemispheric blood flow and metabolism: preliminary clinical observations concerning its use in ischemic cerebrovascular disease. Neurology (Minneap) 1971; 21:691-702.

78. Manley ES, Lawson JW. Effect of beta-adrenergic receptor blockade on skeletal muscle vasodilation produced by isoxsuprine and nylidrin. Arch Int Pharmacodyn Ther 1968; 175:239-50.

79. Weber G, Kreisel T, Peter S, Künzel J. A double-blind placebo controlled cross-over study in patients with peripheral vascular diseases, using a new capillary viscometer. Angiology 1980; 31:1-5.

80. Fazekas JF, Alman RW. Comparative effects of isoxsuprine and carbon dioxide on cerebral hemodynamics. Am J Med Sci 1964; 248:16-9.

81. Coffman JD. Vasodilator drugs in peripheral vascular disease. N Engl J Med 1979; 300:713-7.

82. Meyer JS, Gotoh F, Akiyama M, Yoshitake S. Monitoring cerebral blood flow, oxygen, and glucose metabolism: analysis of cerebral metabolic disorder in stroke and some therapeutic trials in human volunteers. Circulation 1967; 36:197-211.

83. Eisenberg S, Camp MF, Horn MR. The effect of nylidrin hydrochloride (Arlidin) on the cerebral circulation. Am J Med Sci 1960; 240:85-92.

84. Meier-Ruge W, Iwangoff P. Biochemical effects of ergot alkaloids with special reference to the brain. Postgrad Med J 1976; 52: Suppl 1:47-54.

85. Loew DM, Vigouret JM, Jaton AL. Neuropharmacological investigations with two ergot alkaloids, hydergine and bromocriptine. Postgrad Med J 1976; 52: Suppl 1:40-6.

86. Agnoli A, Battistini N, Bozzao L, Fieschi C. Drug action on regional cerebral blood flow in case of acute cerebrovascular involvement. Acta Neurol Scand [Suppl] 1965; 14:142-4.

87. McHenry LC Jr, Jaffe ME, Kawamura J, Goldberg HI. Hydergine effect on cerebral circulation in cerebrovascular disease. J Neurol Sci 1971; 13:475-81.

88. Hughes JR, Williams JG, Currier RD. An ergot alkaloid preparation (Hydergine) in the treatment of dementia: critical review of the clinical literature. J Am Geriatr Soc. 1976; 24:490-7.

89. Allen JA, Connell AM, Harries EHL, Roddie IC. A comparison of the effects of histamine acid phosphate and betahistine hydrochloride on peripheral blood flow and gastric acid secretion in man. J Pharmacol 1971; 2:223-4.

90. Tomita M, Gotoh F, Sato T, et al. Comparative responses of the carotid and vertebral arterial systems of rhesus monkeys to betahistine. Stroke 1978; 9:382-7.

91. Hughes RJD, James IM, Dijane A. The effect of betahistine methane-sulphonate upon cerebral blood flow. Br J Clin Pharmacol 1981; 11:308-10.

92. Rivera VM, Meyer JS, Baer PE, Faibish GM, Matthew NT, Hartmann A. Vertebrobasilar arterial insufficiency with dementia: controlled trials of treatment with betahistine hydrochloride. J Am Geriatr Soc 1974; 22:397-406.

93. Szobor A, Klein M. Ethyl apovincaminate therapy in neurovascular diseases. Arzneimittelforsch 1976; 26:1984-9.

94. Szporny L. Pharmacology of vincamine and its derivatives. Actual Pharmacol (Paris) 1977; 29:87-117.

95. Kohlmeyer K. Zir wirkung von Vincamin auf die Gehirndurchblutung des Menschen im Akutversuch: Untersuchungen mit der ^{133}Xenon-Clearance. Arzneimittelforsch 1977; 27:1285-90.

96. Witzmann HK, Blechacz W. Zur Stellung von Vincamin in der Therapie zerebrovaskulärer Krankheiten und zerebraler Leistungsminderungen. Arzneimittelforsch 1977; 27:1238-47.

97. Levy RI. Drugs used in the treatment of hyperlipoproteinemias. In: Goodman AG, Goodman LS, Gilman A, eds. The pharmacological basis of therapeutics. 6th ed. New York: Macmillan, 1980:839-40.

98. Scheinberg P. The effect of nicotinic acid on the cerebral circulation, with observations on extracerebral contamination of cerebral venous blood in the nitrous oxide procedure for cerebral blood flow. Circulation 1950; 1:1148-54.

99. Boudouresques J, Papy JJ, Daniel F. A long-acting treatment for chronic cerebral circulatory insufficiency. Semaine Therapeutique (Paris) 1970; 46:789-92.

100. Mosher LR. Nicotinic acid side effects and toxicity: a review. Am J Psychiatry 1970; 126:1290-6.

101. Van Neuten JM. Comparative bioassay of vasoactive drugs using isolated perfused rabbit arteries. Eur J Pharmacol 1969; 6:286-93.

Drugs to Decrease Alcohol Consumption

Edward M. Sellers, M.D., Ph.D.,

Claudio A. Naranjo, M.D.,

and John E. Peachey, M.D., M.Sc.

MANY drugs have been used with the expectation of reducing alcohol consumption. A few seem to be associated with a reduction in alcohol use for up to three to six months in some patients, but none is associated with a reduction in alcohol consumption for longer periods.[1,2] In spite of uncertainty about efficacy, over 90 per cent of physicians in private practice prescribe drugs for the treatment of alcoholism.[3] The effectiveness of drug therapies for alcohol-related problems is seriously compromised by the difficulty of characterizing patients according to the cause of their alcohol problems, by the large number of nonpharmacologic modulators of alcohol consumption, by the lack of general agreement on the definition of a successful treatment outcome, and finally by the lack of specific and potent drugs directed at the primary neurochemical antecedent of persistent excessive drinking. Even if a drug has been proved effective during controlled testing, failure of drug treatment to be effective in practice can often be attributed to poor compliance, use in an inappropriate alcoholic population, the lack of a predefined and systematized treatment strategy, or a failure to optimize the conditions under which the drugs are administered.

In defining a successful treatment, one or more of the following variables are used: the amount of alcohol consumed, retention of the patient in treatment, improvement of social and family relations, and financial or employment status. Some therapists and patients believe that abstinence is the only acceptable criterion for therapeutic success.[4,5] However, this goal is challenged by investigators who are developing effective behavioral techniques to achieve controlled drinking as an alternative.[4,5] Many patients also consider abstinence unrealistic. The nature and role of drugs in a treatment whose goal is abstinence are very different from those in a treatment whose goal is controlled drinking.

Pharmacotherapies are used alone or in conjunction with other treatments in patients who have medical or behavioral problems related to excessive alcohol

From the Clinical Pharmacology Program, Addiction Research Foundation, Clinical Institute, and the departments of Pharmacology, Medicine, and Psychiatry, University of Toronto.

Originally published on November 19, 1981 (305:1255-1262).

consumption.[6,7] In this review we discuss only drugs that have a reduction in alcohol consumption as the objective of their use. Such a decrease can be expected to reduce the frequency or severity of alcohol-induced organic disease and to modify behavioral problems that lead to excessive alcohol consumption or result from it.

Aversive Drugs

Regardless of what maintains drinking, an aversive consequence can be used to suppress it. The basic paradigm is that of conditioned aversion: alcohol ingestion is paired either with an emetic agent such as emetine or apomorphine, thereby producing nausea and vomiting, or with an alcohol-sensitizing drug (Table 1), which produces a strong aversive reaction when taken before alcohol.[1,7] Disulfiram and calcium cyanamide (calcium carbimide) are the only agents of the latter type that are widely used and for which there is substantial experimental and clinical information.

Alcohol-Sensitizing Drugs

Of the many compounds that are reported to sensitize the patient to ethanol (Table 1), only disulfiram and carbimide have been used therapeutically in alcoholics. Disulfiram and carbimide inhibit hepatic aldehyde-NAD oxidoreductase (ALDH), causing increases in blood acetaldehyde levels after ethanol administration. Disulfiram's ALDH inhibition develops slowly over 12 hours[8] and is irreversible. Restoration of ALDH activity depends on de novo enzyme synthesis,[9] which occurs over six or more days. Carbimide's ALDH inhibition is maximal one to two hours after drug administration and is reversible, with 80 per cent restoration of ALDH activity occurring within 24 hours. Although disulfiram and carbimide have a similar sensitizing effect in the alcoholic, there are important differences in the onset and duration of this action. The duration of disulfiram-induced inhibition is several days, as compared with that of carbimide (less than one day), and its onset of effect (12 hours) is much slower than that of carbimide (one hour).

Acetaldehyde is implicated in the development of physiologic changes that occur during the disulfiram-acetaldehyde reaction and the carbimide-acetaldehyde reaction induced by ethanol. The appearance and disappearance of flushing, tachycardia, tachypnea, sensations of warmth, palpitations, and shortness of breath coincide with the time of increased blood acetaldehyde concentrations. The intensity and duration of these changes depend on the doses of the drug and of ethanol. After 0.15 g of ethanol per kilogram of body weight (which is equivalent to 36 ml of 40 per cent [80-proof] distilled spirits), alcoholics receiving therapeutic doses of disulfiram (250 mg daily) and carbimide (50 mg twice daily) have detectable effects lasting approximately 30 minutes. When ethanol is taken in amounts greater than 0.2 g per kilogram, the physiologic effects are more severe, and most patients have intense palpitations, dyspnea, nausea, vomiting, and headache that may last up to 90 minutes. In some instances, shock and loss of consciousness can occur.[10] For some alcoholics, the threat of such a reaction alone is a deterrent against drinking.

TABLE 1.   Alcohol-Sensitizing Compounds.

Dithiocarbamates and related compounds
   Thiuram disulfides
      Disulfiram (tetraethylthiuram disulfide, Antabuse)

Carbimide
   Citrated calcium cyanamide (citrated calcium carbimide, Temposil)

Hypoglycemic sulfonylureas
   Chlorpropamide
   Tolbutamide

Other drugs	
Chloramphenicol	Quinacrine
Griseofulvin	Cefoperazone
Phentolamine	Metronidazole
Furazolidone	Pargyline
Tolazoline	

Alcohol-sensitizing mushrooms
   Coprinus atramentarius (inky-cap mushroom)
   Clitocybe clavipes

Other chemicals	
4-Bromopyrazole	Pyrogallol
Hydrogen sulfide	Animal charcoal (amorphous carbon)
Tetraethyllead	

Disulfiram

Metabolism and kinetics.   From 80 to 90 per cent of oral disulfiram is absorbed; peak levels of radioactivity occur one to two hours after drug administration.[11] Disulfiram is reduced to diethyldithiocarbamate (DDC) within one hour and is subsequently metabolized to diethylamine, carbon disulfide, DDC methyl ester, DDC glucuronide, and DDC sulfate.[10] Approximately 50 per cent of the drug and its metabolites are eliminated in urine, feces, and breath within 25 hours, and after six days up to 80 per cent is eliminated. Pharmacokinetic data on disulfiram are incomplete because of difficulties in measuring the drug and its metabolites in biologic fluids.

Efficacy.   Evidence supporting the efficacy of disulfiram is limited. Controlled clinical trials of efficacy show no improvement or short-term improvement only.[1,2,12] Appreciable improvements (abstinence and improved social functioning) reported by chronic alcoholics during the first three months of treatment with therapeutic doses (250 mg daily) and non-therapeutic doses (1 mg daily) probably result from non-specific, nonpharmacologic factors rather than any specific pharmacologic activity of the drug.[2,11] The subsequent decline from early improvement after the first three months of treatment probably reflects both the low potency of the drug and the increased importance of nonpharmacologic factors as determinants of long-term outcomes of treatment.

Disulfiram is most often taken orally; however, in order to improve compliance, eight to 10 100-mg disulfiram tablets (Esperal) are sometimes implanted subcutaneously into the abdominal wall.[13] Blood DDC levels after the disulfiram implantation are much lower than the levels observed after use of oral disulfiram.[14] Blood levels of disulfiram and DDC after the implantation are probably insufficient to exert an important alcohol-sensitizing effect.[15]

Adverse effects. Adverse clinical effects during therapy may result from the disulfiram-acetaldehyde reaction, because of the toxicity of disulfiram or its metabolites or because of an interaction of disulfiram and other drugs.

Medical complications during the disulfiram-acetaldehyde reaction can include marked tachycardia, hypotension, and reversible electrocardiographic changes consisting of T-wave flattening and inversion. Fatalities due to sudden myocardial infarction or cerebrovascular hemorrhage and infarction have been reported.[10] Although most fatal disulfiram-acetaldehyde reactions are associated with disulfiram dosages in excess of 500 mg daily followed by the consumption of more than two drinks of ethanol, deaths have also occurred with lower doses after a single drink (approximately 0.15 g of ethanol per kilogram).[16]

Most reactions to disulfiram or carbimide are self-limited and present no life-threatening risk to the patient.[17] Supportive measures are usually sufficient. However, such reactions should be managed in an emergency room because there are occasional arrhythmias and severe hypotension.

No pathophysiologic rationale or evidence of efficacy for vitamin C, antihistamines, or intravenous iron salts exists; hence, they should not be used. Inhibitors of prostaglandin synthetase (e.g., indomethacin) and H_2 blockers (e.g., cimetidine) may decrease the flushing reaction. However, no therapeutic role in the disulfiram-acetaldehyde reaction has been established.

Various types of toxicity have been associated with disulfiram or its metabolites. Drowsiness and lethargy are commonly reported by alcoholics who are treated with disulfiram.[18] Alcoholics with a history or evidence of depression or schizophrenia can have a relapse or an exacerbation during disulfiram administration.[19,20] Such behavioral toxicity may be the result of altered brain catecholamine levels, since disulfiram and DDC inhibit dopamine-β-hydroxylase (DBH), increasing dopamine levels and decreasing norepinephrine concentrations in the brain and other tissues.[21] Adverse behavioral effects are reported to be more common in alcoholics with low cerebrospinal-fluid DBH activity[22] or low levels of platelet monoamine oxidase and high levels of red-cell catechol-*o*-methyltransferase activities.[23] Peripheral neuropathy, hepatotoxicity, hypertension, increases in cholesterol, and congenital abnormalities have been reported to result from disulfiram treatment.[10] Studies are needed to determine the pathogenesis of disulfiram's behavioral toxicity and to identify clinically useful predictors of patients at risk for toxicity. In any case, substantial evidence suggests that disulfiram is quite toxic. Therefore, systematic prospective monitoring for adverse effects during disulfiram treatment is essential.

Drug-drug interactions are another hazard of disulfiram therapy. Disulfiram inhibits microsomal mixed-function oxidase biotransformation mediated by Phase I reactions but does nt inhibit the glucuronic acid conjugative pathways. Disulfiram decreases the biotransformation of phenytoin,[24] increasing both concentrations and toxicity,[25] and inhibits the biotransformation of antipyrine, warfarin, isoniazid, rifampin, diazepam, and chlordiazepoxide, but not the conjugation of oxazepam and lorazepam.[10]

Clinically serious pharmacodynamic interactions can be anticipated during the disulfiram-acetaldehyde reaction in patients taking other drugs that impair regulation of blood pressure (e.g., α- and β-adrenoceptor-blocking agents and vasodilators), have actions in the central nervous system that are mediated by noradrenaline or dopamine (e.g., tricyclic antidepressants and phenothiazines), or inhibit the same enzymes as disulfiram (e.g., monoamine oxidase inhibitors). Such interactions have been associated with fatal disulfiram-acetaldehyde reactions.[10,26] Conversely, some drugs (e.g., diazepam) may reduce the intensity of the disulfiram-acetaldehyde reaction.[27]

Treatment. Disulfiram is primarily a pharmacologic adjunct in the treatment of alcoholism and should only be used in conjunction with behavioral and psychosocial therapies.[1,7,28]

Obviously, disulfiram should be prescribed only to alcoholics who clearly seek abstinence, who wish to use the drug, and who have no medical or psychosocial contraindications (Table 2). Before treatment commences, the patient should be fully informed of the purpose, procedure, and consequences of disulfiram administration. In particular, the consequences of taking ethanol in any form, including over-the-counter preparations, must be emphasized. A full medical and psychosocial assessment is mandatory before disulfiram treatment, and the patient must agree to return at least monthly during the course of drug administration, for follow-up assessments (Table 3). The patient's willingness to continue disulfiram treatment and changes in desire for abstinence are followed during treatment in order to assess compliance and the potential for a return to drinking. Some reasons for stopping disulfiram therapy include two consecutive missed appointments, noncompliance (as evidenced by taking less than 80 per cent of the prescribed drug), drinking, pregnancy, or changes in liver or cardiac function. The appearance of depressive symptoms can be the prelude to a suicide attempt. There is no experimental evidence to support the efficacy of disulfiram treatment over many months or years. A goal of treatment with the alcohol-sensitizing drugs is to allow the alcoholic to establish the resources necessary to maintain abstinence after the drug treatment is stopped. The durationof disulfiram administration is individualized and is determined by the patient's response or responses to treatment as well as by the development of adverse clinical effects that are related to both the dose and the duration of drug administration. The usual dose of oral disulfiram is 250 mg daily, taken at bedtime to reduce daytime drowsiness. Optimal dosage schedules await adequate knowledge of the pharmacokinetics of the parent drug and its active metabolites in individual patients and in the entire population. A higher dose is associated with more frequent side effects and is not warranted. Drowsiness, lethargy, bothersome body odor, or halitosis can be controlled in most patients by reducing the dosage.

TABLE 2. Contraindications to the Use of the Alcohol-Sensitizing Agents.

Medical and psychiatric contraindications
Myocardial disease
Severe pulmonary insufficiency
Severe liver dysfunction
Chronic renal failure
Organic mental disturbances
Neuropathy
Psychosis
Personality disorders (disorders of impulse control; depressive neuroses with recurrent thoughts of suicide)
Metabolic disorders
Patients receiving other drug treatments (α- and β-adrenoceptor antagonists, vasodilators; sympathomimetic amines; monoamine oxidase inhibitors; tricyclic antidepressants; antipsychotic agents)
Pregnancy

Psychosocial contraindications
Inability or unwillingness to attend monthly medical and psychosocial follow-up assessments and to follow the prescribed regimen

In some jurisdictions and rehabilitation programs, disulfiram can be administered under court order or under coercion. Such mandatory use of disulfiram is problematic in view of the drug's questionable efficacy and known toxicity and the legal and ethical implications of such a procedure.[29]

Calcium Carbimide

Calcium carbimide use is not approved in some countries, including the United States. Clinical trials with carbimide indicate that it may be an alternative alcohol-sensitizing drug, with a milder reaction after ethanol and fewer side effects.[30,31]

Metabolism and kinetics. The absorption of calcium carbimide after oral administration is rapid and may be associated with nausea, headache, and vomiting after high doses. Pharmacokinetic data on calcium carbimide are not available. Calcium carbimide is hydrolyzed in the gastrointestinal tract to carbimide (cyanamide), which is then rapidly absorbed into the portal circulation. In view of the rapid onset (one hour) and short duration (less than one day) of its alcohol-sensitizing action, the biotransformation and elimination of carbimide must be extremely rapid.

TABLE 3. Schedule of Assessment Procedures during Treatment with the Alcohol-Sensitizing Agents.

Procedure or Measurement	Initially	During Treatment		
		at least once monthly	every three months	every six months
Medical examination: function inquiry, physical examination, and assessment of mental status	X	X	—	—
Assessment of drug/alcohol use	X	X	—	—
Reappraisal of treatment goal	X	X	—	—
Psychosocial assessment of family, work, use of leisure time, and legal problems	X	X	—	—
Hemoglobin, erythrocytes, leukocytes	X	—	X	—
Urinalysis	X	—	X	—
Alkaline phosphatase	X	—	X	X
Cholesterol, triglycerides	X	—	—	X
Serum aspartate aminotransferase, gamma-glutamyl transpeptidase	X	—	X	X
Serum electrolytes	X	—	—	X
Creatinine	X	—	—	X
Blood urea nitrogen	X	—	—	X
Total protein, albumin	X	—	—	X
Triiodothyronine, thyroxine	X	—	—	X
Electrocardiogram	X	—	—	X

Efficacy. Carbimide has a short duration of activity, and the intensity and duration of the carbimide-acetaldehyde reaction can vary between alcoholics as well as in the same person on different drinking occasions.[32-35] The intensity of the carbimide-acetaldehyde reaction diminishes after repeated drinks taken in the same drinking session.[36] Such a reduction in the disulfiram-acetaldehyde reaction can also occur after numerous drinks spread over hours or days.[37] Some alcoholics report an ethanol craving during the carbimide-acetaldehyde reaction[32-34] and the disulfiram acetaldehyde reaction.[38] No proper studies of the efficacy of carbimide have been conducted.[2]

Adverse effects. Carbimide produces fewer side effects than disulfiram does during repeated administration. Carbimide does not inhibit DBH and does not usually cause behavioral changes, drowsiness, or lethargy. Peripheral neuropathy has been reported.[39] Hepatocyte inclusion bodies may occur in some alcoholics treated with carbimide,[40] but similar inclusion bodies also occur with disulfiram.[41] The importance of these findings is unclear, since they may be due to ethanol intake, elevated blood acetaldehyde levels, or the alcohol-sensitizing drug that the patient received. Although carbimide exerts substantial antithyroid effects in laboratory animals,[42] thyroid function in alcoholics treated with carbimide is apparently normal.[43] Carbimide does not inhibit the metabolism of phenytoin[26] and may therefore be a preferable agent in alcoholics when inhibition of drug metabolism poses a clinical problem.

Treatment. Until a proper study of this drug's efficacy is conducted, its use should be limited. As with disulfiram therapy, the patient must be made aware of the purpose, plan, and risk of the treatment and told that regular follow-up assignments will be required at least once monthly. Oral carbimide, 50 mg, is taken twice daily because of the short duration of action. Because of the rapid onset and short duration of its effect, carbimide can be taken intermittently in anticipation of situations associated with a substantial risk of renewed drinking. Such an approach is untested, but it could be a useful adjunct to support long-term abstinence in highly motivated patients.

Other Alcohol-Sensitizing Drugs

Some commonly used therapeutic agents exert alcohol-sensitizing activity in human beings (Table 1). Metronidazole has been used to treat alcoholism but is ineffective.[1,2,44] Flushing, tachycardia, and hypotension have been reported to occur after alcohol ingestion in patients receiving cephalosporins, the oral hypoglycemics, pargyline, and chloral hydrate.[10] Alcohol-sensitizing chemicals included 4-bromopyrazole, hydrogen sulfide, tetraethyllead, pyrogallol, and 1-aminocyclopropanol, the active constituent of the inky-cap mushroom (*Coprinus atramentarius*). The pharmacodynamics of these ethanol-drug interactions have not been studied in human beings but appear to be due to an increase in the blood acetaldehyde level after ALDH inhibition.[8]

Other Aversive Drugs

The emetics apomorphine and emetine have been used to produce conditioned aversive reactions to alcohol. The usefulness of this treatment is limited, since effects that appear in a controlled setting cannot be readily extrapolated to everyday living.[1,7] Another conditioning treatment that uses succinylcholine to produce dramatic respiratory paralysis has been largely abandoned.[1,7]

| Reducing the Urge to Drink

Chronic alcoholics are vulnerable to relapse months and possibly years after achieving prolonged abstinence. The specific reasons for such relapses are not known. In general, two explanations are possible: the existence of a protracted withdrawal reaction and the occurrence of subtle external and internal cues that require or stimulate a return to alcohol abuse.[45] Even after the acute withdrawal reaction is complete (three to five days), abstinent chronic alcoholics may continue to have mildly to moderately distressing physiologic and psychological symptoms, which can persist for many months and even years. For example, the sleep pattern may be impaired for as long as four years after abstinence.[46] The protracted alcohol-withdrawal syndrome is characterized by subjective and objective evidence of tremulousness, restlessness, anxiety, respiratory irregularity, depression, impaired autonomic-nervous-system function, and sleep disturbance.[47]

A potential rationale for the use of psychoactive drugs in the long-term treatment of chronic alcoholism would be to reduce protracted withdrawal and thereby provent the need to suppress such symptoms by using ethanol. Such drug use would only maintain abstinence in order to retain the patient in the concurrent means of psychosocial rehabilitation. Methadone maintenance in the treatent of narcotic-dependent persons is analogous. Unfortunately, the existence of a pro-tracted withdrawal syndrome is controversial and does not satisfactorily account for the many alcoholics without such symptoms who nevertheless have relapses, with or without adjunctive therapy.[45]

Irrespective of the rationale for use, anxiolytic agents may reduce the early-dropout rate of alcoholics attending treatment. In one study, unselected skid-row alcoholics had a lower short-term dropout rate with chlordiazepoxide than with placebo, imipramine, thioridazine, or diethylpropion.[48] In another study, chlor-diazepoxide treatment resulted in a greater patient-retention rate than did no medication.[49] In three separate studies in outpatients of low social class who were receiving chlordiazepoxide, an overall improvement of about 23 per cent was reported, as compared with an average recovery rate of about 8 per cent when placebo or other medications were used.[50] However, all this evidence comes from uncontrolled studies in alcoholics of low social class who were not adequately characterized with respect to base-line psychiatric pathologic processes. Hence, the results cannot be generalized, and the evidence should be considered incon-clusive.

Reduction of Alcohol Consumption by Treatment of Psychiatric Problems

Primary alcohol abuse is characterized by excessive alcohol intake with no history of psychiatric illness, whereas secondary alcohol abuse is a consequence of a psychiatric illness such as sociopathic personality disorder, anxiety, or schizophre-nia. Alcohol abuse in this latter context may be a form of self-medication.[51] In primary alcohol abuse, the aim of treatment is to reduce alcohol consumption, with the expectation that improvements in other problem areas will follow. In contrast, in secondary alcohol abuse, amelioration of the underlying disease is expected to diminish alcohol consumption.

Although one might expect a primary psychiatric problem (e.g., depression and schizophrenia) to be associated with increased alcohol consumption, little evidence supports this assumption. Common experience indicates that some patients (e.g., those with phobic or anxiety disorders) decrease their consumption of alcohol when the disorder is treated. Most common are patients with poorly characterized psychological and situational problems. Studies of such patients are difficult and generally of poor quality; however, a short-term reduction in alcohol consumption may be possible with drugs.

Benzodiazepines

Long-term studies of benzodiazepines in patients with anxiety and secondary alcohol abuse have not provided substantial evidence that drug therapy prevents a relapse to drinking or assists in longer-term behavioral adaptation.[7] On the other hand, there is some evidence that over six to eight weeks, chlordiazepoxide (75 mg per day), prazepam, oxazepam, and diazepam are superior to placebo with respect to subjective relief of anxiety or the physician's global rating or both. There was no difference among the various benzodiazepines. At best, the changes were minimal, and contradictory results do exist. In one study, recidivism at six weeks was reduced less with chlordiazepoxide than with thioridazine, methocarbamol, or placebo. In another study in an unselected group of inpatients, therapy with chlorprothixene (60 to 120 mg daily for two weeks), oxazepam (120 to 240 mg daily), or placebo was begun immedaitely on admission. Oxazepam was more effective in reducing the symptoms of anxiety than chlorprothixene, which was more effective than placebo. Chlorprothixene therapy was associated with a greater number of adverse effects than were the other treatments.[7]

Antidepressants

The three classes of tricyclic antidepressant drugs — iminodibenzyls (e.g., imipramine and desipramine), dibenzocycloheptenes (e.g., amitriptyline, nortriptyline, and protriptyline), and dibenzoxepines (e.g., doxepin) — are effective in the treatment of endogenous depression if given in adequate doses. Pharmaceutical claims and clinical preference notwithstanding, all have similar antidepressant activity and would be expected to provide the same symptomatic improvement in chronic alcoholics with depression.

Imipramine was shown to be more effective than placebo in a six-week trial in depressed female alcoholic outpatients and a three-week trial in depressed alcoholic inpatients. In a study of mixed anxiety and depression, doxepin (25 mg three times daily) was more effective than diazepam (5 mg three times daily) after three weeks in male alcoholic inpatients. In a group of 100 unselected patients, both diazepam (5 mg three times daily) and doxepin (50 mg three times daily) appeared to improve the patients' condition, as compared with placebo. However, the placebo group had fewer side effects. Other studies, typically with unselected patients or in outpatient settings with high dropout rates, have failed to show even short-term beneficial effects of tricyclic antidepressants.[7]

Since the benzodiazepines are not effective in endogenous depression and the tricyclic antidepressants are not indicated for anxiety, comparisons between these agents make little sense. Tricyclic antidepressants have a large variety of side effects in the central and autonomic nervous systems and the heart; these effects are especially important and prevalent in older patients. Particularly important are anticholinergic side effects and cardiac arrhythmias. Antidepressants should be used only in chronic alcoholic patients with endogenous depression.[7]

Lithium

There have been many reports on the effects of lithium on alcohol consumption in animals and human beings.[52] In animals, lithium reduces alcohol consumption. The mechanism is not central but involves a modification in the taste of alcohol.[53] Of the few randomized, double-blind, placebo-controlled studies, two recent trials deserve mention. Kline et al.[54] assessed the effects of lithium in patients diagnosed as having "chronic alcoholism associated with nonpsychotic depression." Patients given lithium had fewer drinking bouts than did those given placebo. In the other study,[55] alcoholics without depression responded no better to lithium than to placebo. However, in alcoholics with a Beck depression score of 15 or higher, lithium was superior to placebo in reducing the total number of days during which patients were incapacitated by drinking. In interpreting the results of lithium therapy in reducing alcohol consumption, a high attrition rate must be considered, since the differences between lithium and placebo disappear when the dropouts are included.

Miscellaneous Agents

Propranolol. In addition to its peripheral β-adrenoceptor-blocking action, propranolol has effects in the central nervous system. Results with propranolol in the treatment of chronic alcoholism are conflicting. Some studies suggest a short-term global amelioration of symptoms, but others indicate no influence on the effect of drinking or on the level of consumption.[7,56]

Phenothiazines. Several studies suggest that some phenothiazines control the symptoms of anxiety, but these drugs have never been shown to be effective and safe in chronic alcoholics.[7]

Lysergide (lysergic acid diethylamide or LSD). Even though some uncontrolled studies showed transient short-term benefits with lysergide, no studies have demonstrated long-term effects.[1,51]

Other agents. Vitamins continue to be investigated as a potential treatment for chronic alcoholism. In a five-year uncontrolled study of massive niacin (nicotinic acid) therapy in 507 alcoholics, improvements in mood stabilization and reductions in drinking recidivism were reported.[57] However, such claims require confirmation by controlled studies.

Many other agents have been studied in reasonably well-controlled investigations. There is no evidence to justify the use of carbamazepine, mephenoxalone, cyproheptadine, tybamate, nialamide, phenaglycodol, or hydroxyzine in the rehabilitation of chronic alcoholics.[7]

Other Neuropharmacologic Approaches to Decreasing Alcohol Consumption

Alcohol consumption is maintained by reinforcement, which has a neurochemical basis.[58] Pharmacotherapy could alter the neurochemical changes associated with the reinforcement afforded by alcohol. Data in animals suggest that such a direct effect is possible.[58-60] However, the development of such specific pharmacologic interventions has been hampered by the lack of a full understanding of the modulation of ethanol consumption.[61] Recent studies indicate that alcohol consumption is mediated or regulated by several interacting central neurotransmitter systems,[62] including central catecholaminergic[59] and serotoninergic mechanisms.[62,63] Drugs that increase the availability of serotonin in the synaptic cleft by blocking serotonin reuptake[63] and inhibitors of dopamine-β-hydroxylase have markedly decreased ethanol intake in rats.[59,60] In contrast, ventricularly infused tetrahydropapaveroline may increase ethanol consumption in rats.[64]

Numerous substances have been tested in animal models of alcohol consumption. A reduction of intake has often been reported, but biologically pertinent levels of alcohol consumption have usually not been reached.[61] Thus the relevance of these studies is unknown. In the absence of appropriate animal models the identification of potentially useful drugs will continue to be exclusively dependent on the serendipitous observations of astute clinicians or researchers.[61]

| Conclusions

Drugs are unlikely ever to have a primary role in the rehabilitation of the chronic alcoholic. A number of precautions seem judicious for future studies of drug efficacy. The therapeutic goal of a drug regimen must be defined. Studies must be appropriately controlled and should be double-blind wherever possible. Groups of patients must be adequately characterized and representative of the affected population. Patients should receive drugs that are appropriate to therapeutic goals as well as to their psychological status. Alcohol consumption must be measured as a dependent variable. A measure of compliance with the instructions for medication must be included. Measurements of drug concentrations in blood or plasma should be included wherever possible. Adverse effects of drugs must be monitored in detail. Only with these precautions, among others, will we be able to define more exactly the adjunct role of drug therapies and ensure that effective drug therapies are not judged inadequate and discarded because of faulty trial design, and that myths of efficacy do not continue in perpetuity.

Of all the drugs mentioned in this review, only disulfiram and possibly calcium carbimide have current therapeutic applications in primary alcoholics.

On the other hand, in primary affective disorders, the short-term usefulness of anxiolytics and antidepressants may maximize the patient's ability to participate in other programs. Evidence of this is scant. Therapists' and patients' claims notwithstanding, no drug is available that has a sufficiently predictable and powerful therapeutic effect, combined with adequate safety, to encourage its widespread use as a deterrent to alcohol. The scientific evidence supports only the systematic but selective and carefully monitored use of disulfiram and calcium carbimide, and until proper studies of these drugs are conducted, their use should also be limited. New agents with actions directed at the neurochemical disturbances present in patients with alcohol problems are urgently needed. Even when such agents become available, they too will only be adjuncts to behavioral and social therapies directed at stabilizing all aspects of a patient's function.

We are indebted to Mrs. D. McKenzie and Ms. C. Van Der Giessen for assistance in preparing this manuscript.

| References

1. Mottin JL. Drug-induced attenuation of alcohol consumption: a review and evaluation of claimed, potential or current therapies. Q J Stud Alcohol 1973; 34:444-72.
2. Naranjo CA. A methodological analysis of drug trials with the alcohol sensitizing drugs. In: Peachey JE, Brien JF, eds. Alcohol sensitizing drugs: current status in alcoholism treatment. Toronto: Addiction Research Foundation. (in press).
3. Jones RW, Helrich AR. Treatment of alcoholism by physicians in private practice: a national survey. Q J Stud Alcohol 1972; 33:117-31.
4. Miller WR, Caddy GR. Abstinence and controlled drinking in the treatment of problem drinkers. J Stud Alcohol 1977; 38:986-1003.
5. Pattison EM. A critique of alcoholism treatment concepts: with special reference to abstinence. Q J Stud Alcohol 1966; 27:49-71.
6. Cronkite RC, Moos RH. Evaluating alcoholism treatment programs: an integrated approach. J Consult Clin Psychol 1978; 46:1105-19.
7. Sellers EM, Kalant H. Pharmacotherapy of acute and chronic alcoholism and alcohol withdrawal syndrome. In: Clarke NG, del Guidice J, eds. Principles of psychopharmacology. New York: Academic Press, 1978:721-40.
8. Marchner H, Tottmar O. A comparative study on the effects of disulfiram, cyanamide and 1-aminocyclopropanol on the acetaldehyde metabolism in rats. Acta Pharmacol Toxicol (Copenh) 1978; 43:219-32.
9. Deitrich RA, Erwin VG. Mechanism of the inhibition of aldehyde dehydrogenase *in vivo* by disulfiram and diethyldithiocarbamate. Mol Pharmacol 1971; 7:301-7.
10. Peachey JE, Brien JF, Roach CA, Loomis CW. A comparative review of the pharmacological and toxicological properties of disulfiram and calcium carbimide. J Clin Psychopharmacol 1981; 1:21-6.
11. Eldjarn L. The metabolism of tetraethyl thiuramdisulphide (Antabus, Aversan) in the rat, investigated by means of radioactive sulphur. Scand J Clin Lab Invest 1950; 2:198-201.
12. Fuller RK, Roth HP. Disulfiram for the treatment of alcoholism: an evaluation in 128 men. Ann Intern Med 1979; 90:901-4.

13. Wilson A. Disulfiram implantation in alcoholism treatment: a review. J Stud Alcohol 1975; 36:555-65.

14. Boss D, Sauter A, Cornu F. Abstinenzverhalten und Disulfiram-Plasmakonzentration bei Alkoholikern nach Espéral-Implantation. Schweiz Med Wochenschr 1976; 106:1074-7.

15. Kitson TM. On the probability of implanted disulfiram's causing a reaction to ethanol. J Stud Alcohol 1978; 39:183-6.

16. Guarnaschelli JJ, Zapanta E, Pitts FW. Intracranial hemorrhage associated with the disulfiram-alcohol reaction. Bull Los Angeles Neurol Soc 1972; 37:19-23.

17. Peachey JE, Maglana S, Robinson GM, Hemy M, Brien JF. Cardiovascular changes during the calcium carbimide-ethanol interaction. Clin Pharmacol Ther 1981; 29:40-6.

18. Lemere F. Disulfiram as a sedative in alcoholism. Q J Stud Alcohol 1953; 14:197-9.

19. Heath RG, Nesselhof W Jr, Bishop MP, Byers LW. Behavioral and metabolic changes associated with administration of tetraethylthiuram disulfide (Antabuse). Dis Nerv Syst 1965; 26:99-105.

20. Nasrallah HA. Vulnerability to disulfiram psychosis. West J Med 1979; 130:575-7.

21. Goldstein M, Nakajima K. The effect of disulfiram on catecholamine levels in the brain. J Pharmacol Exp Ther 1967; 157:96-102.

22. Major LF, Lerner P, Ballenger JC, Brown GL, Goodwin FK, Lovenberg W. Dopamine-β-hydroxylase in the cerebrospinal fluid: relationship to disulfiram-induced psychosis. Biol Psychiatry 1979; 14:337-44.

23. Major LF, Murphy DL, Gershon ES, Brown GL. The role of plasma amine oxidase, platelet monoamine oxidase, and red cell catechol-O-methyl transferase in severe behavioral reactions to disulfiram. Am J Psychiatry 1979; 136:679-84.

24. Olesen OV. The influence of disulfiram and calcium carbimide on the serum diphenyl-hydantoin: excretion of HPPH in the urine. Arch Neurol 1967; 16:642-4.

25. Kiørboe E. Phenytoin intoxication during treatment with Antabuse® (disulfiram). Epilepsia 1966; 7:246-9.

26. Smolik J. Pripad umrti pri lecebnem pouziti Antikolu [A case of death after Antikol administration]. Protialkoholicky Obzor 1969; 4:97-100.

27. MacCallum WAG. Drug interactions in alcoholism treatment. Lancet 1969; 1:313.

28. Peachey JE. A review of the clinical use of disulfiram and calcium carbimide in alcoholism treatment. J Clin Psychopharmacol. (in press).

29. Marco CH, Marco JM. Antabuse: medication in exchange for a limited freedom — is it legal? Am J Law Med 1980; 5:295-330.

30. Levy MS, Livingston BL, Collins DM. A clinical comparison of disulfiram and calcium carbimide. Am J Psychiatry 1967; 123:1018-22.

31. Marconi J, Solari G, Gaete S. Comparative clinical study of the effects of disulfiram and calcium carbimide. II. Reaction to alcohol. Q J Stud Alcohol 1961; 22:46-51.

32. Glatt MM. Disulfiram and citrated calcium carbimide in the treatment of alcoholism. J Ment Sci 1959; 105:476-81.

33. Mellor CS, Sims ACP. Citrated calcium carbimide/alcohol reaction — its severity and effectiveness as a deterrent. Br J Addict 1971; 66:123-8.

34. Minto A, Roberts FJ. "Temposil": a new drug in the treatment of alcoholism. J Ment Sci 1968; 106:288-95.

35. Brien JF, Peachey JE, Loomis CW. Calcium carbimide-ethanol interaction. Clin Pharmacol Ther 1980; 27:426-33.

36. *Idem*. Intraindividual variability in the calcium carbimide-ethanol interaction. Eur J Clin Pharmacol 1980; 18:199-205.

37. Peachey JE, Zilm DH, Cappell H. "Burning off the antabuse": fact or fiction? Lancet 1981; 1:943-4.

38. Chevens LCF. Antabuse addiction. Br Med J 1953; 1:1450-1.

39. Reilly TM. Peripheral neuropathy associated with citrated calcium carbimide. Lancet 1976; 1:911-2.

40. Vázquez JJ, Cervera S. Cyanamide-induced liver injury in alcoholics. Lancet 1980; 1:361-2.

41. Vázquez JJ, Pardo-Mindan J. Liver cell injury (bodies similar to Lafora's) in alcoholics treated wtih disulfiram (Antabuse). Histopathology 1979; 3:377-84.

42. Benitz K-F, Kramer AW Jr, Dambach G. Comparative studies on the morphologic effects of calcium carbimide, propylthiouracil, and disulfiram in male rats. Toxicol Appl Pharmacol 1965; 7:128-62.

43. Brunner-Orne M. Evaluation of calcium carbimide in the treatment of alcoholism. J Neuropsychiatry 1962; 3:163-7.

44. Linton PH, Hain JD. Metronidazole in the treatment of alcoholism. Q J Stud Alcohol 1967; 28:544-6.

45. Mendelson JH, Mello NK. Biological concomitants of alcoholism. N Engl J Med 1979; 301:912-91.

46. Wagman AMI, Allen RP. Effects of alcohol ingestion and abstinence on slow wave sleep of alcohol. Adv Exp Med Biol 1977; 59:453-66.

47. Kissin B. Biological investigations in alcohol research. J Stud Alcohol [Suppl] 1979; 8:146-81.

48. Ditman KS. Evaluation of drugs in the treatment of alcoholics. Q J Stud Alcohol [Suppl] 1961; 1:107-16.

49. Rosenberg CM. Drug maintenance in the outpatient treatment of chronic alcoholism. Arch Gen Psychiatry 1974; 30:373-7.

50. Kissin B. The use of psychoactive drugs in the long-term treatment of chronic alcoholics. Ann NY Acad Sci 1975; 252:385-95.

51. Baekeland F. Evaluation of treatment methods in chronic alcoholism. In: Kissin B, Begleiter H, eds. The biology of alcoholism: treatment and rehabilitation of chronic alcoholics. New York: Plenum Press, 1977:385-440.

52. Schou M. Lithium in the treatment of other psychiatric and nonpsychiatric disorders. Arch Gen Psychiatry 1979; 36:856-9.

53. Boland FJ, Stern MH. Suppression by lithium of voluntary alcohol intake in the rat: mechanism of action. Pharmacol Biochem Behav 1980; 12:239-48.

54. Kline NS, Wren JC, Cooper TB, Varga E, Canal O. Evaluation of lithium therapy in chronic and periodic alcoholism. Am J Med Sci 1974; 268:15-22.

55. Merry J, Reynolds CM, Bailey J, Coppen A. Prophylactic treatment of alcoholism by lithium carbonate: a controlled study. Lancet 1976; 2:481-2.

56. Carlsson C. Propranolol in the treatment of alcoholism: a review. Postgrad Med J 1976; 52: Suppl 4:166-7.

57. Smith RF. Five-year field trial of massive nicotine acid therapy of alcoholics in Michigan. J Orthomol Psychiatry 1974; 3:327-31.

58. Meisch RA. Ethanol self-administration: infra-human studies. In: Thompson T, Dews PB, eds. Advances in behavioral pharmacology. Vol. 1. New York: Academic Press, 1977:36-84.

59. Amit Z, Levitan DE, Brown ZE, Sutherland EA. Catecholaminergic involvement in alcohol's rewarding properties: implications for a treatment model for alcoholics. Adv Exp Med Biol 1977; 85A:486-94.
60. Davis WM, Werner TE, Smith SG. Reinforcement with intragastric infusions of ethanol: blocking effect of FLA 57. Pharmacol Biochem Behav 1979; 11:545-8.
61. Naranjo CA, Cappell H, Sellers EM. Pharmacological control of alcohol consumption: tactics for the identification and testing of new drugs. Addict Behav 1981; 6:261-9.
62. Myers RD. Psychopharmacology of alcohol. Annu Rev Pharmacol Toxicol 1978; 18:125-44.
63. Rockman GE, Amit Z, Carr G, Brown ZW, Ögren S-O. Attenuation of ethanol intake by 5-hydroxytryptamine uptake blockade in laboratory rats. I. Involvement of brain 5-hydroxytryptamine in the mediation of the positive reinforcing of ethanol. Arch Int Pharmacodyn Ther 1979; 241:245-59.
64. Myers RD, Melchior CL. Alcohol drinking: abnormal intake caused by tetrahydro-papaveroline in brain. Science 1977; 196:554-6.

Correspondence

Drugs to Decrease Alcohol Consumption*

To the Editor:

In reference to the paper by Sellars et al. in the November 19 issue,† the basic paradigm for the use of disulfiram is not conditioned aversion. With currently accepted methods of disulfiram administration, the successfully treated patient will never have a disulfiram-alcohol reaction. A close analogy to the mode of action of disulfiram is the placebo effect. It is the patient's expectation of a pharmacologic reaction that is in fact the therapeutic effect. This anticipation of an unpleasant experience seems not only to assist many patients in avoiding impulsive drinking but also to facilitate the dismissal of thoughts of drinking, freeing the mind for more positive activity. Because of this mode of action, controlled, double-blind studies have limited meaning, since the drug and place-bo would be expected to have the same effect.

I agree with Sellars et al. about the importance of appropriate selection and monitoring of patients receiving disulfiram therapy. I believe that the authors have overemphasized the toxicity of this drug, however. That side effects and idiosyncratic reactions occur is well documented, but the frequency of reports of serious reactions is certainly low for a drug that has been in relatively widespread use for 33 years.

I find that the proposed schedule for examination and laboratory testing of patients on disulfiram therapy is markedly in excess of usual practice and unwarranted by reports in the scientific literature. The proposed protocol would be

*Originally published on March 25, 1982 (306:747-748).

†Sellars EM, Naranjo CA, Peachey JE. Drugs to decrease alcohol consumption. N Engl J Med 1981; 305:1255-62.

suitable for an investigational drug, but as a standard of practice it would cause further unnecessary increases in health-care costs.

DONALD M. GRAGG, M.D., PH.D.
Kaiser–Permanente Medical Center
Los Angeles, CA 90027

To the Editor:

Sellars et al. provide an interesting overview of drugs used to decrease alcohol consumption. Unfortunately, they convey a somewhat pessimistic view of the use of existing psychopharmacologic techniques to modify drinking behavior. Both antidepressants and lithium hold greater promise for some alcoholics than the review article implies.

Clinically important depressions occur in 8.6 to 25 per cent of persons diagnosed as alcoholics.[1,2] The latter figure refers to those with primary depression and secondary alcoholism diagnosed in a general population. In over 90 per cent of patients with major nondelusional depression, relief of the depression is achieved with adequate doses of imipramine.[3] These data offer the potential for effective treatment of a considerable number of alcoholics with primary affective disorders. The dexamethasone-suppression test for diagnosis of endogenous depression during periods of sobriety should further aid physicians in delineating this neglected subgroup of patients.[4]

The use of lithium in the treatment of primary alcoholism also remains an open question. Rather than assuming that differences between lithium and placebo groups disappear because of a high dropout rate, one might consider that high dropout rates are a common problem in most alcohol studies. Such dropout rates, in fact, would probably make it difficult to demonstrate the efficacy of penicillin or insulin.

JOHN C. KUEHNLE, M.D.
McLean Hospital
Belmont, MA 02178

1. Keeler MH, Taylor CI, Miller WC. Are all recently detoxified alcoholics depressed? Am J Psychiatry 1979; 136:586-8.
2. Weissman MM, Myers JK. Clinical depression in alcoholism. Am J Psychiatry 1980; 137:372-3.
3. Glassman AH, Perel JM, Shostak M, Kantor SJ, Fleiss JL. Clinical implications of imipramine plasma levels for depressive illness. Arch Gen Psychiatry 1977; 34:197-204.
4. Carroll BV, Feinberg M, Greden JF, et al. A specific laboratory test for the diagnosis of melancholia. Arch Gen Psychiatry 1981; 38:15-22.

To the Editor:

I would like to point out an omission in the list of alcohol-sensitizing compounds in the article by Sellars et al. The general class of monoamine oxidase inhibitors should be included. They have general enzyme-inhibiting properties that can interfere with the detoxification of many substances, including ethanol.[1] A member of this class that should be mentioned specifically is procarbazine. By virtue of its ability to inhibit acetaldehyde dehydrogenase, this drug may produce erythematous facies, headache, and diaphoresis with alcohol ingestion.[2] This is important when one is counseling patients receiving cancer chemotherapy who wish to drink alcohol.

MARY A. SIMMONDS, M.D.
Pennsylvania State University College of Medicine
Hershey, PA 17033

1. Jarvik ME. Drugs used in the treatment of psychiatric disorders. In: Goodman LS, Gilman A, eds. The pharmacologic basis of therapeutics. 4th ed. New York: MacMillan, 1970:184.
2. Spivack SD. Procarbazine. Ann Intern Med 1981; 81:795-800.

The above letters were referred to the authors of the article in question, who offer the following reply:

To the Editor:
A recent controlled study found no differences between pharmacologic doses of disulfiram (250 or 500 mg per day) and nonpharmacologic doses (1 mg per day),[1] suggesting that the threat of an aversive reaction has as much therapeutic effect as the reaction itself. In our experience and that of other workers,[1,2] alcoholics frequently drink while taking disulfiram or shortly after discontinuing the drug. Thus, a sizable proportion of patients have an aversive reaction. Consequently, the small therapeutic effect of disulfiram is due to both conditioned avoidance (because of the fear of an aversive reaction) and conditioned aversion (because of the actual experience of an aversive reaction). More important is the fact that disulfiram use is associated with risks considerably greater than those associated with treatment with a placebo. In addition to the disulfiram-acetaldehyde reaction, a wide range of toxic effects are associated with the parent compound, its metabolites, and possibly acetaldehyde.[3] No systematic studies of the frequency and determinants of such toxicity are available. Since the full extent of disulfiram toxicity is not known, and since its efficacy is questionable, we cannot acept Dr. Gragg's suggestion that "usual practice" is the appropriate standard of care. The full assessment of patients before they enter therapy and at monthly follow-up visits is mandatory.[4] Frequent follow-up visits may incidentally serve as important contributors to treatment by preventing relapse.

A low dropout rate among patients receiving treatment for alcoholism (including drug therapy) is itself a good measure of therapeutic efficacy.[5] In fact, the relation between a high compliance rate and a favorable outcome of treatment in alcoholics is well documented.[1,6] Exclusion of dropouts, as suggested by Dr. Kuehnle, will introduce a profound bias in results, because regardless of the treatment, subjects who comply with therapy are destined to have a substantially better outcome than noncompliant patients.[7]

We agree with Dr. Simmonds that the monoamine oxidase inhibitors should be included in the list of inhibitors of acetaldehyde dehydrogenase.

E. M. SELLERS, M.D., PH.D.
C. A. NARANJO, M.D.
J. E. PEACHEY, M.D., M.SC.
Addiction Research Foundation
Toronto, ON M5S 2S1, Canada

1. Fuller RK, Roth HP. Disulfiram for the treatment of alcoholism: an evaluation in 128 men. Ann Intern Med 1979; 90:901-4.
2. Wilson A, Davidson WJ, Blanchard R. Disulfiram implantation: a trial using placebo implants and two types of controls. J Stud Alcohol 1980; 41:429-36.
3. Peachey JE, Naranjo CA. The use of disulfiram and other alcohol-sensitizing drugs in the treatment of alcoholism. In: Israel Y, Glaser FB, Kalant H, Popham RE, Schmidt W, Smart R, eds. Research advances in alcohol and drug problems. Vol. VII. New York: Plenum Press. (in press).
4. Sellers EM, Naranjo CA, Peachey JE. Drugs to decrease alcohol consumption. N Engl J Med 1981; 305:1255-62.
5. Sellers EM, Cappell HD, Marshman JA. Compliance in the control of alcohol abuse. In: Hayes RB, Taylor DW, Sackett DL, eds. Compliance in health care. Baltimore: Johns Hopkins Press, 1979:223-43.
6. Baekeland F, Lundwall L. Dropping out of treatment: a critical review. Psychol Bull 1975; 82:738-83.
7. Feinstein AR. Clinical biostatistics. XXX. Biostatistical problems in compliance bias. Clin Pharmacol Ther 1974; 16:846-57.

Metoclopramide

Konrad Schulze-Delrieu, M.D.

IN 1964 Justin-Besançon and his co-workers described a new compound that depressed the vomiting center and stimulated gut motility.[1] Metoclopramide (Fig. 1) (*meth*oxy*chl*o*ro*procain*amide* [Reglan]) resulted from efforts to alter the procaine molecule so that its antiemetic properties would equal those of the phenothiazines.[1,2] Like the phenothiazines, metoclopramide acts on the brain by blocking dopamine receptors: it induces extrapyramidal symptoms and stimulates prolactin secretion but has at best weak antipsychotic properties. Since metoclopramide and its congeners sulpiride, sultopride, and tiapride differ in some clinical and pharmacologic respects from other antipsychotic drugs, it has been suggested that these substituted benzamides act on a specific subpopulation of cerebral dopamine receptors.[3]

Metoclopramide can be shown to block some actions of dopamine on tissues of the alimentary canal, but many of its peripheral effects are explained more easily by alternative mechanisms. In contrast to the phenothiazines, which have anticholinergic effects, metoclopramide has powerful cholinergic stimulant effects. Curiously, its cholinergic effects are largely restricted to the musculature of the proximal gut and require some background cholinergic activity.[4]

The actions of metoclopramide are unique and so diverse that they have generated hopes for improved diagnostic and therapeutic measures in many fields of medicine.[2] The increased prolactin secretion caused by this drug has been suggested as a means to test pituitary function or to improve lactation in the postpartum period.[5,6] Its effect on gastric motility is considered a bonus in attempts to treat nausea and vomiting, particularly in clinical settings with a threat of aspiration.[2,7] Metoclopramide has been used to improve the effectiveness of oral medication when the medication or the patient's underlying condition slows gastric emptying.[2,8] Symptoms of reflux esophagitis, gastric stasis, and postoperative ileus have been improved by metoclopramide.[9-11] It has even been tried against hiccups, vertigo, and orthostatic hypotension.[2,12] In the United States the use of metoclopramide remains restricted to two diagnostic indications (as of January 1981). Single intravenous injections may be given to adults and children in whom attempts to intubate the duodenum have failed or in whom delayed

From the Department of Medicine, University of Iowa, Iowa City.

Supported by a grant (AM 00519-03) from the National Institute of Arthritis, Metabolism, and Digestive Diseases.

Originally published on July 2, 1981 (305:28-33).

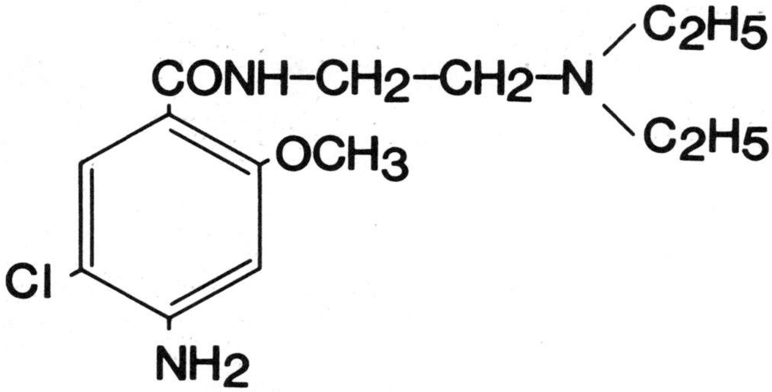

$$CONH-CH_2-CH_2-N \underset{C_2H_5}{\overset{C_2H_5}{<}}$$

OCH₃

Cl

NH₂

Figure 1. Structural Formula for Metoclopramide.

This configuration results when a 2-methoxy group and a 5-chloro group are added to a molecule of procainamide. Metoclopramide is the prototype of the selective dopamine antagonists called substituted benzamides.

gastric emptying has rendered the radiographic examination of the stomach and intestines difficult. Parenteral metoclopramide is used throughout Europe and Japan for intrapartum and emergency anesthesia. Oral metoclopramide is used for syndromes of gastric stasis and reflux esophagitis.

Gastrokinetic and Prokinetic Properties

The terms "gastrokinetic" and "prokinetic" have been proposed to describe the effects of drugs like metoclopramide on movements of the walls and of the luminal contents in the proximal gut. The gastrokinetic effects of metoclopramide consist of an increase of the resting muscle tension, most notably as increased pressure in the lower esophageal sphincter and the gastric fundus; an increase in the size of the contractions of the peristaltic ring in the esophagus, gastric antrum, and small intestine; and an increased coordination of mechanical activity of various gut segments, as exemplified by relaxation of the pylorus and duodenum during contraction of the stomach.[4,13-18] All these gastrokinetic actions are likely to contribute to the prokinetic effects of metoclopramide: hastened esophageal clearance, accelerated gastric emptying of liquids and solids, and shortened transit through the small bowel. The increased resting tension should promote aboral movement of luminal contents, by preventing reflux and by decreasing the luminal diameter of the proximal gut.[19] The increased amplitude of ring contractions should improve the sweeping effect of peristalsis. The increased coordination should facilitate flow over long segments of gut and across organ boundaries.

The gastrokinetic and prokinetic effects of metoclopramide resemble the fronts of mechanical activity that spread periodically over the gut during fasting and that are credited with clearing residual contents.[16] These "housekeeper" fronts are thought to originate in some central nervous center, and they are suppressed by food and some diseases.[16] Perhaps metoclopramide simply interferes with such central suppression[1,17] and therefore elicits "housekeeper" activity whenever this activity is not already present. The impact that metoclopramide has on gut motility is known to vary with the degree of mechanical activity preceding its administration,[4,18] but identity of its motor effects with the "housekeeper" activity has not been established.

An alternative explanation for the gastrokinetic effect of this drug is enhancement of the peristaltic reflex.[4] Distention of the gut generates increased resting tension in longitudinal muscle and propagated ring contraction in circular muscle. By lowering the threshold for the reflex,[20] metoclopramide may produce increased motor activity and propulsion through a chain of local reflexes.

Dopamine Antagonism

The antiemetic properties of metoclopramide result from its antagonism of cerebral dopamine receptors and from its effect on the stomach. Apomorphine, hydergine, and levodopa — after decarboxylation to dopamine — all excite dopamine receptors in the chemoreceptor trigger zone, and dopamine antagonists such as metoclopramide block their effect.[2,3] In the stomach, immobility, dilatation, and reverse motility accompany the vomiting reflex. Metoclopramide prevents the gastric immobility produced by small doses of apomorphine and seems to reinforce an antegrade motility gradient in the gut.[4,13] Dopamine decreases the size of esophageal-ring contractions, relaxes the proximal stomach, and reduces gastric secretion. Metoclopramide blocks these inhibitory effects of dopamine.[14] Nevertheless, the role of dopamine in the peripheral control of gut motility and secretion seems minor, and it is likely that metoclopramide's therapeutic activity resides largely in its cholinergic actions.[4]

Cholinergic Properties

Most actions of metoclopramide on gut motility have also been observed with cholinergic drugs such as bethanechol, and are blocked by atropine and opioids but not by vagotomy.[21,22] There is evidence that metoclopramide sensitizes gut muscle to the action of acetylcholine[23]; this effect explains why metoclopramide, unlike conventional cholinergic compounds, requires background cholinergic activity to be effective. Postsynaptic activity results also from the capacity of metoclopramide to release acetylcholine from cholinergic nerve terminals.[24] The density of cholinergic innervation is higher in the musculature of the proximal gut than in that of the distal gut. Local variations in cholinergic control may explain the apparent paradox that in intact subjects metoclopramide is most active on the stomach, but that in excised human tissue, it is most active on the colon.[15,23] Perhaps even its relative ineffectiveness on other visceral muscle and glands can be explained on similar grounds.

Cholinergic mechanisms seem to be responsible for most excitatory motor phenomena in the gut. Lack of cholinergic stimulation accounts for many abnormalities of the vagotomized stomach, and failure of vagal cholinergic stimulation has also been considered responsible for the occurrence of reflux in some patients with idiopathic esophagitis.[25] Metoclopramide should therefore be useful in all motor abnormalities of the gut in which cholinergic activity is diminished but not abolished.

The antiemetic and gastrokinetic effects of metoclopramide have frequently overshadowed consideration of its other properties. Under certain conditions smooth muscle from the bladder, the colon, the biliary tract, and the vascular system will respond to metoclopramide.[26] The observation that metoclopramide helps in the passage of kidney stones by restoring ureteral peristalsis needs confirmation.[27] Metoclopramide has quinidine-like antiarrhythmic properties and local anesthetic effects.[28]

Clinical Uses

Nausea and Vomiting

In various conditions associated with nausea and vomiting, metoclopramide has been found to be equal or superior to the established antiemetics prochlorperazine and trimethobenzamide.[2,7,29] It is particularly useful in anesthesia for emergencies and for labor and delivery, in which its gastrokinetic effect may reduce the risk of aspiration of gastric contents. It should be remembered, however, that the usefulness of metoclopramide may be diminished in anesthesia, because of the drug's short duration of action and the possibility of prior administration of atropine.[2,30] Early use of metoclopramide to prevent the nausea and vomiting associated with chemotherapy gave disappointing results, but according to some pilot studies, doses of up to 1 to 2 mg per kilogram of body weight may be effective.[31]

Diagnostic Radiography and Intubation

The originators of metoclopramide first suggested that it might be helpful in diagnostic radiology. Relaxation of the pylorus and duodenal bulb is desirable during examination of the upper gastrointestinal tract. Unlike atropine and glucagon, which are commonly used for this purpose, metoclopramide has the advantage of shortening the duration of small-bowel transit, thus saving time and reducing radiation exposure.[17,32]

Metoclopramide reduces the time required to pass tubes into the small bowel, at least in normal persons.[33] It has been used during endoscopy, particularly when blood and other gastric contents have restricted the visual field, but this use is not covered by FDA regulations.

Gastroesophageal Reflux and Esophagitis

Testing of metoclopramide in reflux was motivated by the discovery that the drug increased the resting pressure of the lower esophageal sphincter. Decreased resting pressure in this organ has probably been overrated as a factor in reflux. Changes in salivation, swallowing, esophageal clearance, gastric emptying, and relaxation of the lower esophageal sphincter may all be important, and metoclopramide is known to influence at least some of these mechanisms favorably. In patients with chronic gastroesophageal reflux, metoclopramide reduces the incidence of heartburn more than standard medical management (e.g., elevation of the head of the bed, loose clothes, weight reduction, and regular use of antacids). A few patients with esophagitis have complete clinical remission while taking metoclopramide, and the remission seems to outlast the period of drug administration by a few weeks.[9,10]

More effective palliation of heartburn is, however, only one of the goals in treatment of reflux esophagitis. Furthermore, it may be argued that symptomatic benefits relate to metoclopramide's central effects, since it remains to be demonstrated that its gastrokinetic effects lead to an objective improvement of esophagitis. In a recent study, bethanechol was found to lessen the inflammatory changes in the esophagus that are due to reflux.[34] It is to be hoped that metoclopramide will also be shown to promote healing of esophageal lesions. Still, the complications of gastroesophageal reflux take years or decades to develop, and temporary suppression of reflux esophagitis is no guarantee against eventual formation of strictures, epithelial metaplasia, and neoplasia. Operative intervention in the form of fundoplication decreases or at least postpones these risks, and standard medical treatment does not.[35]

Prevention of late complications from a condition that is often lifelong calls for the design of treatment modes that are effective, safe, and inexpensive. Intermittent treatment of symptomatic exacerbations may be sound: the inflammatory changes of reflux depress esophageal motor activity, and a drug that counteracts reflux may help to break the cycle in which damage from reflux perpetuates reflux.

Gastric Motor Failure

Testing of metoclopramide has revealed that serious impairment of the ability of the stomach to handle food is a comparatively common disorder and that it is not restricted to the occasional patient with advanced diabetes or vagotomy. Metoclopramide relieves but does not abolish early satiety, epigastric discomfort, nausea, and vomiting in patients unable to digest solid food, as demonstrated by delayed emptying of barium from the stomach when this radiotracer is given after a meal of hamburger. This treatment seems to be effective irrespective of the cause (vagotomy, diabetes, gastritis, gastric ulcers, or preceding viral illness) of the gastric motor failure.[11]

Testing of metoclopramide in patients with gastric motor failure was prompted by the finding that the drug accelerated the rate of gastric evacuation.

Gastric stasis, however, is not the only mechanical abnormality of the stomach after vagotomy or in diabetes (Table 1). Failure of fundic relaxation results in poor storage capacity and may be accompanied by the precipitous emptying of fluids called dumping. Absence of antral grinding or, alternatively, of the "housekeeper" activity has been considered responsible for delayed evacuation of solids and recurrent bezoar formation.[16,36] An ideal drug would restore grinding activity, storage capacity, and "housekeeper" activity to a failing stomach rather than merely speed up its evacuation. That speedy evacuation alone may cause problems is indicated by the poor absorption of digoxin when it is given with metoclopramide.[37]

Some investigators have found metoclopramide to be superior to carbachol in treating gastric stasis after vagotomy, and others have found it to be ineffective without bethanechol.[38,39] Conflicting results may be due to differences in the timing, route, and amount of drug given. Blood levels of the drug that are sufficient for gastrokinetic effects have not been achieved in many normal volunteers receiving 10 mg by mouth,[40] and these levels may be further depressed if the drug is retained in the stomach.[4]

Differences in the severity and the duration of the gastric abnormality are another source of problems. Drug effects are typically measured by the scoring of symptoms such as bloating, epigastric discomfort, and nausea. These scores bear little relation to the severity of gastric motor failure. A classification system is needed that takes into account pathophysiologic consequences and other prognostic features of these failures. Otherwise, it will remain unclear whether metoclopramide is of symptomatic benefit only or whether it is potent enough to prevent weight loss, bezoar formation, and gastric dilatation in severely affected patients.

Drug Absorption, Metabolism, and Excretion

Metoclopramide is rapidly absorbed from the gut, and peak plasma concentrations are achieved within 40 to 120 minutes. When the drug is given by mouth, its bioavailability has been found to vary from 30 to 100 per cent. The majority of patients achieve therapeutic ranges of 40 to 80 ng per milliliter of plasma after taking a 10-mg tablet before meals, but occasionally it is difficult to establish the proper dose and timing of the oral drug.

Metoclopramide is weakly bound to serum proteins and is rapidly and widely distributed in most tissues. Its plasma half-life is about four hours; most of it (80 per cent) is excreted in the urine unchanged or as the sulfate and the glucuronide conjugates of nonmetabolized drug, within 24 hours.[4] Impairment of renal function prolongs the half-life.[40] Renal and hepatic failure were present in one patient who died with dystonic reactions from metoclopramide.[41]

Side Effects, Contraindications, and Toxicity

Metoclopramide is a comparatively safe drug. Overdoses and antipsychotic doses up to 100 times the recommended dose have been tolerated without serious side

TABLE 1. Effects of Gastric Motor Failure and Metoclopramide.

Mechanical Failure	In Gastric Motor Failure	Mechanism	After Metoclopramide	Mechanism
Fundic pressure	Increased	Failure of vagal inhibition	Increased	Blockage of inhibitory mechanisms
Antral contractions (amplitude)	Decreased	Failure of cholinergic excitation	Increased	Cholinergic activity
Antroduodenal coordination	Decreased	Unknown	Increased	Unknown
Pyloric pressure	Unknown	—	Controversial	—
Response to cholinergic drugs	Normal	Cholinergic	Increased	Cholinergic sensitization
Retention of solid contents	Increased	Inefficient grinding or absence of "house-keeper" activity	Decreased	Pyloric relaxation, increased peristalsis, or restored fasting "housekeeper" activity
Dumping of gastric contents	Increased	Decreased storage capacity	Unknown	—
Chyme formation	Possibly decreased	Poor antral peristalsis	Unknown	—

effects. The most common side effects arise in the central nervous system and include nervousness, somnolence, and dystonic reactions.[2] Akathisia, a feeling of unease and restlessness of the lower limbs, seems to be related to peak plasma concentrations over 100 ng per milliliter.[40] Drowsiness may be of some benefit when metoclopramide is being used as an antiemetic and when diagnostic procedures are being performed, but may be harmful when alertness is required. The concomitant use of other drugs with sedative effects is therefore not advisable. Also, because of possible aggravation of extrapyramidal symptoms, metoclopramide should not be used in patients receiving phenothiazines, butyrophenones, or thioxanthines. Dyskinesias, including trismus, torticollis, facial spasms, opisthotonos, and oculogyric crisis, occur particularly in children and typically respond immediately to administration of diazepam or benztropine or remit within a day or so on drug withdrawal.

Metoclopramide is likely to cross the placenta and to be excreted in milk; its safety for the growing fetus and the nursing child has not been established. Gastric lavage or induction of vomiting are recommended for overdosage. Drugs such as benztropine may be needed to suppress dystonic reactions. Metoclopramide blocks the dopamine inhibition of aldosterone secretion,[42] and the possibility of sodium retention and hypokalemia should be considered in patients with edema. Current concern about prolonged use of metoclopramide stems from its effect on prolactin secretion. Galactorrhea and menstrual disorders have been reported to occur during drug administration but are typically reversible on drug withdrawal.[43] The possible role of prolactin in breast cancers, pituitary tumors, and cardiac arrhythmias remains a threat, however.

Dosage and Administration

Metoclopramide is available in the United States as Reglan Injectable (A.H. Robins Co.), a solution of the monohydrochloride monohydrate of metoclopramide at a concentration of 5 mg per milliliter of solution. The cost recently quoted to our pharmacy is $2.05 per 2-ml ampule.

A dose of 10 to 20 mg should be injected intravenously (slowly, in order to avoid anxiety) shortly before attempts at duodenal intubation or contrast examination of the gut. The dosage in children should be calculated at 0.1 mg of drug per kilogram of body weight.

Conclusions

Metoclopramide is a substituted benzamide with antiemetic and gastrokinetic effects. Central and peripheral effects combine to make it a particularly useful antiemetic in conditions in which nausea and vomiting are due to gastric stasis or in which residual gastric contents increase the risk of aspiration. The gastrokinetic effects of metoclopramide are also helpful in administering oral drugs for whose effectiveness prompt gastric emptying is critical, as well as in lessening symptoms related to reflux esophagitis and gastric motor failure. This agent's effect on the prognosis of these disorders is unclear, however. To date, the FDA has approved only the use of parenteral metoclopramide for diagnostic intubation and radiographic examination of the proximal gut.

References

1. Justin-Besançon L, Laville C, Thominet M. Le métoclopramide et ses homologues: introduction à leur étude biologique. C R Acad Sci (Paris) 1964; 258:4384-6.
2. Pinder RM, Brogden RN, Sawyer PR, Speight TM, Avery GS. Metoclopramide: a review of its pharmacological properties and clinical use. Drugs 1976; 12:81-131.
3. Jenner P, Marsden CD. The substituted benzamides — a novel class of dopamine antagonists. Life Sci 1979; 25:479-85.
4. Schulze-Delrieu K. Metoclopramide. Gastroenterology 1979; 77:768-79.
5. Guzmán V, Toscano G, Canales ES, Zárate A. Improvement of defective lactation by using oral metoclopramide. Acta Obstet Gynecol Scand 1979; 58:53-5.
6. Vázquez-Matute L, Canales ES, Alger M, Zárate A. Clinical use of metoclopramide test in the diagnosis of women with hyperprolactinemia. Horm Res 1979; 10:207-12.
7. McGarry JM. A double-blind comparison of the anti-emetic effect during labour of metoclopramide and perphenazine. Br J Anaesth 1971; 43:613-5.
8. Nimmo WS. Drugs, diseases and altered gastric emptying. Clin Pharmacokinet 1976; 1:189-203.
9. Johnson AG. Controlled trial of metoclopramide in the treatment of flatulent dyspepsia. Br Med J 1971; 2:25-6.
10. McCallum RW, Ippoliti AF, Cooney C, Sturdevant RAL. A controlled trial of metoclopramide in symptomatic gastroesophageal reflux. N Engl J Med 1977; 296:354-7.
11. Perkel MS, Moore C, Hersh T, Davidson ED. Metoclopramide therapy in patients with delayed gastric emptying: a randomized, double-blind study. Am J Dig Dis Sci 1979; 24:662-6.
12. Kuchel O, Buu NT, Gutkowska J, Genest J. Treatment of severe orthostatic hypotension by metoclopramide. Ann Intern Med 1980; 93:841-3.
13. Ramsbottom N, Hunt JN. Studies of the effect of metoclopramide and apomorphine on gastric emptying and secretion in man. Gut 1970; 11:989-93.
14. Valenzuela JE. Dopamine as a possible neurotransmitter in gastric relaxation. Gastroenterology 1976; 71:1019-22.
15. Eisner M. Effect of metoclopramide on gastrointestinal motility in man: a manometric study. Am J Dig Dis 1971; 16:409-19.
16. Malagelada J-R, Rees WDW, Mazzotta LJ, Go VLW. Gastric motor abnormalities in diabetic and postvagotomy gastroparesis: effect of metoclopramide and bethanechol. Gastroenterology 1980; 78:286-93.
17. Justin-Besançon OL, Grivaux N, Wattez E. L'épreuve au métoclopramide en radiologie digestive. Bull Soc Med Hop (Paris) 1964; 115:721-6.
18. Johnson AG. Gastroduodenal motility and synchronization. Postgrad Med J 1973; Suppl 4:29-33.

19. Matuchansky C, Huet PM, Mary JY, Rambaud JC, Bernier JJ. Effects of cholecysto-kinin and metoclopramide on jejunal movements of water and electrolytes on the transit time of luminal fluid in man. Eur J Clin Invest 1972; 2:169-75.

20. Okwuasaba FK, Hamilton JT. The effect of metoclopramide on intestinal muscle responses and the peristaltic reflex in vitro. Can J Physiol Pharmacol 1976; 54:393-404.

21. Jacoby HI, Brodie DA. Gastrointestinal actions of metoclopramide: an experimental study. Gastroenterology 1967; 52:676-84.

22. Stadaas J, Aune S. The effect of metoclopramide (Primperan®) on gastric motility before and after vagotomy in man. Scand J Gastroenterol 1971; 6:17-21.

23. Eisner M. Gastrointestinal effects of metoclopramide in man: in vitro experiments with human smooth muscle preparations. Br Med J 1968; 4:679-80.

24. Hay AM, Man WK. Effect of metoclopramide on guinea pig stomach: critical depend-ence on intrinsic stores of acetylcholine. Gastroenterology 1979; 76:492-6.

25. Heatley RV, Collins RJ, James PD, Atkinson M. Vagal function in relation to gastro-oesophageal reflux and associated motility changes. Br Med J 1980; 280:755-7.

26. Marmo E, Di Mezza F, Imperatore A, Di Giacomon S. Metoclopramid und die Muskulatur von Ösophagus, Magen, Darm, Milz, Trachea, Gallen- und harnblase: Untersuchungen in vitro. Arzneimittelforsch 1970; 20:18-27.

27. Schelin S. Observations of the effect of metoclopramide (Primperan®) on the human ureter: a preliminary communication. Scand J Urol Nephrol 1979; 13:79-82.

28. Cheymol G, Mouillé P. Étude des effects anti-arythmisants de dérivés du métoclopra-mide. Arch Int Pharmacodyn Ther 1975; 215:150-9.

29. Dobkin AB, Evers W, Israel JS. Double-blind evaluation of metoclopramide (MK 745, Sinemet®), trimethobenzamide (Tigan®) and a placebo as postanaesthetic anti-emetics following methoxyflurane anaesthesia. Can Anaesth Soc J 1968; 15:80-91.

30. Assaf RAE, Clarke RSJ, Dundee JW, Samuel IO. Studies of drugs given before anaesthesia. XXIV. Metoclopramide with morphine and pethidine. Br J Anaesth 1974; 46:514-9.

31. Kahn T, Elias EG, Mason GR. A single dose of metoclopramide in the control of vomiting from cis-dichlorodiammineplatinum(II) in man. Cancer Treat Rep 1978; 62:1106-7.

32. Pearson MC, Edwards D, Tate A, et al. Comparison of the effects of oral and intrave-nous metoclopramide on the small bowel. Postgrad Med J 1973; Suppl 4:47-50.

33. Arvanitakis C, Gonzalez G, Rhodes JB. The role of metoclopramide in peroral jejunal biopsy: a controlled randomized trial. Am J Dig Dis 1976; 21:880-4.

34. Thanik KD, Chey WY, Shah AN, Gutierrez JG. Reflux esophagitis: effect of oral bethanechol on symptoms and endoscopic findings. Ann Intern Med 1980; 92:805-8.

35. Behar J, Sheahan DG, Biancani P, Spiro HM, Storer EH. Medical and surgical management of reflux esophagitis: a 38-month report on a prospective clinical trial. N Engl J Med 1975; 293:263-8.

36. Schulze-Delrieu K. The study of gastric stasis: static no longer. Gastroenterology 1980; 78:867-80.

37. Johnson BF, O'Grady J, Bye C. The influence of digoxin particle size on absorption of digoxin and the effect of propantheline and metoclopramide. Br J Clin Pharmacol 1978; 5:465-7.

38. McCelland RN, Horton JW. Relief of acute, persistent postvagotomy atony by meto-clopramide. Ann Surg 1978; 188:439-45.

39. Sheiner HJ, Catchpole BN. Drug therapy for postvagotomy gastric stasis. Br J Surg 1967; 63:608-11.

40. Bateman DN, Davies DS. Pharmacokinetics of metoclopramide. Lancet 1979; 1: 166.

41. Reasbeck PG, Hossenbocus A. Death following dystonic reaction to oral metoclopramide. Br J Clin Pract 1979; 33:31-3.

42. Carey RM, Thorner MO, Ortt EM. Effects of metoclopramide and bromocriptine on the renin-angiotensin-aldosterone system in man: dopaminergic control of aldosterone. J Clin Invest 1979; 63:727-35.

43. Aono T, Shioji T, Kinugasa T, Onishi T, Kurachi K. Clinical and endocrinological analyses of patients with galactorrhea and menstrual disorders due to sulpiride or metoclopramide. J Clin Endocrinol Metab 1978; 47:675-80.

Correspondence

Metoclopramide*

To the Editor:
Schulze-Delrieu[1] has described the following initial FDA-approved use for injectable metoclopramide: to facilitate small-bowel intubation when necessary, and to stimulate gastric emptying and intestinal transit of barium when delayed emptying interferes with radiologic examination of the upper gastrointestinal tract.

More recently, however (on December 30, 1980), the FDA approved the use of metoclopramide tablets for the relief of symptoms associated with acute and chronic gastric motor failure due to diabetic gastroparesis. The role of gastric dysfunction in patients with diabetes has achieved renewed prominence since Aylett demonstrated an inverse correlation between blood sugar levels and gastric motility.[2]

It seems appropriate to update the Schulze-Delrieu article by pointing out that New Drug Applications are now undergoing review by the FDA for the use of high-dose intravenous metoclopramide in the prophylaxis of vomiting associated with cancer-chemotherapy regimens that include the highly emetogenic cisplatin, and also as a short-term adjunct to conventional therapy for gastroesophageal reflux disease when other methods of treatment have failed.

It is evident that the potential additional indications fall well within the drug's broad pharmacologic profile, which has been so amply documented by Schulze-Delrieu.

S.A. TISDALE, JR., M.D.
JAMES H. BRINCKERHOFF, B.S.
A.H. Robins Company
Richmond, VA 23220

*Originally published on October 29, 1981 (305:1093).

1. Schulze-Delrieu K. Drug therapy: metoclopramide. N Engl J Med 1981; 305:28-33.
2. Aylett P. Gastric emptying and change of blood glucose level, as affected by glucagon and insulin. Clin Sci 1962; 22:171-8.

To the Editor:

One aspect that was ignored in the otherwise complete review on metoclopramide by Dr. Schulze-Delrieu is the effect of the "gastrokinetic" action of this compound on the availability of oral medications given at the same time.

Since acidic drugs are absorbed at the stomach level or in the first portion of the duodenum, it is likely that any accelerated gastric emptying will decrease the bioavailability of these drugs. This phenomenon has been demonstrated for penicillin V[1] and digoxin,[2] but not for isoniazid,[3] a basic compound.

This potential "side effect" should be kept in mind when one gives oral medications with metoclopramide.

MARC H. BLANC, M.D.
University Hospital
1211 Geneva 4, Switzerland

1. Blanc MH, Berthoud S, Rudhardt M, et al. Pénicilline V et interactions médicamenteuses. Praxis 1973; 62:861-7.
2. Maaminen V, Apajalahti A, Melin J, et al. Altered absorption of digoxin in patients given propantheline and metoclopramide. Lancet 1973; 1:398-400.
3. Savio E, Pontiggia P. Metoclopramide e assorbimemto intestinale di isoniazide. Ann Med Sondalo 1965; 13:1-6.

Parkinsonism and Tardive Dyskinesia Associated with Long-Term Metoclopramide Therapy*

To the Editor:

Dr. Schulze-Delrieu has recently reviewed the status of metoclopramide (July 2 issue).[1] He notes that the drug is now approved only for limited, single-dose intravenous use in the United States. Metoclopramide has been available for oral use in Canada since 1974 and was released much earlier in England.

In 1978, the first reports of parkinsonism and chronic tardive dyskinesia secondary to long-term metoclopramide therapy appeared.[2,3]

Over the past three years in our movement-disorders clinic, metoclopramide-induced parkinsonism and tardive dyskinesia have become frequent diagnoses. Detailed observations and two years of follow-up have been documented in 14 patients.[4]

Twelve patients (average age, 67 years) had parkinsonism after using metoclopramide (average dose, 29.5 mg) daily for an average of 8.7 months. Tardive dyskinesia was seen in seven patients (five in the group with parkinsonism and

*Originally published on December 3, 1981 (305:1417).

two others) after they had received the drug for an average of 2.5 years. Parkinsonism was reversible with discontinuation of metoclopramide. Tardive dyskinesia was chronic after 15 months of follow-up in three patients. Six of the 12 patients with parkinsonism had been previously misdiagnosed as having classical Parkinson's disease and were already receiving levodopa.

I continue to see new patients with these metoclopramide-induced disorders at a rate of at least one every two months, and I have now had experience with 19 cases of parkinsonism and 10 of tardive dyskinesia.

Because the disorders for which metoclopramide is indicated are frequently chronic, I have observed a great tendency to continue long-term therapy once initial relief of symptoms has been obtained.

Therefore, because of its ability to block central dopamine receptors, metoclopramide, if used over the long term, is capable of causing reversible parkinsonism and potentially irreversible tardive dyskinesia. These neurologic complications of long-term therapy should be seriously considered when treatment regimens with oral metoclopramide are being planned.

J. DAVID GRIMES, M.D.
1081 Carling Ave., Suite 304
Ottawa, ON K1Y 4G2, Canada

1. Schulze-Delrieu K. Metoclopramide. N Engl J Med 1981; 305:28-33.
2. Lavy S, Melamed E, Penchas S. Tardive dyskinesia associated with metoclopramide. Br Med J 1978; 1:77-8.
3. Kataria M, Traub M, Marsden CD. Extrapyramidal side-effects of metoclopramide. Lancet 1978; 2:1254-5.
4. Grimes JD, Hassan MN, Preston DN. Adverse neurological effects of metoclopramide. Can Med Assoc J (in press).

Metronidazole

Peter Goldman, M.D.

METRONIDAZOLE provided the first effective cure for trichomoniasis, a disease that until 20 years ago was said to cause more suffering than cancer.[1] The drug was placed under a cloud, however, when, after nearly 15 years of widespread use, attention was called to observations indicating that metronidazole was a mutagen of bacteria and an oncogen in animals.[2] In this situation proved clinical benefits had to be reconciled with laboratory evidence that suggested human risk. The search for such a reconciliation cannot be avoided. Alternative therapies are either ineffective or use drugs with similar structures and similar laboratory properties.

In judgments about metronidazole, it is reasonable that certain kinds of evidence receive greater emphasis and that the emphasis may change as new evidence becomes available. Solely on the basis of its laboratory properties, metronidazole would probably be considered to have too great a risk for human use.[3] However, shortly after the worrisome laboratory properties were discovered, studies in human beings placed the laboratory data in a new context. By then, not only had the clinical benefits been amply documented but it was also possible to survey previously exposed patients to obtain a direct estimate of risk. In this context one can rely more on data from tests in human beings and less on those from the laboratory, in the clinical evaluation of this useful drug.

Trichomonal Vaginitis

The eradication of the trichomonad and the symptoms that it causes remains the most important benefit of metronidazole. Some physicians treat only women who are symptomatic, and may or may not simultaneously treat their partners. Others treat all women with evidence of infestation. Advocacy of treatment in the absence of symptoms is based on the view that the parasite will sooner or later cause symptoms and that in the meantime its presence may confuse the interpretation of routine cervical cytology.[4] The decision to treat the asymptomatic patient therefore depends as much on perceptions about the value of cervical cytology and the natural history of trichomoniasis as on the risk to the patient of treatment with metronidazole.

From the Division of Clinical Pharmacology, Department of Pharmacology, Harvard Medical School, and from the Charles A. Dana Research Institute and the Harvard–Thorndike Laboratory of Beth Israel Hospital, Department of Medicine, Beth Israel Hospital, Boston.

Originally published on November 20, 1980 (303:1212-1218).

Various dosage schedules have been used to treat trichomoniasis, and several are approximately 90 per cent effective both in relieving symptoms and in eradicating the parasite. The current package insert recommends a dosage schedule of 250 mg three times daily for seven days. However, five days of this program[5,6] appears to be equally effective. The package insert also notes the effectiveness of a single dose of as little as 2 g.[7,8]

Inadequate compliance with medication is probably a common cause of treatment failure; if the physician suspects that noncompliance will occur, treatment with a single 2-g dose may be offered at the time of diagnosis. Inadequate drug absorption seems unlikely as a cause of treatment failure, since all oral preparations tested have good bioavailability[9] and absorption seems generally to be quite complete.[10]

Because trichomoniasis is transmitted by sexual contact, a case of trichomonal vaginitis that appears to be intractable may simply be reinfection either from the same partner or another one. The package insert suggests treating the partner simultaneously with the patient, particularly in cases of recurrence. Such treatment is advisable because it is seldom possible to obtain evidence of infection in men. The need to treat the partner is suggested by some observations[8] but not by others.[11]

Since both aerobic and anaerobic bacteria inactivate metronidazole,[12] concomitant bacterial vaginitis could theoretically prevent maintenance of an adequate trichomonicidal concentration of the drug.

Strains of trichomonads that are somewhat resistant to metronidazole have recently been isolated, suggesting another possible cause of intractable trichomoniasis. Such disease should be readily treatable since these strains appear to be responsive when the dose is increased.[13] Resistant strains have only been documented in a few cases, however, and it would be desirable to establish their prevalence in order to formulate a therapeutic strategy for patients whose disease is refractory to standard treatment.

Amebiasis

For acute intestinal amebiasis the package insert recommends a 250-mg dose three times daily for five to 10 days; this dose may be doubled or tripled for treatment of amebic abscess. Many authorities consider it the drug of choice.[14]

Giardiasis

Several studies indicate that metronidazole is effective in the treatment of giardiasis, and it is regarded as an alternative agent for this purpose.[14] Unfortunately, however, this use is not approved by the Food and Drug Administration. Although metronidazole may not be as effective as equal doses of a structurally related drug, tinidazole,[15] tinidazole is not available in the United States. Therefore the choice for American patients and physicians in treating giardiasis is between quinacrine and metronidazole, and there appears to be little difference in the effectiveness of the two drugs. Published comparisons have tested metronidazole under various dosage schedules, e.g., 2 g daily for three days,[16] 250 mg twice daily for 10 days, or, as prescribed by some British and American physicians, either 200 or 250 mg three times daily for a week.[17] Although the two drugs are equally effective, many physicians prefer quinacrine because they are concerned about the laboratory evidence of metronidazole's mutagenicity and carcinogenicity. It should be recognized, however, that quinacrine reacts with DNA so avidly that it is used as a chromosomal stain.[18] Neither drug is without laboratory properties suggestive of risk to human beings.

| Anaerobic Bacterial Infections

The largely successful results obtained with metronidazole in anaerobic infections at sites such as the abdomen, pelvis, and chest and in the treatment of bacteremia, endocarditis, and meningitis have been reviewed.[19] Some of these infections are so uncommon that systematic evaluation of their treatment by various agents is not easy. However, the value of metronidazole both in common infections and in bacterial prophylaxis has been the subject of systematic investigation.

Studies based on historical controls suggest a role for the drug in the treatment of acute diverticulitis[20] and in the management of septic shock from intraabdominal infection.[21] Randomized clinical trials show that "nonspecific" vaginitis due to Haemophilus vaginalis is very effectively treated with 400 to 500 mg twice daily for a week.[22,23]

Controlled trials also indicate that metronidazole, either alone or in combination with another antibiotic, provides effective prophylaxis in surgical operations in which the risk of postoperative anaerobic infection is high. Anaerobic bacterial infections after appendectomy were eliminated when either intravenous or rectal administration of metronidazole was begun in the preoperative period.[24,25] Treatment was continued for up to a week in one study,[24] but a single 500-mg dose administered intravenously just before operation also seemed to lower the incidence of infection.[26] The incidence of infection after appendectomy was decreased more by a combination of a metronidazole suppository and intravenous cefazolin than by either drug alone.[27]

Metronidazole also decreases the incidence of infection after colon surgery. In two studies the incidence of infection was decreased at least fourfold when the drug was administered preoperatively and continued for either one or seven days postoperatively.[28,29] Some studies have demonstrated successful prophylaxis when metronidazole was used in combination with another antibiotic, e.g., gentamicin,[28] neomycin, or kanamycin.[30] It is not clear, however, that better results are achieved with the additional antibiotic than are possible with metronidazole alone. One study found that the incidence of postoperative infection was lower with a combination of neomycin and metronidazole than with metronidazole alone.[31] In this study, however, antibiotics were administered only in the pre-operative period, and thus the added benefit of neomycin might have been obtained simply by more prolonged treatment with metronidazole by itself.

Metronidazole decreases the risk of postoperative infection after both vaginal and abdominal hysterectomy,[32-34] but it may be no more effective for this purpose than a cephalosporin.[32] Metronidazole and cephradine were compared for effectiveness in preventing infection after cesarean section; both drugs decreased the infection rate from approximately 26 per cent to approximately 5 per cent.[35] Most of the studies that demonstrate the efficacy of metronidazole in preventing postoperative bacterial infection have administered the drug either as an intravenous infusion or as a rectal suppository.[24-31,33-35] Neither of these preparations is currently available in the United States, but approval for an intravenous preparation is being sought.

Metronidazole also may have value in dental surgery; it was found in one series to decrease the incidence of anaerobic infection after the removal of impacted wisdom teeth from approximately 3 per cent to less than 1 per cent.[36]

It seems likely that metronidazole will soon gain formal approval from the FDA for at least some of these antibacterial indications. Physicians will then have to decide between metronidazole and some of the newer cephalosporins for the treatment and prophylaxis of anaerobic infections.

Possible Additional Therapeutic Properties

Metronidazole enhances the sensitivity of anaerobic tissue-culture cells to x-rays, and it has been used experimentally as a radiation sensitizer in animals and patients.[37] Its use for this purpose is limited, however, because peripheral neuropathy occurs at the high doses of metronidazole that are necessary to maintain adequate concentrations of drug in the tumor during a course of radiation therapy. Compounds structurally related to metronidazole may have more promise as radiation sensitizers.

Another use of metronidazole is suggested by the observation that it is more effective than other antibiotics in an animal model of colitis.[38] Accordingly, the drug has been used in several small trials in the treatment of Crohn's disease. Although overall results are not encouraging, benefit was noted in one series for patients with Crohn's disease confined to the colon.[39]

Adverse Effects

Most of the adverse side effects of metronidazole are self-limited and readily tolerated at the doses needed to treat either protozoal or bacterial infections or to effect bacterial prophylaxis. Side effects include strange taste, nausea, and a curious intolerance to alcohol, which is similar to that occurring with disulfiram. Although the package insert recommends obtaining total and differential leukocyte counts both before and after the drug is administered, the scarcity of reports of noteworthy leukopenia in the usual brief treatment period seems to make this precaution unnecessary. When the drug is used for more prolonged periods in the treatment of infections, it is likely that leukocyte counts will be obtained anyway. A serious side effect is peripheral neuropathy, but this is rarely a problem unless the dose is large. Fortunately, manifestations such as paresthesias are generally reversible if treatment is stopped when symptoms first occur.[40]

Other concerns about toxicity are not based on tests in human beings but are derived entirely from evidence obtained in the laboratory. On a balance sheet of metronidazole's assets and liabilities, these concerns might be assigned to the category of "contingent liabilities."

Metronidazole and Cancer

Several studies confirm that long-term feeding of metronidazole in high doses causes an increase in pulmonary tumors and sometimes other tumors in laboratory mice.[40] Similar studies also indicate that hepatocarcinomas as well as mammary tumors and other tumors develop in rats,[40,41] but no tumors have been reported in hamsters.[40]

Neither of two studies[42,43] indicates that the incidence of cancer is increased in patients previously exposed to metronidazole. However, these studies were conducted in relatively small numbers of patients who were followed for periods that may have been too short to encompass the latency period necessary for chemical carcinogenesis in human beings. Thus, the evidence in human beings is only adequate to exclude a large excess risk of cancer that might become manifest within approximately 10 years of exposure to a trichomonicidal dose of metronidazole. The dose to which patients were exposed (probably 7.5 g in 10 days) is greater than that now considered necessary to treat trichomoniasis and is also greater than that necessary to provide effective bacterial prophylaxis. The drug is currently used mostly at doses below those whose effects are examined in this kind of surveillance.

Mutagenicity

The dominant lethal test in rats or the detection of either unscheduled DNA synthesis or chromosomal abnormalities are the usual means of assessing whether a compound is mutagenic for mammalian cells. These tests, although not necessarily exhaustive or sufficiently sensitive, have not implicated metronidazole as a mammalian mutagen.[44,45] One study reports chromosomal abnormalities in patients with Crohn's disease previously treated with metronidazole, but a more carefully designed study performed by the same investigators did not find chromosomal damage after treatment with 800 mg daily for four months.[46]

The occurrence of congenital defects in infants born to women who were treated with metronidazole during pregnancy has been examined in several small studies. None of these investigations indicate any increased teratological risk even when exposure occurred during the first trimester.[11,40,47,48] Although there are several such reports, the number of patients examined in a systematic way is insufficient to exclude completely a relatively small risk to the fetus. It seems prudent, therefore, to be guided by the warning in the package insert that metronidazole be avoided during pregnancy.

Although metronidazole is mutagenic for a variety of bacteria, its mutagenicity for the Ames histidine auxotrophs of *Salmonella typhimurium*[48] has attracted particular attention because of an apparent correlation between a compound's mutagenicity for these bacteria and its carcinogenicity in animals.[49] As a result of this apparent correlation, the Ames test may assume importance beyond that relating to bacterial mutagenicity. With regard to metronidazole, the test has relatively little value in view of the availability of other evidence. Metronidazole is a carcinogen for animals and therefore a potential carcinogen for human beings. A measure of any human carcinogenicity is what we really want, and this information can only be estimated from epidemiologic studies such as the two mentioned previously.[42,43]

Metabolism and Pharmacokinetics

Either of the two side chains of metronidazole (Fig. 1, I) can be oxidized, presumably in the liver, to form either the "alcohol" (II) or the "acid" (III) metabolite. These major metabolites, along with metronidazole itself, are found in the urine,[50] but only the alcohol metabolite is found in serum when renal function is normal.[51,52] Like the parent compound, the two metabolites have both antibacterial and mutagenic activity. The alcohol metabolite is a more potent mutagen than the parent compound,[50] but its antibacterial activity is not as great.[51] Unfortunately, many of the earlier studies of the pharmacokinetics of metronidazole are faulty because the drug was assayed either by its antibacterial activity or through polarography. Neither of these methods distinguishes between metronidazole and metabolites such as II and III.

In spite of some inconsistencies that may be attributed to imprecise assay methods,[53] it is possible to conclude that metronidazole is generally absorbed well after administration by mouth but more slowly and variably after administration by rectum.[54-56] It is only weakly bound to serum protein and achieves a volume of distribution similar to that of total body water.[9,53] Bactericidal concentrations equal to that in serum have been demonstrated in cerebrospinal fluid,[53] bile,[57] bone,[36] and pelvic tissues.[54] As expected, the drug also appears in human milk.[19,53] Studies using a specific chromatographic assay have shown that metronidazole has a half-life of approximately seven hours.[56] Drug clearance is not changed in the anuric patient, but it is doubled in patients undergoing hemodialysis.[52]

Although metronidazole concentrations have not been measured in the human vagina, studies of concentrations in other sites in human beings and studies in animals indicate that vaginal concentrations should be similar to those

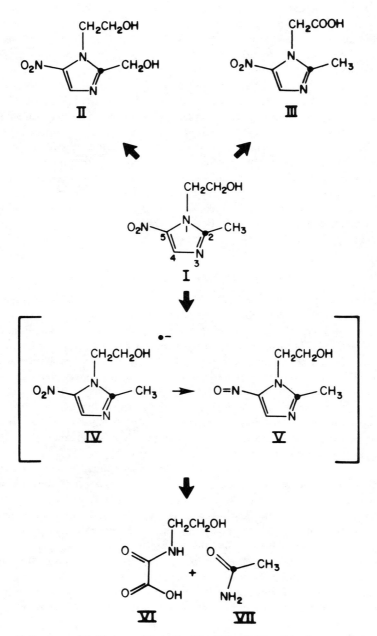

Figure 1. Summary of Oxidative and Reductive Metabolism of Metronidazole (I), Including Postulated Intermediates.

For details of pharmacokinetics and mechanism of action, see text.

of serum. A vaginal suppository of metronidazole is ineffective for trichomoniasis[6] and is no longer available in the United States.

Mechanism of Action

Apparently all metronidazole's biologic activities are related to reduction of its nitro group. Mutagenicity, for example, which is detected in a strain of the Ames histidine auxotrophs of *S. typhimurium*, is diminished in a mutant bacterium that lacks nitroreductase activity.[48] Similarly, a rare strain of *Bacteroides fragilis* that is relatively resistant to metronidazole has been found to have greatly diminished nitroreductase activity.[58] The concept that nitro-group reduction is essential for metronidazole's activity is supported by studies of structure and activity that compare metronidazole's properties with those of other nitroheterocyclic compounds. Such studies show a strong correlation between a compound's electron affinity and its potency for cytotoxicity,[59] mutagenicity,[60] and radiation sensitization.[61] It appears, therefore, that the biologic properties of metronidazole and compounds like it may be mediated by a partially reduced intermediate that binds to critical sites in susceptible cells.[62,63] DNA is disrupted by chemically reduced metronidazole in a reaction that may serve as a prototype of the biologic action of metronidazole.[64,65]

Electron-spin resonance studies indicate that the radical anion (Fig. 1, IV) is formed in both mammalian and bacterial enzyme preparations.[66,67] Under anaerobic conditions bacteria form metabolites such as N-(2-hydroxyethyl) oxamic acid (VI) and acetamide (VII), which indicate cleavage of the imidazole ring.[68,69] These reactions may proceed through partially reduced intermediates such as IV and V,[66-69] which may be the actual mediators of metronidazole's biologic actions. Reactions resulting in ring cleavage have been detected in vivo only as a result of the activity of the intestinal flora,[68,69] raising the possibility that a reactive intermediate may form in the flora and affect the mammalian host. A speculation like this one is difficult to substantiate,[3] but the concept might explain why metronidazole may benefit patients with Crohn's disease only in the colon, where the concentration of the flora is high.[39]

The formation of acetamide has other possible implications, because prolonged feeding of high doses of this compound to rats, like feeding of high doses of metronidazole itself, causes hepatocarcinoma.[41,70] Very small amounts of acetamide are also found in the urine of patients taking metronidazole.[71]

Arriving at Conclusions When Studies in Human Beings and Laboratory Data Appear Incompatible

How is one to evaluate this kind of laboratory data in making decisions about the clinical use of this very effective drug? If it had been known before 1960 that metronidazole formed acetamide, it could reasonably have been argued that trials in human beings should be initiated with an analogue of metronidazole that did

318 / Drug Therapy

not yet yield this weak carcinogen as a metabolite. Today, however, the risk associated with the drug may be estimated directly from past experience, and laboratory evidence of possible risk accordingly assumes less importance. Human studies indicate that the risk of teratogenicity and cancer is almost certainly not large and is probably negligible. This risk may be even more precisely defined in the future as a result of studies of past exposure. We do not know, nor are we likely to know for decades, the risk associated with alternative forms of effective therapy. Data from the laboratory may provide insight into the mechanism responsible for metronidazole's many biologic actions. However, these data cannot be considered comparable to clinical data on risk and benefit when clinical decisions are being formulated.

References

1. Gardner HL. Trichomoniasis. Obstet Gynecol 1962; 19:279-81.
2. Anonymous. Is Flagyl dangerous? Med Lett 1975; 17:53-4.
3. Goldman P. Metronidazole: proven benefits and potential risks. Johns Hopkins Med J 1980; 147:1-9.
4. Frost JK. Cytology of benign conditions. Clin Obstet Gynecol 1961; 4:1075-96.
5. Nicol CS, Barrow J, Redmond A. Flagyl (8823 RP) in the treatment of trichomoniasis. Br J Vener Dis 1960; 36:152-3.
6. Pereyra AJ, Lansing JD. Urogenital trichomoniasis: treatment with metronidazole in 2002 incarcerated women. Obstet Gynecol 1964; 24:499-508.
7. Csonka GW. Trichomonal vaginitis treated with one dose of metronidazole. Br J Vener Dis 1971; 47:456-8.
8. Dykers JR Jr. Single-dose metronidazole for trichomonal vaginitis: patient and consort. N Engl J Med 1975; 293:23-4.
9. McGilveray IJ, Midha KK, Loo JCK, Cooper JK. The bioavailability of commercial metronidazole formulations. Int J Clin Pharmacol 1978; 16:110-5.
10. Amon I, Amon K, Huller H. Pharmacokinetics and therapeutic efficacy of metronidazole at different dosages. Int J Clin Pharmacol 1978; 16:384-6.
11. Peterson WF, Stauch JE, Ryder CD. Metronidazole in pregnancy. Am J Obstet Gynecol 1966; 94:343-9.
12. Chrystal EJT, Koch RL, McLafferty MA, Goldman P. The relationship between metronidazole metabolism and bactericidal activity. Antimicrob Agents Chemother 1980; 18:566-73.
13. Muller M, Meingassner JG, Miller WA, Ledger WJ. Three metronidazole-resistant strains of *Trichomonas vaginalis* from the U.S.A. Am J Obstet Gynecol. (in press).
14. Anonymous. Metronidazole (Flagyl). Med Lett 1979; 21:89-90.
15. Bakshi JS, Ghiara JM, Nanivadekar AS. How does tinidazole compare with metronidazole?: A summary report of Indian trials in amoebiasis and giardiasis. Drugs 1978; 15: Suppl 1:33-42.
16. Wright SG, Tomkins AM, Ridley DS. Giardiasis: clinical and therapeutic aspects. Gut 1977; 18:343-50.
17. Anonymous. Giardiasis. Br Med J 1974; 2:347-8.
18. Gottesfeld JM, Bonner J, Radda GK, Walker IO. Biophysical studies on the mechanism of quinacrine staining of chromosomes. Biochemistry 1974; 13:2937-45.

19. Brogden RN, Heel RC, Speight TM, Avery GS. Metronidazole in anaerobic infections: a review of its activity, pharmacokinetics and therapeutic use. Drugs 1978; 16:387-417.

20. Pashby NL. Metronidazole in the management of acute diverticular disease. In: Phillips I, Collier J, eds. Metronidazole. London: Academic Press, 1979:63-8. (Royal Society of Medicine International Congress and Symposium series no. 18).

21. Goodwin NM. The use of intravenous metronidazole in the treatment of serious intraabdominal infections. In: Phillips I, Collier J, eds. Metronidazole. London: Academic Press, 1979:59-62. (Royal Society of Medicine International Congress and Symposium series no. 18).

22. Pheifer TA, Forsyth PS, Durfee MA, Pollock HM, Holmes KK. Nonspecific vaginitis: role of *Haemophilus vaginalis* and treatment with metronidazole. N Engl J Med 1978; 298:1429-34.

23. Balsdon MJ, Taylor GE, Pead L, Maskell R. Corynebacterium vaginale and vaginitis: a controlled trial of treatment. Lancet 1980; 1:501-4.

24. Willis AT, Ferguson IR, Jones PH, et al. Metronidazole in prevention and treatment of bacteroides infections after appendicectomy. Br Med J 1976; 1:318-21.

25. Rodgers J, Ross D, McNaught W, Gillespie G. Intrarectal metronidazole in the prevention of anaerobic infections after emergency appendicectomy: a controlled clinical trial. Br J Surg 1979; 66:425-7.

26. McMahon MJ, Greenall MJ, Cooke EM. The prevention of wound infection after appendicectomy by intravenously administered metronidazole. In: Phillips I, Collier J, eds. Metronidazole. London: Academic Press, 1979:133-6. (Royuald Society of Medicine International Congress and Symposium series no. 18).

27. Morris WT, Ellis-Pegler RB, Innes DB. The influence of metronidazole and cefazolin on post-appendicectomy wound sepsis. In: Phillips I, Collier J, eds. Metronidazole. London: Academic Press, 1979:129-31. (Royal Society of Medicine International Congress and Symposium series no. 18).

28. Willis AT, Ferguson IR, Jones PH, et al. Metronidazole in prevention and treatment of bacteroides infections in elective colonic surgery. Br Med J 1977; 1:607-10.

29. Eykyn SJ, Jackson BT, Lockhart-Mummery HE, Phillips I. Prophylactic preoperative intravenous metronidazole in elective colorectal surgery. Lancet 1979; 2:761-4.

30. Willis AT, Jones PH. The prophylactic role of metronidazole in colorectal surgery. In: Phillips I, Collier J, eds. Metronidazole. London: Academic Press, 1979:137-48. (Royal Society of Medicine International Congress and Symposium series no. 18).

31. Vallance S, Jones B, Arabi Y, Keighley MRB. A comaprison of the prophylactic effect of oral metronidazole and neomycin with metronidazole in colonic surgery. In: Phillips I, Collier J, eds. Metronidazole. London: Academic Press, 1979:155-9. (Royal Society of Medicine International Congress and Symposium series no. 18).

32. Hamod KA, Spence MR, Rosenshein NB, Dillon MB. Single-dose and multidose prophylaxis in vaginal hysterectomy: a comparison of sodium cephalothin and metronidazole. Am J Obstet Gynecol 1980; 136:976-9.

33. Jackson P, Ridley WJ, Pattison NS. Single dose metronidazole prophylaxis in gynaecological surgery. NZ Med J 1979; 89:243-5.

34. Hughes TBJ, Frampton J, Begg HB, Khan MS. The prophylactic effect of a short course of intravenous metronidazole during gynaecological surgery. In: Phillips I, Collier J, eds. Metronidazole. London: Academic Press, 1979:207-10. (Royal Society of Medicine International Congress and Symposium series no. 18).

35. Vaughan JE. Comparison of metronidazole and cephradine in the prevention of wound sepsis following Caesarean section. In: Phillips I, Collier J, eds. Metronidazole. London: Academic Press, 1979:203-5. (Royal Society of Medicine International Congress and Symposium series no. 18).

36. Rood JP, Collier J. Metronidazole levels in alveolar bone. In: Phillips I, Collier J, eds. Metronidazole. London: Academic Press, 1979:45-7. (Royal Society of Medicine International Congress and Symposium series no. 18).

37. Chapman JD. Hypoxic sensitizers — implications for radiation therapy. N Engl J Med 1979; 301:1429-32.

38. Onderdonk AB, Hermos JA, Dzink JL, Bartlett JG. Protective effect of metronidazole in experimental ulcerative colitis. Gastroenterology 1978; 74:521-6.

39. Blichfeldt P, Blomhoff JP, Myhre E, Gjone E. Metronidazole in Crohn's disease: a double blind cross-over clinical trial. Scand J Gastroenterol 1978; 13:123-7.

40. Roe JFC. A critical appraisal of the toxicology of metronidazole. In: Phillips I, Collier J, eds. Metronidazole. London: Academic Press, 1979:215-22. (Royal Society of Medicine International Congress and Symposium series no. 18).

41. Rustia M, Shubik P. Experimental induction of hepatomas, mammary tumors, and other tumors with metronidazole in noninbred Sas: MRC(WI)BR rats. J Natl Cancer Inst 1979; 63:863-7.

42. Beard CM, Noller KL, O'Fallon WM, Kurkland LT, Dockerty MB. Lack of evidence for cancer due to use of metronidazole. N Engl J Med 1979; 301:519-22.

43. Friedman GD. Cancer after metronidazole. N Engl J Med 1980; 302:519.

44. Bost RG. Metronidazole: mammalian mutagenicity. In: Finegold SM, ed. Metronidazole: proceedings of the International Metronidazole Conference. Amsterdam: Excerpta Medica, 1977:126-31.

45. Lambert B, Lindblad A, Ringborg U. Absence of genotoxic effects of metronidazole and two of its urinary metabolites on human lymphocytes in vitro. Mutat Res 1979; 67:281-7.

46. Mittelman F, Strombeck B, Ursing B. No cytogenic effect of metronidazole. Lancet 1980; 1:1249-50.

47. Morgan IFK. Metronidazole treatment in pregnancy. In: Phillips I, Collier J, eds. Metronidazole. London: Academic Press, 1979:245-7. (Royal Society of Medicine International Congress and Symposium series no. 18).

48. Rosenkranz HS, Speck WT. Mutagenicity of metronidazole: activation by mammalian liver microsomes. Biochem Biophys Res Commun 1975; 66:520-5.

49. McCann J, Ames BN. Detection of carcinogens as mutagens in the Salmonella/microsome test: assay of 300 chemicals. Proc Natl Acad Sci USA 1976; 73:950-4.

50. Connor TH, Stoeckel M, Evrard J, Legator MS. The contribution of metronidazole and two metabolites to the mutagenic activity detected in urine of treated humans and mice. Cancer Res 1977; 37:629-33.

51. Wheeler LA, De Meo M, Halula M, George L, Heseltine P. Use of high-pressure liquid chromatography to determine plasma levels of metronidazole and metabolites after intravenous administration. Antimicrob Agents Chemother 1978; 13:205-9.

52. Gabriel R, Page CM, Weller IVD, et al. The pharmacokinetics of metronidazole in patients with chronic renal failure. In: Phillips I, Collier J, eds. Metronidazole. London: Academic Press, 1979:49-54. (Royal Society of Medicine International Congress and Symposium series no. 18).

53. Templeton R. Metabolism and pharmacokinetics of metronidazole: a review. In: Finegold SM, ed. Metronidazole: proceedings of the International Metronidazole Conference. Amsterdam: Excerpta Medica, 1977:28-49.

54. Elder MG, Kane JL. The pelvic tissue levels achieved by metronidazole after single or multiple dosing — oral and rectal. In: Phillips I, Collier J, eds. Metronidazole. London: Academic Press, 1979:55-8. (Royal Society of Medicine International Congress and Symposium series no. 18).

55. Houghton GW, Templeton R. Statistical analysis of serum metronidazole levels in patients receiving the drug mainly by suppository. J Antimicrob Chemother 1978; 4: Suppl C:91-6.

56. Houghton GW, Thorne PS, Smith J, Templeton R, Cook PJ, James IM. Plasma metronidazole concentrations after suppository administration. In: Phillips I, Collier J, eds. Metronidazole. London: Academic Press, 1979:41-4. (Royal Society of Medicine International Congress and Symposium series no. 18).

57. Lykkegaard Nielsen M, Justesen T. Excretion of metronidazole in human bile: investigations of hepatic bile, common duct bile, and gallbladder bile. Scand J Gastroenterol 1977; 12:1003-8.

58. Tally FP, Snydman DR, Shimell MJ, Goldin BR. Mechanisms of antimicrobial resistance of *Bacteroides fragilis*. In: Phillips I, Collier J, eds. Metronidazole. London: Academic Press, 1979:19-27. (Royal Society of Medicine International Congress and Symposium series no. 18).

59. Adams GE, Clarke EC, Jacobs RS, et al. Mammalian cell toxicity of nitro compounds: dependence upon reduction potential. Biochem Biophys Res Commun 1976; 72:824-9.

60. Chin JB, Sheinin DMK, Rauth AM. Screening for the mutagenicity of nitro-group containing hypoxic cell radiosensitizers using *Salmonella typhimurium* strains TA 100 and TA 98. Mutat Res 1978; 58:1-10.

61. Adams GE, Flockhart IR, Smithen CE, Stratford IJ, Wardman P, Watts ME. Electron-affinic sensitization. VII. A correlation between structures, one-electron reduction potentials, and efficiencies of nitroimidazoles as hypoxic cell radiosensitizers. Radiat Res 1976; 67:9-20.

62. Lindmark DG, Müller M. Antitrichomonad action, mutagenicity, and reduction of metronidazole and other nitroimidazoles. Antimicrob Agents Chemother 1976; 10:476-82.

63. Ings RMJ, McFadzean JA, Ormerod WE. The mode of action of metronidazole in *Trichomonas vaginalis* and other micro-organisms. Biochem Pharmacol 1974; 23:1421-9.

64. LaRusso NF, Tomasz M, Muller M, Lipman R. Interaction of metronidazole with nucleic acids *in vitro*. Mol Pharmacol 1977; 13:872-82.

65. Knight RC, Skolimowski IM, Edwards DI. The interaction of reduced metronidazole with DNA. Biochem Pharmacol 1978; 27:2089-93.

66. Perez-Reyes E, Kalyanaraman B, Mason RP. The reductive metabolism of metronidazole and ronidazole by aerobic liver microsomes. Mol Pharmacol 1980; 17:239-44.

67. Peterson FJ, Mason RP, Hovsepian J, Holtzman JL. Oxygen-sensitive and -insensitive nitroreduction by *Escherichia coli* and rat hepatic microsomes. J Biol Chem 1979; 254:4009-14.

68. Koch RL, Goldman P. The anaerobic metabolism of metronidazole forms N-(2-hydroxyethyl)-oxamic acid. J Pharmacol Exp Ther 1979; 208:406-10.

69. Koch RL, Chrystal EJT, Beaulieu BB Jr, Goldman P. Acetamide — a metabolite of metronidazole formed by the intestinal flora. Biochem Pharmacol 1979; 28:3611-5.
70. Jackson B, Dessau FI. Liver tumors in rats fed acetamide. Lab Invest 1961; 10:909-23.
71. Koch RL, Beaulieu BB, Chrystal EJT, Goldman P. Metabolites of metronidazole in human urine and their risk. Science. (in press).

| Correspondence

Correction: Metronidazole Dose for Amebiasis*

To the Editor:

An error in my Drug Therapy article on metronidazole (November 20 issue) has been called to my attention, and I would like to have it noted.

For the treatment of acute intestinal amebiasis the dose of metronidazole recommended in the package insert is 750 mg three times daily.

PETER GOLDMAN, M.D.
Harvard Medical School
Boston, MA 02215

Metronidazole†

To the Editor:

In his excellent article on metronidazole in the November 20 issue, Dr. Goldman suggests that strains of *Trichomonas vaginalis* with increased tolerance of metronidazole should be readily eradicated by simply increasing the drug dosage. Although this may be true of organisms with only minor to moderate alterations in susceptibility to metronidazole, it is not true of organisms demonstrating marked resistance to the drug. To date, the laboratory minimal lethal concentrations (MLCs) that correlate with potential treatment efficacy versus treatment failure have not been defined.

My colleagues and I have treated a woman with trichomonas vulvovaginitis that proved to be totally refractory to repeated treatment with high dosages of metronidazole (up to 6 g daily for five days in the hospital). Although treatments have consistently resulted in clinical improvement, we have not eradicated the organism at any time. Reinfection was virtually excluded as a possible cause. Pharmacokinetic studies revealed high serum drug levels, thereby excluding malabsorption as a possible variable. This *T. vaginalis* strain demonstrated MLC levels of 7.5 μg per milliliter according to the tube-dilution method. MLC values were 22.5 μg in anaerobic wells and 525 μg in aerobic wells. In studies of

*Originally published on February 26, 1981 (304:547).

†Originally published on March 19,1981 (304:735).

subcutaneous inoculations of mice with the organism, 100 to 300 mg per kilogram of body weight three times a day was required to eradicate infection — 10 to 30 times the dose of metronidazole required to cure clinically susceptible strains.

Metronidazole-resistant strains of *T. vaginalis* that cannot be eradicated with large doses of metronidazole by mouth unquestionably exist in the United States. Although their prevalence is currently undefined and undoubtedly small, no predictably effective alternative therapeutic treatment is available for these patients. Similar treatment-resistant strains have been reported in Sweden and England.[1,2] The development of resistance to metronidazole by *T. vaginalis* indicates a need to develop other effective treatments for this very common and troublesome disorder.

Joseph G. Lossick, D.O.
Columbus Health Department
Columbus, OH 43215

1. Forsgren A, Forssman L. Metronidazole resistant *Trichomonas vaginalis*. Br J Vener Dis 1979; 55:351-3.
2. Heyworth R, Simpson D, McNeillage GLC, et al. Isolation of *Trichomonas vaginalis* resistant to metronidazole. Lancet 1980; 2:476-8.

The above letter was referred to Dr. Goldman, who offers the following reply:

To the Editor:

As Dr. Lossick indicates, the available data do not permit an estimate of the prevalence of intractable trichomoniasis due to organisms with resistance to metronidazole. Such an estimate will require a more systematic study of the problem than has been reported so far. Patients such as the one whom Dr. Lossick describes may be treated successfully in the future, however, with one of the many drugs that are structurally related to metronidazole. We find that one such drug, the 2-nitroimidazole misonidazole, is more potent that metronidazole and other 5-nitroimidazoles against *T. vaginalis* in vitro and is equally potent against strain IR-78 of *T. vaginalis,* which is relatively resistant to metronidazole.* At the moment, however, misonidazole is an experimental drug approved for human use only as a radiosensitizer in clinical trials.

Peter Goldman, M.D.
Beth Israel Hospital
Boston, MA 02215

*Meingassner JG, Thurner J. Strain of *Trichomonas vaginalis* resistant to metronidazole and other 5-nitroimidazoles. Antimicrob Agents Chemother 1979; 15:254.